PROTEASOME INHIBITORS IN CANCER THERAPY

CANCER DRUG DISCOVERY AND DEVELOPMENT

BEVERLY A. TEICHER, SERIES EDITOR

PROTEASOME INHIBITORS IN CANCER THERAPY

Edited by

JULIAN ADAMS, PhD

Infinity Pharmaceuticals Inc., Cambridge, MA

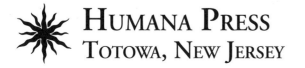

HUMANA PRESS
TOTOWA, NEW JERSEY

Cover illustration: Figure 1C from Chapter 3, "Structures of the Yeast Proteasome Core Particle in Complex with Inhibitors," by Michael Groll and Robert Huber.

Cover design by Patricia F. Cleary.

This publication is printed on acid-free paper. ∞
ANSI Z39.48-1984 (American National Standards Institute)
Permanence of Paper for Printed Library Materials

For additional copies, pricing for bulk purchases, and/or information about other Humana titles, contact Humana at the above address or at any of the following numbers: Tel.:973-256-1699; Fax: 973-256-8341; Email: humanapr.com; or visit our Website: http://humanapress.com

Printed in the United States of America. 10 9 8 7 6 5 4 3 2 1

Library of Congress Cataloging-in-Publication Data
Proteasome inhibitors in cancer therapy / edited by Julian Adams.
                        p. ; cm. — (Cancer drug discovery and development)
    Includes bibliographical references and index.
    ISBN 1-58829-250-9 (alk. paper) eISBN 1-59259-794-7
    1. Protease inhibitors—Therapeutic use. 2. Cancer—Chemotherapy.
    [DNLM: 1. Neoplasms—drug therapy. 2. Clinical Trials. 3. Drug Design. 4. Drug Evaluation, Preclinical. 5. Protease Inhibitors—therapeutic use. QZ 267 P967 2004] I. Adams, Julian, 1954- II. Series.
    RC271.P74P76 2004
    616.99'4061—dc22   2003027863

PREFACE

The proteasome field has exploded in the years since the proteasome's discovery in the early 1990s. The proteasome is a highly conserved multicatalytic protease that is responsible for cellular protein turnover, and by definition governs critical processes in cell biology. This field is no less complex and exciting than the more trodden path of transcription and protein synthesis. The unique biochemistry of the proteasome as one of nature's most fascinating proteases has allowed chemists to develop synthetic inhibitors of this most intriguing enzyme. While chemists applied their skills to develop mechanism-based inhibitors, it was also revealed that Mother Nature had evolved her own inhibitors, natural products, secondary metabolites, all with origins in bacteria.

Although all these investigations represent an enzymologist's dreamscape for academic investigation, the development of "tool drugs" to inhibit the proteasome has allowed an even more impressive number of studies in cell biology to interrogate the function of the ubiquitin proteasome pathway in numerous cell lines. Such research has allowed the determination of the function, temporal presence of short-lived proteins, antigen presentation, cell cycle regulation, transcriptional activation, cell adhesion, and apoptosis, to name a few processes.

One common feature was inevitably revealed. Inhibition of the proteasome in cultured cells, mostly of tumor origin, produced profound stabilization of hundreds, if not thousands, of proteins, ultimately turning on the programmed cell death machinery, at concentrations that directly correlated to the intrinsic inhibition constant of the proteasome. Such observations begged further investigation of proteasome inhibition in the treatment of human cancers. At first consideration, it would appear that it should be "illegal" to inhibit the proteasome and that a reasonable therapeutic index could simply not be achieved. Indeed, there was much reasonable skepticism in the scientific community that proteasome inhibitors could be safely used in animal studies, much less to treat human patients with cancer. No responsible scientist could fault such a negative view of the use of proteasome inhibitors in vivo. However, as we will see revealed in the chapters of *Proteasome Inhibitors in Cancer Therapy*, there is indeed a well-developed body of empirical evidence that the proteasome is a viable target to treat human diseases. *Proteasome Inhibitors in Cancer Therapy* focuses on the role of the proteasome inhibitors in cancer, for that is the most advanced body of knowledge to date, but as we shall see there are hints and data that the proteasome can also treat vascular diseases, viral infections, and possibly other maladies. Whether any of these investigations eventually lead to a practical treatment in human patients remains to be seen. At the time of this writing, the data seem to be mounting that the treatment of hematological diseases, especially multiple myeloma, would indicate a potential for the introduction of a novel important contribution to these deadly cancers.

The compelling reason for editing and contributing to this compilation of scientific studies of the proteasome arose from our desire to assemble a set of chapters describing the discovery of the basic enzymology and cell biology, combined with the creativity of medicinal chemistry, to take a field of limited academic interest and show that in less than a decade drug candidates are testing the practical utility of proteasome inhibition in cancer. The story flies in the face of conventional wisdom. Moreover, some of the chemical matter embedded in these inhibitors also represents a break from conventional drug substances. Mechanism-based inhibitors are rare in the pharmacopoeia, but the proteasome begs to be inhibited by such odd substances as boronic acid peptides, β-lactone natural products, peptide epoxides, and complex depsipeptide structures. The boronic acid PS-341 (bortezomib) represents the most advanced of these agents and a following Phase III randomized clinical trial in an international multicenter, has recently been approved by the FDA for use in multiple myeloma. This molecule features prominently in many of the chapters as being the first, and ground breaking, drug, but I expect that it is but the beginning of many exciting therapeutics in the field.

Proteasome Inhibitors in Cancer Therapy is divided into four parts: The first part addresses the broader issues of the complexities and challenges of drug development for new cancer agents, in an ever competitive market, with changing standards of care and treatment combinations. Greene provides a most insightful analysis of the world of oncology addressing very practical and economic considerations.

The next chapters address the basic biochemistry and early discoveries in cell biology. Alfred Goldberg, one of the early pioneers, and founder of Myogenics (later becoming ProScript) teaches us in his chapter the history and mechanism of the proteasome. Subsequent chapters address natural product and synthetic inhibitors, which enabled the brilliant work of Robert Huber and his colleagues to define the three-dimensional structure of this awesome proteolytic machine. Subsequent contributions reveal the role of the proteasome in the cell cycle and apoptosis. The National Cancer Institute played a formidable public service in the comprehensive assessment of the inhibition of the proteasome in their 60-tumor cell panel and used sophisticated informatics to correlate proteasome inhibition and inhibition of cell growth and apoptosis. One may argue that the proteasome inhibition is a sledge hammer approach to blocking cellular protein turnover. Read and Brownell teach us that using proteasome inhibitors as tools, we may reveal more important medicinal targets in the ubiquitination machinery to target a subset of proteins that govern very restricted functions in cells.

The third part of the book addresses the very empirical and practical development of rationales to test proteasome inhibitors in cancer models. A major contribution, originally made by Maniatis, Goldberg, and colleagues at Harvard, and subsequently extended by Cusack and Baldwin and others, was elucidating of the role of the proteasome in NF-κB activation. DNA damage leads to a profound activation of the transcription factor that can be abrogated by proteasome inhibitors. This part of the book documents the generality of combining conventional chemotherapy and radiation with proteasome inhibition, notably PS-341. Schubert has extended the possibility that proteasome inhibitors may provide a new method of inhibiting viral maturation and budding by targeting the supporting cellular structures that assist retrovirus release from infected cells. Another remarkable contribution from Groettrup and colleagues reveals that the HIV protease inhibitor, ritonavir, is itself a proteasome inhibitor and may be part of its proven efficacy in the treatment of AIDS. Though ProScript, now a part of Millennium Pharmaceuticals, was the first to introduce a proteasome inhibitor into human trials, we note that other pharmaceutical companies have been active in the field and this is documented by García-Echeverría, from Novartis.

Part IV of this book represents a work in progress, documenting the development of bortezomib (VELCADE™) in clinical trials. The preclinical development allowed for the selection of doses and schedules that could be translated to human patients. Perhaps the most important element was the use of a pharmacodynamic assay to monitor proteasome inhibition in the blood to ensure that partial and temporal inhibition was maintained in a manner that could be tolerated by patients. The Phase I investigations are a joint effort of Millennium-sponsored trials together with the NCI extramural sites. The important contribution by Anderson, considered one of the leading authorities in multiple myeloma research and treatment, describes the activity of bortezomib in a multicentered Phase II clinical trial in patients with relapsed and refractory myeloma. Proteasome inhibition in myeloma and other diseases is also being pioneered using modern pharmacogenomic tools to assess which patients will be predicted to respond to therapy. Ross and colleagues describe the potential for such techniques to accompany proteasome inhibitor therapy.

Proteasome inhibition has certainly consumed my life for almost a decade and I feel privileged and fortunate to have been part of the emergence of this field, and participate in what I believe to be a fertile arena for many future discoveries, which my instincts tell me will provide much relief of suffering and extend quality life to patients afflicted with cancer and other debilitating diseases. I hope *Proteasome Inhibitors in Cancer Therapy* can provide some useful teachings for students, professors, and industry researchers alike.

Julian Adams, PhD

CONTENTS

CONTRIBUTORS

JULIAN ADAMS, PhD • *Chief Scientific Officer, Infinity Pharmaceuticals Inc., Cambridge, MA*

KENNETH C. ANDERSON, MD • *Dana-Farber Cancer Institute, Harvard Medical School, Boston, MA*

PAGE BOUCHARD • *Millennium Pharmaceuticals Inc., Cambridge, MA*

GEOFFREY BOWERS, BS • *Department of Neurosurgery, Emory University School of Medicine, Atlanta, GA*

JEFFREY BROWN, PhD • *Millennium Pharmaceuticals Inc., Cambridge, MA*

CRAIG M. CREWS, PhD • *Molecular, Cellular and Developmental Biology, Yale University, New Haven, CT*

JAMES C. CUSACK, JR., MD • *Division of Surgical Oncology, Harvard Medical School, Massachusetts General Hospital, Boston, MA*

JIM DEEDS • *Millennium Pharmaceuticals Inc., Cambridge, MA*

RITA DE GIULI • *Research Department, Cantonal Hospital, St. Gallen, Switzerland*

WILLIAM DEGRAFF, PhD • *Radiation Biology Branch, National Cancer Institute, National Institutes of Health, Bethesda, MD*

PETER J. ELLIOTT • *Combinatorx, Boston, MA*

DIXIE-LEE W. ESSELTINE, MD, FRCPC • *Senior Director, Clinical Research, Millennium Pharmaceuticals Inc., Cambridge, MA*

CARLOS GARCÍA-ECHEVERRÍA, PhD • *Oncology Research, Novartis Pharma AG, Basel, Switzerland*

GEOFFREY S. GINSBURG, MD, PhD • *Millennium Pharmaceuticals Inc., Cambridge, MA*

ALFRED L. GOLDBERG, MD • *Department of Cell Biology, Harvard Medical School, Boston, MA*

BARRY GREENE • *Chief Operating Office, Alnylam Pharmaceuticals, Cambridge, MA*

MARCUS GROETTRUP, PhD • *Division of Immunology, Department of Biology, University of Constance, Konstanz, Germany*

MICHAEL GROLL, MD • *Abteilung Strukturforschung MPI für Biochemie, Planegg-Martinsried, Germany*

SUSAN L. HOLBECK, PhD • *Developmental Therapeutics Program, Information Technology Branch, National Cancer Institute, Bethesda, MD*

ROBERT HUBER, MD • *Physical Chemistry Institute, University of Zürich, Zürich, Switzerland*

OSCAR KASHALA, MD • *Millennium Pharmaceuticals Inc., Cambridge, MA*

MICHAEL KAUFFMAN, MD, PhD • *CEO, Predix Pharmaceuticals, Woburn, MA*

KYUNG BO KIM, PhD • *Department of Pharmaceutical Sciences, College of Pharmacy, University of Kentucky, Lexington, KY*

LEONARD LIEBES, MD • *New York University School of Medicine, New York, NY*

GERALD P. LINETTE, MD, PhD • *Millennium Pharmaceuticals Inc., Cambridge, MA*

YI-HE LING, PhD • *Department of Oncology, Albert Einstein College of Medicine, Bronx, NY*

WILLIAM H. MCBRIDE, MD • *Department of Radiation Oncology, UCLA Medical Center, Torrance, CA*

DAVID J. MCCONKEY, MD • *M.D. Anderson Cancer Center, University of Texas, Houston, TX*

EDWARD G. MIMNAUGH • *Urologic Oncology Branch, National Cancer Institute, National Institutes of Health, Rockville, MD*

JAMES B. MITCHELL, PhD • *Chief, Radiation Biology Branch, National Cancer Institute, National Institutes of Health, Bethesda, MD*

REBECCA MOSHER, MD • *Millennium Pharmaceuticals Inc., Cambridge, MA*

GEORGE MULLIGAN, PhD • *Millennium Pharmaceuticals Inc., Cambridge, MA*

LEONARD M. NECKERS, MD • *Urologic Oncology Branch, National Cancer Institute, National Institutes of Health, Rockville, MD*

BRUCE NG, MS • *NYU Cancer Institute, New York, NY*

JEFFREY J. OLSON, MD • *Department of Neurosurgery, Emory University School of Medicine, Atlanta, GA*

ROBERT Z. ORLOWSKI, MD, PhD • *Division of Hematology/Oncology, University of North Carolina at Chapel Hill, Chapel Hill, NC*

FRANK PAJONK • *Division for Clinical and Experimental Radiation Biology Research, Department of Radiation Oncology, University Clinic Freiburg, Freiburg, Germany*

ROMAN PEREZ-SOLER, MD • *Albert Einstein College of Medicine, Montefiore Medical Center, Bronx, NY*

JEFFREY S. ROSS, MD • *Scientific Fellow Oncology Molecular Medicine, Millennium Pharmaceuticals Inc., Cambridge, MA, and Chairman, Department of Pathology and Laboratory Medicine, Albany Medical College, Albany, NY*

EDWARD A. SAUSVILLE, MD, PhD • *Developmental Therapeutics Program, National Cancer Institute, Rockville, MD*

THOMAS J. SAYERS, PhD • *SAIC-Frederick, National Cancer Institute-Frederick, Frederick, MD*

DAVID P. SCHENKEIN, MD • *Vice President and Head of Oncology Clinical Development, Millennium Pharmaceuticals Inc, Cambridge, MA*

GUNTER SCHMIDTKE, MD • *Department of Biology, Division of Immunology, University of Constance, Konstanz, Germany*

ULRICH SCHUBERT, PhD • *Institute for Clinical and Molecular Virology, University of Erlanger–Nürnberg, Erlanger, Germany*

JAMES STEC • *Millennium Pharmaceuticals Inc., Cambridge, MA*

JOHN B. SUNWOO, MD • *Tumor Biology Section, Head and Neck Surgery Branch, National Institute on Deafness, and Other Communication Disorders, National Institutes of Health, Bethesda, MD*

WILLIAM TREPICCHIO, PhD • *Millennium Pharmaceuticals Inc., Cambridge, MA*

CARTER VAN WAES, MD, PhD • *Tumor Biology Section, Head and Neck Surgery Branch, National Institute on Deafness and Other Communication Disorders, National Institutes of Health, Bethesda, MD*

SIMON A. WILLIAMS, MD • *Department of Oncology, The Sidney Kimmel Comprehensive Cancer Center at Johns Hopkins, Baltimore, MD*

ZHAOBIN ZHANG, BA • *Department of Neurosurgery, Emory University School of Medicine, Atlanta, GA*

Color Illustrations

The color insert includes the following illustrations (follows page 240):

I | Cancer Drug Development

1

Cancer Drug Development

Challenges in a Competitive Market

Barry Greene and Michael Kauffman

ABSTRACT

In the 1940s, a leak from a leftover canister of mustard gas prompted scientists to take a closer look at the myelosuppressive implications of nitrogen mustard for treating acute leukemia (then deemed a fatal disease). A new era of hope and possibility started with a mere accident, an inadvertent gas leak from a canister of nitrogen mustard. The era of genotoxic drug development had begun. Subsequent decades would herald remarkable advances in oncology medicine—in molecular understanding, scientific method, diagnostic tools, and therapeutic options.

Improved techniques and better diagnostic tools were enabling doctors to detect more cancers earlier. Improvements in the diagnosis and treatment of infectious and cardiovascular diseases were increasing the number of patients living long enough to contract cancer. An aging population contributed to a greater incidence of cancer and, consequently, higher therapeutic demand. Both the number of patients on cancer medicines and the duration of their treatment were growing. The "war on cancer," as declared by President Nixon, and the increased public perception of the "Big C" was further fueling the demand for anticancer agents. Genomically based, targeted therapies had begun to offer real hope: better efficacy and tolerability were providing the potential to live longer.

Between 1991 and 1995 the number of drugs in oncology development grew rapidly. One company, Bristol-Myers Squibb, demonstrated the opportunity to gain commercial success in a market once thought of as strictly niche.

From: *Cancer Drug Discovery and Development: Proteasome Inhibitors in Cancer Therapy*
Edited by: J. Adams © Humana Press Inc., Totowa, NJ

Apparent breakthroughs and frustrations, and emergent challenges and unmet needs, motivated and confounded a pharmaceutical industry that recognized the extraordinary opportunity inherent in the development of anticancer agents and the difficulties associated with turning such theoretical opportunities into a thriving, viable business.

With the common belief that cancer was a growing issue that had to be solved, biopharmaceutical companies seemed particularly well positioned to capture a significant proportion of a market in which traditional cytotoxic and hormonal therapies were expected to yield to targeted and novel therapeutics in the coming years.

In the early 2000s, many companies found that the promise of genomics was feasible, but not all approaches, and, in fact, few approaches, would actually work—there was a dose of reality. Bortezomib/Velcade is a case study of a company, Millennium, taking a completely new approach to treating cancer and bringing a novel drug, with a new mechanism of action to approval and market launch.

KEY WORDS

Cancer; reality of cancer drug development; circumventing the pitfalls in cancer development; bortezomib; velcade; oncology; commercial; cancer team composition; cancer development collaborative approach; FDA; drug approval.

1. INTRODUCTION

In the 1940s, a leak from a leftover canister of mustard gas prompted scientists to take a closer look at the myelosuppressive implications of nitrogen mustard for treating acute leukemia (then deemed a fatal disease) *(1)*. A new era of hope and possibility started with a mere accident, an inadvertent gas leak from a canister of nitrogen mustard. The era of genotoxic drug development had begun. Subsequent decades would herald remarkable advances in oncology medicine—in molecular understanding, scientific method, diagnostic tools, and therapeutic options *(1)* .

Improved techniques and better diagnostic tools (better mammography, helical computed tomographic scans, and magnetic resonance imaging; serum-based screening tests such as prostate-specific antigen, CA-125, and α-fetoprotein; and molecular pathology testing) were enabling doctors to detect more cancers earlier. Improvements in the diagnosis and treatment of infectious and cardiovascular diseases were increasing the number of patients living long enough to contract cancer. An aging population contributed to a greater incidence of cancer and, consequently, higher therapeutic demand. Both the number of patients on cancer medicines and the duration of their treatment were growing. The "war on cancer," as declared by President Nixon, and the increased public perception of the "Big C" were further fueling the demand for anticancer agents *(2)*. Genomically based, targeted therapies had begun to offer real hope: better efficacy and tolerability were providing the potential to live longer.

By 1991, 126 oncology compounds were in development in laboratories around the world. By 1995, that number had grown to 302, with 138 companies managing oncology clinical pipelines (Millennium, data on file). Still, difficult questions challenged the nascent genotoxic drug development industry. Paclitaxel (Taxol®), which went on to become the top-selling oncology drug in history, generated $1.5 billion in sales in 1999. Bristol-Myers Squibb (BMS) had proved that launching a blockbuster oncology product was possible, despite the small and increasingly fragmented cancer-patient population *(3)*. (BMS also developed carboplatin, which generated $700 million in sales in 2001 *[4]*). Taxol was the right product for the right time providing proof that oncology drug development was just a viable commercial opportunity.

Apparent breakthroughs and frustrations, as well as emerging challenges and unmet needs, both motivated and confounded a pharmaceutical industry that recognized the extraordinary opportunity inherent in the development of anticancer agents and the difficulties associated with turning such theoretical opportunities into a thriving, viable business.

With forecasters projecting 8 million cancer patients in the United States, Europe, and Japan by 2008, and an oncology market of $17 billion by 2005 (Millennium, data on file), building an organizational platform around oncology research and development seemed less like a "pipe dream" and more like an imperative. Biopharmaceutical companies seemed particularly well positioned to capture a significant proportion of a market in which traditional cytotoxic and hormonal therapies were expected to yield to targeted and novel therapeutics in the coming years (Millennium, data on file).

1.1. Barriers to Entry

Barriers to entry were attractively low, in comparison with other therapeutic areas. In theory, the failure rate of anticancer drugs is lower than the failure rate of drugs used to treat diseases such as high blood pressure, diabetes, or reflux disease. The reason is simple: a dry cough associated with a blood pressure product may be annoying, a disincentive that prompts patients and physicians alike to look for other therapeutic options, but with anticancer drugs, a patient often has only one real choice—to endure the nausea, diarrhea, headache, fatigue, pain, or dizziness so often associated with such powerful agents, or to face the more deadly consequences of the disease itself.

In oncology drug development, the number of cancer patients enrolled in clinical studies is far lower—on the order of 10–100 times fewer—than the number enrolled in studies designed for products in other therapeutic areas (Millennium, data on file). The fewer enrollees a study has, the fewer resources that study taps—fewer investigators and hospitals are typically required, for example, and less product has to be prepared for distribution. Although the more lengthy and complex Case Report Forms represent a major investment, the overall investment is well worth the tradeoff.

Millennium is conducting the largest randomized clinical trial in multiple myeloma, in which total enrollment is more than 600 patients. Although this is huge by the standards of hematologic cancer clinical trials, the size of this study pales in comparison with the 60,000 patients enrolled in trials for the hypertension product felodipine (Plendil®) a few years ago (Millennium, data on file).

When a company is launching a product that has potential application for a large percentage of a population, it is compelled to canvas all potential prescribing physicians with a large, and thus expensive, sales force (Millennium, data on file). Oncology products, however, are prescribed only by hematologists and oncologists and require a far smaller sales force (the smallest territory cut for oncology is 80 compared with 500 for primary care; Millennium, data on file).

2. A DOSE OF REALITY

In the summer of 2002, more than 500 compounds, a full half of which involved novel mechanisms and pathways, were under development in the United States (Millennium, data on file). Breakthrough products such as imatinib mesylate (Gleevec®; Glivac® in Europe), a Novartis product designed to treat chronic myelogenous leukemia *(5)*, and trastuzumab (Herceptin®) *(6)*, a Genentech product for the treatment of metastatic breast cancer, fueled talk of the possibility of a cancer cure. Patient advocacy groups were clamoring for more and better drugs—faster. Optimism, not to mention ambition, was everywhere; the lure of oncology drug development was strong.

However, of the hundreds of products in development, most would fail and never reach the market, costing pharmaceutical companies billions in unrecoverable research dollars. Failed products also caused distractions in the marketplace: patients were drawn into studies from which they would not benefit, and physicians seeking reliable information were confused by therapeutic options. Doubt was cast on the ability of pharmaceutical companies to locate that entirely too elusive cancer cure, and demands for sophistication and foresight on the part of sponsor companies increased. Excitement regarding possible breakthoughs was followed by announcements of rejection of regulatory approval, sending companies back to their proverbial "drawing boards."

Cetuximab (Erbitux®) is a therapeutic antibody developed by ImClone in partnership with BMS in the United States, and Merck, KGA, in Europe and Japan. Developed to treat epithelial diseases like colon cancer and, potentially, lung cancer, cetuximab was found to have little activity on its own and was combined with irinotecan (Camptosar®), a Pharmacia product, during clinical trials. A single-arm phase II study of cetuximab plus irinotecan in patients with colon cancer who had previously received irinotecan (and yet had progressive disease) found a response rate of around 20%. This was enough, ImClone believed, to go to the Food and Drug Administration (FDA) to seek approval for the drug *(7)*. Unfortunately for the patients the drug was designed to treat, the data were neither conclusive nor persuasive. First, it was unclear from the data derived from this single-arm trial design whether the responses observed were due to cetuximab or whether the same or better response rates would have been achieved with irinotecan alone. Although the patients in this phase II study had previously received irinotecan alone, the data collected in the trial did not provide enough information regarding pretrial resistance rates to irinotecan *(7)*. This is a crucial point: in some oncology patients, when a tumor has previously progressed under treatment with a certain agent, retreatment with the same agent can lead to a response, although the response—tumor shrinkage in this case—is often short lived *(7)*. Although better characterization of the patients entering the trial was also needed, the FDA postponed evaluation of the clinical data until a control trial had been completed *(7)*. Erbitux was approved over a year later.

In a single-arm, single-center phase II clinical trial of thalidomide (Thalomid®), which in clinical trials has shown activity in patients with multiple myeloma, patients with one or two prior therapies for multiple myeloma were treated with escalating doses of thalidomide. The trial ultimately showed a response rate of 32% and an average duration of response of between 3 and 4 mo *(8)*. During their review of thalidomide, the FDA required Celgene, the sponsoring company, to design and undertake an entirely new supplemental clinical trial that would effectively compare the efficacy of thalidomide with another agent meant to treat patients with multiple myeloma (Millennium, data on file). Although the specifics about the thalidomide submission are not available, it is likely that Celgene encountered FDA concerns relating to dosing, ambiguities surrounding prior patient therapies and resistance, and the fact that a single-center study is inevitably subject to center bias. Celgene announced submitting an SNDA in early 2004. The FDA has not approved a drug for the specific treatment of multiple myeloma since it approved melphalan (Alkeran®), and it is believed that the FDA is not likely to approve such a drug until data prove that there is indeed a benefit to the experimental drug, including a persuasive response rate and duration of response. Those working in oncology recognize that response rates, or tumor shrinkage, are becoming increasingly *unfavorable on their own* as regulatory endpoints. From a regulatory—and patient's—perspective, it is as or more important for an anticancer agent to *prevent the progression* of disease. There are many cases in which anticancer agents shrink tumors initially, but the tumors rapidly regrow at a rate that may negate the initial size reduction (Millennium, data on file). Merely marginal response rates will never be enough: it is essential to prove that the drug is better than something else or, indeed, better than nothing at all.

When the FDA or the European Agency for the Evaluation of Medicinal Products (EMEA) does not approve a cancer product or when a company has to go back and conduct a new pivotal trial, it faces an additional expense of between $10 and $30 million (Millennium, data on file). Also, every day that a product is kept off the market, anywhere between $500,000 and $2 million of potential revenues are lost (Millennium, data on file).

3. CIRCUMVENTING THE PITFALLS

Many companies, looking at complex development cycles, believe that they can shorten the time of the process by conducting concurrent phase I/phase II trials or conducting large phase II studies with the hope that the regulatory agencies will find the response rates so significant that the phase III study will be merely confirmatory. However, skimming time from the process is wasted if the process is itself inherently flawed, if the wrong datasets are pursued, if the wrong combination drugs are investigated, or if the wrong emphasis is placed on identifying the ideal dose or conducting the most scientifically eloquent (but ultimately irrelevant) studies.

Many companies put too much emphasis on ancillary, irrelevant studies, focusing unduly on validating early scientific targets, for example, or going far off the beaten track with poorly conceived safety studies. These kinds of studies are of paramount importance in other therapeutic areas, but they are less relevant in oncology. *Pharmacokinetics*, the action of drugs in the body over a period of time (and on the related processes of absorption, distribution, excretion), is a fascinating field of study and highly pertinent in many therapeutic areas (e.g., β-blockers) in which there is a true correlation between the amount of drug in the serum level and the body's response. However, the relationships among drug levels, dosing intervals, and efficacy are still unclear for the vast majority of anticancer agents *(9)*. The relationship between peak or trough serum levels of anticancer agents and side effects in any *individual patient* is tenuous at best, yet companies still succumb to the dictatorship of pharmacokinetics, seeking to understand the drug levels in serum and to correlate these with antitumor response.

For anticancer agents that are designed to change the way cells live or die, the real issue is *pharmacodynamics*, or the biochemical impact of the therapeutic agent and its mechanisms of action *(9)*. Pharmacodynamics studies answer the questions: Is the drug hitting its target? Is it having a true biochemical impact? Is that impact the one for which the drug was designed? A good pharmacodynamic marker will enable a company to assess how well modulation of a specific target in a human actually corresponds to modulation of that same target in the animal model system. For example, if the animal studies that were used to justify the move into human studies showed efficacy at a certain pharmacodynamic level, then achieving that same pharmacodynamic level in humans is a reasonable goal. If it so happens there is no or marginal efficacy in humans at the pharmacodynamic effect level seen in the animal models, then the efficacy justification for moving into humans is essentially flawed. Thus, having a good pharmacodynamic marker that can be used in animals and humans—and can be used to "communicate" between the model systems and the patients—is crucial to determining when to expect to see results and when to halt drug development.

Dosing issues have also proved to be a stumbling block for many organizations developing anticancer agents. Identifying the most efficacious dose possible often comes down to giving the most amount of drug one can without seriously harming the patient, rather than obsessing over identifying the ideal dosage. In cancer, response rates and time to progression can take upward of a year while dosing regimens undergo constant refinements and improvements. Identifying the perfect dose could theoretically take a dozen years, but the focus must be to find a dose that works, rather than the dose that works the best.

Beating the odds in cancer therapy also means being extremely careful about choosing combination drugs. Combination therapies will become increasingly common, complicating clinical trial design, regulatory approval, and physician understanding. In recent cancer therapy, the approach to combinations has been less than scientific, as companies and oncologists tended simply to take two drugs, put them together, and hope for at least additive efficacy without excessive toxicity. It is a strategy that may have worked when there were only 15 drugs to choose from, but with some 50 products in development, every company must have a scientific rationale relying on both in vitro (with the focus on mechanistic/biochemical implications) and in vivo (with the focus on enhanced efficacy with nonadditive side effects) data for the combination therapies it chooses to investigate. Designing nonclinical and clinical trials around a well-defined drug approval strategy is key.

From the project's very onset, it is important to pay close attention to market uptake issues. What must and should the product label say? What educational messages are imperative? What data will have to be made available in order for physicians to make informed choices about using the product being developed? Articulating a market uptake strategy early in the development cycle is crucial, particularly in cancer therapy, in which drugs are often used by physicians in a manner not always outlined on the label (10). They are prescribed by physicians who believe in the mechanism or target, or are demanded by patients with diseases that have failed to respond to every other known product and insist on being given one last chance. To ensure proper scientific (publication-driven) use, one must design studies yielding data that lead to informed decision making.

It is a well-understood reality in drug development that to ensure approval by the FDA all one must really do is prove that a drug works safely and works better than placebo. Any company, for example, is free to develop a proton pump inhibitor and take the risk as to whether it will receive a commercial return. In developing anticancer agents, the stakes are far higher. Here one must prove that the agent is *better* than the accepted standard of care—a requirement that puts every enterprise at risk. Standards of care are always subject to change, increasingly so as more agents appear on the market. Consequently, many companies could conceivably face the challenge of having to redesign phase III studies midcourse to ensure that their product is being assessed against the appropriate comparison arms. A vigilant and relentless analysis of ongoing development trends is extremely important throughout the long development cycle.

There is one way to succeed in this increasingly competitive industry: keeping one's eye on the goal line. In most cancer therapies, the goal line comprises time to progression and survival. There are a number of proven guiding principles and firm strategic footholds to meet this goal: pursuing the development of anticancer agents with a thorough understanding of, and healthy respect for, current and emerging market situation, unmet medical needs, demographics of the patient population, physician use and practice, and promises and pitfalls inherent in all scientific discovery.

- Between phase I (safety), phase II (dosing), and phase III (testing the experimental drug against the standard of care in, traditionally, a randomized, well-controlled, multicenter pivotal trial or series of trials), a company will probably spend 4.5 yr developing a drug and another 6–12 mo seeking regulatory approval (Millennium, data on file).
- The clinical trials need to be designed to answer expeditiously all pertinent questions about the compound's efficacy, safety, and relationship to the current standard of care in certain patient populations.
- Effective clinical trials will play an emphatic role in the drug's market uptake after launch by providing data that lead to informed decision making and help ensure proper scientific (publication-driven) use.
- Most clinical trials focus on a compound's response rate. With hematological cancers, that may in fact be the most relevant measure of a compound's value, but for most solid tumors, response rate alone is simply not an acceptable measure; in many instances, response rate does not correlate with survival, or even with time to progression. The shrinking of a tumor defined radiographically (usually on a computed tomographic or magnetic resonance scan) does not automatically imply a cure, or even a benefit. What matters is when and if the tumor returns, how fast, and when it begins to grow larger.

A company on the verge of taking an experimental compound into the clinic must be able to plan for what the regulatory agencies will require in order to approve the drug. It must be able to design trials yielding the data that will answer pressing questions about response rate, time to progression, and survival. If time to progression becomes the most important "surrogate" endpoint for survival, compounds that are *tolerable* when taken chronically will automatically have an edge. A company must be willing to enroll patients in early studies who will be able to provide historical controls as the later data roll in, and it must be willing to provide drugs to patients *without progression* indefinitely. It must be willing to forego elegant studies that will yield little more than interesting fodder for scientific publications. Finally, it must never lose sight of the absolute importance of demonstrating efficacy in humans as early and as consistently as possible.

4. BORTEZOMIB: A CASE STUDY

Developing and marketing anticancer agents requires a highly developed talent for making the right decisions in a conclusive and timely manner. At Millennium, we have taken an assertive approach to managing bortezomib (Velcade; formerly known as PS-341), a proteasome inhibitor that in laboratory studies interrupts the cell cycle and induces apoptosis in cancer cells. Currently being studied for use in the treatment of various solid tumors and hematologic malignancies, bortezomib is, at present, being evaluated in a number of clinical trials for time to disease progression, response rate, and survival. Our strategies throughout the design and execution of the clinical trials have been fueled by a tremendous faith in our data.

In preliminary trials, bortezomib dosing was guided by biologic and antitumor activity and a pharmacodynamic assay that was designed to study the percentage of proteasome inhibition seen in various tissues. The pharmacodynamic (proteasome-inhibition) assay was developed for use with human whole blood, providing a relatively simple and straightforward method of assessing the drug's biochemical effects. The proteasome-inhibition assay was also carried out in all the animal models tested, including those in which combination therapy was used. Going into phase I first in human studies, we expected to see anticancer activity of bortezomib when greater than 60% peak proteasome inhibition was achieved. Antitumor activity was observed in phase I studies of patients with multiple myeloma at doses of bortezomib that provided 60–80% peak proteasome inhibition. When early reports from clinical trials suggested that biologically active doses of bortezomib might be associated with antitumor activity, retardation of disease progression, and manageable toxicity in multiple myeloma patients, Millennium proceeded with multicenter trials of bortezomib as monotherapy and in combination with dexamethasone in patients with multiple myeloma, and also with phase II studies of bortezomib in combination with standard chemotherapeutic agents for other cancers.

From very early on, our philosophy was to pay serious attention to the first few patients dosed with the drug. We believed that a handful of patients provides some insight into the future of this compound—that if the first three to five patients were not showing a response or at least stabilization of disease, for example, we could comfortably conclude that we were not in possession of a very active agent. Certainly many agents are developed and evaluated in up to 12–14 patients before response assessment is made. But as the "bar" gets higher, the chances are minimal that an agent producing only 1 response in 12 will ultimately represent a significant breakthrough.

In the case of bortezomib in multiple myeloma clinical trials, in a phase I trial, there was one complete response rate, two satisfactory response rates, several patients with stable disease, and a few patients for whom the drug did not appear to have an effect. These data were sufficiently encouraging to justify the launch of a 75-person phase II clinical trial. (Typical phase II trials study between 25 and 40 patients, particularly in hematologic malignancies.) It was a decision we felt comfortable making because we wanted to know—with as much precision as possible—what the full capabilities of our product were. Moreover, if bortezomib was not a powerful agent, we wanted to know that as well, so that we could potentially discontinue development as rapidly as possible.

Preliminary data from patients with relapsed, refractory, *and* progressive disease in the phase II multiple myeloma clinical trials with bortezomib show that the response rate was 10% CR and 59 OR (35% CR/PR), the time to progression was 6 mo, and the median survival rate was greater than 6 mo. The patients in this trial had had an average of five prior therapies. It was with enormous optimism, therefore, that we launched the 612-patient phase III trial of bortezomib in patients with multiple myeloma that is currently under way.

5. TEAM COMPOSITION

Decisions are driven by data, but they are made by people, and the development of cancer agents depends on the existence and management of a team of individuals knowledgeable in biology, chemistry, clinical development, finance, marketing, regulation, and project leadership, not to mention manufacturing and technology transfer. Oncology drug development requires people who know what "good" data look like in cancer—capable people who can think out of the box and foresee the future of oncology research, an entire team that is willing to "read all the early tea leaves" and set the project on a viable course.

The success of a team does not revolve exclusively around its composition. A team cannot win unless it is also fully aligned around clear goals, objectives, roles, and responsibilities and it is fully integrated to meet the project goals. Infighting will hurt a team sooner than murky data ever will, and success or failure often hinges on communication and cooperation between and among functional experts. Leaders, consequently, are key, and in anticancer drug development, team leaders must be skilled at articulating the project goals early on and ensuring that only activities contributing to those goals are effectively pursued. This entails focus; leaders must drive their teams with the products in mind, recognizing that mere functional excellence is never enough. Team leaders must ensure that the internal goals are both aggressive and consistent, that extraordinary work gets rewarded, that fires are lit over the course of the long development cycle so that the work never flags or falters or gets stuck in damaging ruts. They must also guard against making irresponsible promises to a marketplace and a patient population that must be given good reason to trust what they hear.

Perhaps most importantly, team leaders must also be adept at keeping priorities straight for the many team members as they seek to address and satisfy the competing voices, dreams, and demands placed on them by their multiple customers. Thought leaders and physicians, regional and local oncologists, patient advocates, regulatory authorities, oncology nurses, Wall Street analysts, patients, internal managers, and boards of directors all pull and push at the development process, clamoring to have their voices heard. It is the responsibility of the team, as managed by its leader, to keep the focus on the two most essential outcomes: getting the best possible drug approved and ensuring its uptake by the market.

6. A COLLABORATIVE ENTERPRISE

Collaboration is essential in oncology drug development; every new genomic and molecular breakthrough represents a win not just for the company itself, but for humanity, and no individual company has the resources to pursue the science entirely on its own. From now until the conceivable future, cancer therapy will rely on combination treatments, drugs from different laboratories that collectively slow, arrest, and ultimately eradicate the disease. Systemic cytotoxics, metastasis inhibitors, selective apoptosis inducers, anti-angiogenesis agents, cancer vaccines, antibody-targeted therapy, signal transduction inhibitors, tumor suppressor replacement, and hormonal therapies will all be part of the treatment portfolio going forward, each new breakthrough informing the next, each new approved product elevating the standard of care, each new therapeutic agent changing the profile of "good" in cancer drugs.

The urge to be first, the corporate imperative to seize a share of the market and to protect intellectual property makes collaboration a prickly matter, a land mine all its own. The key, it seems, is to focus the company on what it does best, to engage others to fill in the spaces, and to build relationships in which everyone involved can win. At Millennium, we tend to spend much time with our collaborators—forming real partnerships, intelligently structuring contracts, sharing the right data freely, and at the same time never losing sight of the fact that we cannot control our partners; we can only develop a relationship in which both sides see the benefit in learning from each other. We recognize, at Millennium, that we all share a common goal: to bring new cancer therapeutics to the marketplace as expeditiously as possible.

Patient advocacy groups, the Cancer Therapy Evaluation Program of the National Cancer Institute (CTEP/NCI), the European Organization for Research and Treatment of Cancer (EORTC), clinical investigators, and scientific investigators all play a crucial role in the work we do and the decisions we make; all advance our internal programs and help bring our products to market sooner. Lead investigators who have sought and received permission for use of our drugs in their own animal studies have heightened our own understanding of the molecular biology of our compounds. Patient advocates who have asked to be kept abreast of our work and who have accepted our invitations to sit in on our own internal discussions and review our clinical development plans have later played pivotal roles in knowledgably informing patients about other treatment options, clinical trials, and the interpretation of clinical data.

Oncology drug development is not a pursuit in which one roots for one's competitors to fail. Knowledge feeds knowledge. Success feeds success. Clean science, smart clinical trials, carefully prepared submissions for marketing authorization (such as New Drug Applications, Biological License Applications, and EMEA Applications) speed the approval process, free up scarce regulatory resources, and expand the portfolio of combination alternatives. The lone scientist does not win in oncology. The collaborative effort does. Certainly without the great support and collaboration we at Millennium have established with many groups, a good number of which are highlighted in the pages to come, we would not have made the progress we have made, nor would the future of oncology look as bright as it now does.

REFERENCES

1. Baguley BC. A brief history of cancer chemotherapy. In: Baguley BC, Kerr DJ, eds. *Anticancer Drug Development*. San Diego: Academic Press, 2001:1–11.
2. Grammer E. Researchers march on in war on cancer. Washington, DC: American Association for the Advancement of Science. www.aasa.org, accessed July 3, 2003.
3. *Making a Difference for All Time: 1999 Bristol-Myers Squibb Annual Report*. New York: Bristol-Myers Squibb. 2003:1–56.
4. Top pharmaceuticals companies report. *Contract Pharm*. July/August 2002. www.contractpharmac.com, accessed July 3, 2003.
5. FDA approves Gleevec for leukemia treatment; Gleevec also produces complete remission in GIST cancer. Washington, DC: US Food and Drug Administration, May 14, 2001. www.HIVand Hepatitis.com, accessed April 4, 2003.
6. Package insert. Herceptin. Trastuzumab anti-HER monoclonal antibody. *Physician's Desk Reference 2003*, 57th ed. Montvale, NJ: Thomson PDR, 2003:1399–1402.
7. Jerian S. Conversation with cancer patient advocates. Cetuximab (Erbitux) presentation, sponsored by ImClone, October 10, 2002.

8. Singhal S, Mehta J, Desikan R, et al. Antitumor activity of thalidomide in refractory multiple myeloma. *N Engl J Med* 1999;341:1565–1571.
9. Sparreboom A, Loos WJ, de Jonge MJ, Verweij J. Clinical trial design: incorporation of pharmacokinetic, pharmacodynamic, and pharmacogenetic principles. In: Baguley BC, Kerr DJ, eds. *Anticancer Drug Development*. San Diego: Academic Press, 2001:329–351.
10. Abeloff MD. Off-label uses of anticancer drugs. *JAMA* 1992;267:2473–2474.

II CHEMISTRY AND CELL BIOLOGY OF THE PROTEASOME

2 Introduction to the Proteasome and its Inhibitors

Biochemistry and Cell Biology

Alfred L. Goldberg

CONTENTS

ABSTRACT

The development of proteasome inhibitors for treatment of multiple myeloma and probably other cancers has followed an unusual course but is clearly linked to recent basic advances in our understanding of intracellular protein breakdown. After the discovery of the ATP-dependent pathway for protein degradation in the 1970s, ATP was shown necessary for the conjugation of ubiquitin to cell proteins, which marks them for degradation by the 26S proteasome. Its 19S regulatory complex uses ATP to unfold proteins and to inject them into the 20S core proteasome where proteins are digested to small peptides. The active sites in the 20S proteasome function by a novel threonine-based mechanism which allows their selective inhibition (e.g., by the boronate, Velcade). Surprisingly, we initially organized a biotechnology company to develop inhibitors of the ubiquitin–proteasome pathway not for cancer therapy, but with the goal of reducing the excessive proteolysis seen in atrophying muscle or cachexia, as well as inhibition of MHC class I antigen presentation, both of which depend on proteasome function. The availability of proteasome inhibitors has greatly advanced our understanding of the many functions of the proteasome, such as its key role in the activation of the transcription factor NF-κB, which led to a recognition that proteasome inhibitors might have anti-inflammatory and antineoplastic actions. The unexpected discovery that these inhibitors cause apoptosis selectively in neoplastic cells led to systematic studies and clinical trials against cancer. Amongst their multiple actions, proteasome inhibitors (1) cause the accumulation of

From: *Cancer Drug Discovery and Development: Proteasome Inhibitors in Cancer Therapy*
Edited by: J. Adams © Humana Press Inc., Totowa, NJ

abnormal proteins, which can trigger apoptosis; (2) stabilize tumor suppressors (p53, p27); (3) inhibit production of NF-κB, which is antiapoptic and generates important growth factors and cell adhesion molecules. However, the actual importance of these mechanisms in vivo in combating cancer remains uncertain.

KEY WORDS

Proteasome inhibitors; proteasome mechanisms; proteasome functions; NF-κB; Velcade (PS-341); cancer.

1. INTRODUCTION

Although there can be many frustrations in a life devoted to biomedical research, there can also be unique rewards, especially the satisfaction that comes from seeing one's work lead to a greater understanding of living organisms and even, on occasion, to improvements in medical care. Consequently, those of us whose research has focused on the mechanisms of intracellular protein breakdown and the functions of the proteasome view with particular satisfaction and some parental pride the exciting emergence of proteasome inhibitors in the treatment of various cancers. Also highly gratifying has been the enormous utility that proteasome inhibitors have had as research tools that have greatly expanded our knowledge of the importance of the ubiquitin–proteasome pathway in cell regulation, immune surveillance, and human disease.

The research that led up to the synthesis of bortezomib (Velcade™; formerly known as PS-341) and its introduction for the treatment of cancer has had a curious, unpredictable history that is very much linked to the multiple strands of my own research career. In this chapter, I review the scientific findings that led to the development of bortezomib, which is now showing such exciting promise in clinical trials against cancer. Interestingly, this research, and even the organization of a biotechnology company whose primary program was to generate inhibitors of the ubiquitin–proteasome pathway, were not undertaken to find new cancer therapies. However, advances in biochemistry and drug development often do not follow predictable paths, and new insights in this area, as in others, have often come about by unexpected routes. This chapter, in addition to explaining the scientific background and rationale for the preclinical development of proteasome inhibitors, attempts to summarize our present understanding of the proteasome's function that has emerged from 25 yr of biochemical studies and studies using proteasome inhibitors.

1.1. Why Did We Want to Generate Inhibitors of the Proteasome?

The research paths leading to bortezomib and our decision in 1992 to undertake an effort to synthesize proteasome inhibitors for possible therapeutic applications derived not from the field of cancer biology, but from more arcane studies I had initiated almost 40 yr ago as a medical-graduate student to clarify the mechanisms of muscle atrophy, such as that occurring with denervation, disuse, and many major systemic diseases, including cancer cachexia, sepsis, renal failure, and AIDS (1,2). That early work demonstrated that this loss of cell protein following denervation was caused not by a simple reduction in muscle protein synthesis (as we had expected), but rather by an acceleration of the rate of protein breakdown (3). This finding was the first evidence that overall rates of protein breakdown in mammalian cells are regulated and can be of major importance in human disease.

At the time, virtually nothing was known about the pathways for protein catabolism in cells *(4,5)*. Therefore, in starting my own laboratory in 1969, I decided to focus my research on elucidating this degradative pathway through biochemical studies, not in muscle, but rather in simpler cells, initially *Escherichia coli* (because of the opportunity to use genetic approaches) and then mammalian reticulocytes. In the 1970s and 1980s, these studies led to the discovery of the soluble ATP-dependent proteolytic system and of the roles of the 26S proteasome and ubiquitin in this pathway. Although seemingly unrelated to muscle wasting or cancer therapy, these very basic studies have eventually influenced both areas. Ten years ago, these biochemical discoveries and parallel findings about muscle protein degradation suggested to us that selective pharmacologic inhibition of the ubiquitin–proteasome pathway might be feasible and could provide a rational approach toward developing agents to combat muscle wasting and cachexia. Although that therapeutic goal has not been achieved, in pursuing that objective, many important scientific insights have been obtained, and, most excitingly, bortezomib has emerged.

1.2. Discovery of the Ubiquitin–Proteasome Pathway

A major motivation for our undertaking to study protein degradation in bacteria and reticulocytes was that these cells lack lysosomes, which were then believed to be the site of protein breakdown in cells. However, I had become convinced that these organelles could not account for the extreme selectivity and regulation of intracellular proteolysis. Our present understanding of this process emerged from a series of developments, first through key in vivo findings and then in vitro studies of their biochemical basis.

Of particular importance was my finding that bacteria, which were long believed not to degrade their own proteins, could not only activate intracellular proteolysis when starved for amino acids or aminoacyl tRNA *(6)*, but that even during exponential growth, these cells rapidly degraded proteins with abnormal structures, such as those that may arise by mutation or postsynthetic damage *(7)*. Reticulocytes were also shown to carry out the degradation of abnormal proteins, which further suggested to us the existence of a nonlysosomal system for selective protein breakdown in eukaryotic cells *(5)*.

We showed that a key feature of this process was that it required ATP *(5,7)*, which clearly distinguished this intracellular process from known proteolytic enzymes and implied novel biochemical mechanisms. This energy requirement, in fact, was the critical clue to our finding and elucidation of the responsible degradative system and was, at the time, most puzzling, because there was clearly no thermodynamic necessity for energy to support peptide bond hydrolysis and no ATP requirement for the function of known proteases. Although studies in mammalian cells in the 1960s and early 1970s, especially by Schimke, Tomkins, and co-workers, had indicated that many tightly regulated enzymes were rapidly degraded in vivo *(4)*, this process ceased when cells were broken open, in large part because of this energy requirement for intracellular proteolysis *(8)*. It had been speculated that energy might be required for lysosomal function; however, our finding of a similar ATP requirement in bacteria and reticulocytes indicated that another explanation must apply.

On this basis, Joseph Etlinger and I searched for such a system in cell-free extracts of reticulocytes and were able to demonstrate a soluble, nonlysosomal (neutral pH optimum) proteolytic system that carried out the selective degradation of abnormal proteins when provided with ATP in a similar fashion to intact cells *(9)*. The biochemical dissection of this degradative system focused on an attempt to understand the molecular basis for this mysterious ATP requirement.

A fundamental advance was the discovery by Avram Hershko and Aaron Ciechanover of the involvement in this process of a small, heat-stable protein, subsequently identified by others to be the polypeptide ubiquitin, which was known to be linked in vivo to certain histones *(10,11)*. Their seminal work, together with that of Ernie Rose (1979–1982), established that ATP was necessary for covalent linkage chains of ubiquitin to protein substrates, which marks them for rapid degradation by the 26S proteasome. These workers also identified the three types of enzymes that are involved in the activation (E1), transfer (E2), and ligation (E3) of the ubiquitin. Mammalian cells appear to contain at least 20–30 different E2s and hundreds of distinct ubiquitination ligases, which provide the selectivity to this degradative pathway and are already emerging as very attractive drug targets *(10,11)*.

In parallel studies of protein breakdown in *E. coli* and mitochondria, we discovered a very different explanation of the ATP requirement for proteolysis. The bacteria and these organelles were shown to contain a soluble ATP-dependent proteolytic system for degradation of abnormal proteins. However, in exploring the basis for this requirement, we discovered a new type of proteolytic enzyme, very large proteolytic complexes (20–100 times the size of typical proteases) that are both proteases and ATPases (Figs. 1 and 2) *(12,13)*. Bacteria and mitochondria lack ubiquitin or a similar substrate-marking system. Instead, selective protein breakdown involves several ATP-dependent proteolytic complexes (in *E. coli* named Lon or La, ClpAP or Ti, ClpXP, HslUV, or FtsH) that hydrolyze ATP and proteins in a linked process and are selective for different kinds of substrates.

These investigations thus initially suggested two very different explanations for the ATP requirement for proteolysis, ubiquitin ligation in eukaryotes and ATP-dependent proteases in prokaryotes. However, subsequent work indicated that both mechanisms must also function in mammalian cells and that the degradation of ubiquitinated proteins and certain non-ubiquitinated substrates must be by an ATP-dependent protease *(12,14)*. In 1987, in fact, we had found such an ATP-stimulated proteolytic activity very early, but its isolation, characterization, and precise role took many years to clarify *(15)*. Finally, Rechsteiner's *(16)* and our group *(17)* were able to isolate a very large complex that degraded ubiquitin-conjugated proteins in an ATP-dependent process, the complex we subsequently named the 26S proteasome. These ATP-dependent proteases appear to function through similar ATP-dependent mechanisms as the 26S proteasome. In fact, one of these ATP-dependent proteases, HslUV, in eubacteria and the homologous proteasomes of archaebacteria and actinomyces appear to be the evolutionary ancestors of the eukaryotic 26S proteasome. Thus, proteasomes evolved quite early, before protein breakdown became linked to ubiquitin conjugation, which clearly provided opportunities for greater selectivity and regulation.

Initially, this proteolytic complex appeared to be very different from the 600-kDa proteolytic complex, which we now call the 20S proteasome (20S and 26S refer to their sedimentation rates). This structure, containing multiple peptidases, had been discovered in the early 1980s in several contexts—as a peptidase complex that hydrolyzes neuropeptides by Wilk and Orlowski *(18)*, as a nonproteolytic "ribonucleoprotein" particle by Scherrer, and as a major cytosolic endoprotease by DeMartino, our lab, and others. In the literature, there were actually at least 17 different names and multiple functions proposed

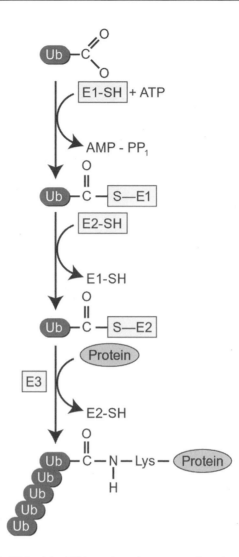

Fig. 1. Ubiquitin (Ub) conjugation to protein substrates.

for this complex. Eventually, we were able to show that these different structures corre-sponded to the same particle, which we named the 20S proteasome to indicate that it was a particle with protease function *(19)*. The next critical step was the demonstration by immunoprecipitation that the 20S proteasome was essential in the ubiquitin-dependent degradation of proteins in reticulocytes *(20)*. Finally, we *(21)* and Hershko's lab *(22)* were able to show that in the presence of ATP, the 20S particle was incorporated into the larger 26S (2.2-kDa) complex that degrades ubiquitin conjugates, which we then named the 26S proteasome (Fig. 3).

1.3. The Path to Proteasome Inhibitors and Bortezomib

These major biochemical advances did not by themselves provide the therapeutic rationale for an effort to synthesize proteasome inhibitors. In addition to these biochemi-

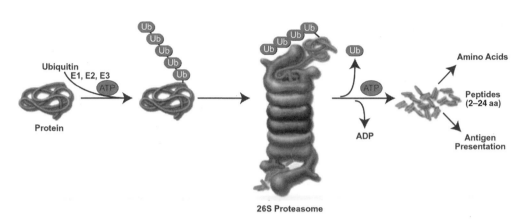

Fig. 2. The ubiquitin (Ub)–proteasome pathway.

cal studies, my lab continued to pursue physiologic studies of the control of protein breakdown in muscle in normal and disease states. A major advance was the development of simple in vitro techniques for precise measurement of rates of protein breakdown in incubated rodent muscles, which enabled us in the 1970s and 1980s to demonstrate that protein breakdown in muscle was accelerated in various diseases (e.g., cancer cachexia, renal failure, sepsis) in which muscle wasting is prominent (for reviews, see refs. **1** and **2**). Initially, it was assumed that this general acceleration of proteolysis was due to activation of the lysosomal (autophagic) pathway for proteolysis or the Ca^{2+}-activated proteases (calpains). However, blocking their function in isolated muscles had no effect on the excessive proteolysis, and, with time, we were able to demonstrate that the increased protein degradation was primarily due to an activation of the ubiquitin–proteasome pathway. This finding was surprising, since it had been generally assumed that this system primarily degraded the short-lived proteins in cells (e.g., abnormally folded polypeptides or regulatory molecules) *(10,11)* and not the long-lived proteins (e.g., contractile proteins), which comprise the bulk of cell proteins. In fact, it is now clearly established that atrophying muscles (whether due to fasting, denervation, cancer, sepsis, or diabetes) undergo a common series of transcriptional adaptations that enhance its capacity for proteolysis *(1,2)*, including increased expression of ubiquitin, proteasomes, and key new ubiquitination enzymes (E3s) *(23,24)*.

These insights led me to propose that it might be of major benefit to an enormous number of patients to be able to retard pharmacologically this degradative pathway in muscle, especially since only a relatively small increase in overall proteolysis (two- to threefold) appeared to be responsible for the rapid muscle atrophy. Therefore, our initial goal in undertaking to synthesize proteasome inhibitors was to partially inhibit the proteasome and thus to reduce muscle proteolysis to its normal rate in these catabolic states. On that basis, I convinced a group of Harvard colleagues to form a Scientific Advisory Board and to help found a biotechnology company whose primary goal would be to try to control the debilitating loss of muscle in these diseases by retarding the ubiquitin–proteasome pathway. Founding a company was attractive, because in a university setting, in which research programs are restricted by individuals' grants, it is really impossible to bring together chemists, biologists, and pharmacologists to work as a team toward a common goal. Venture-capital backing was obtained, and a biotechnology

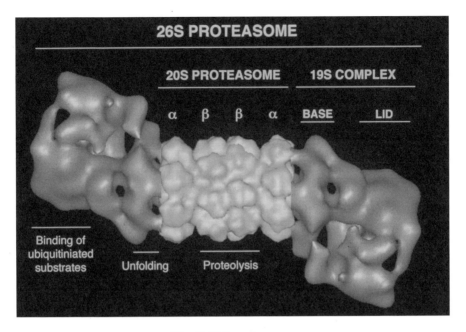

Fig. 3. 26S proteasome.

company was founded in 1993 and named MyoGenics to indicate our goal of preventing debilitating loss of muscle. Its first target was to develop inhibitors of the proteasome. With financial backing, we eventually assembled a talented team of enzymologists (led by Ross Stein), chemists (led by Julian Adams), and cell biologists (led by Vito Palombella), whose efforts led eventually to the development of the proteasome inhibitors bortezomib and PS-519, now in clinical trials.

This company was unusual in its close collaboration with academia; in fact, its scientific board met almost monthly, and the early scientific knowledge developed rapidly through fruitful collaborations between several of us Harvard-based founder-scientists and the talented enzymologists and biochemists in the company. For example , as soon as the first inhibitors were available, their effects on cells were analyzed in my lab and Kenneth Rock's (25,26), and subsequent studies on nuclear factor-κB (NF-κB) were pursued in collaboration between company scientists and Tom Maniatis's laboratory at Harvard (27).

Perhaps the most fundamental finding from our own initial studies at Harvard in collaboration with Ken Rock was that reducing or blocking proteasome function in vivo did not immediately kill cells or interfere with their normal functions, both of which were theoretical possibilities. In fact, my real fear in initiating this company was that inhibition of the proteasome would rapidly lead to an accumulation of short-lived cell proteins in inactive ubiquitin-conjugated forms and thus be highly toxic. However, the presence in cells of a large number of enzymes that remove ubiquitin from proteins (i.e., isopeptidases) means that only a small fraction of cell proteins accumulate in the ubiquitinated form, even after marked inhibition of proteasomes. In other words, cells could function quite well for hours or even days with significantly reduced proteasomal capacity, as became clearly evident from subsequent animal studies and recent clinical trials.

An important motivation (at least for me, personally) for generating such inhibitors was purely scientific—the recognition that the availability of inhibitors that could enter cells and block proteasome function would be of tremendous value in clarifying its various physiologic roles. However, venture capitalists, stockholders, and company managers are not solely motivated by their interest in advancing biological science, for understandable reasons. Thus, this motivation was a hidden agenda of mine, although it has proved to be a major legacy of MyoGenics/ProScript, because their introduction of proteasome inhibitors greatly advanced our understanding of this area of biology *(28–30)*. In fact, very few biotechnology or pharmaceutical companies have had such a marked effect on an area of science. Moreover, this company did distribute some inhibitors freely to academic investigators, whose efforts rapidly advanced our knowledge of their effects. For example, early academic studies with these inhibitors remarkably altered our knowledge of the proteasome's importance in cancer, apoptosis, inflammation, and antigen presentation. At the same time, these studies ruled out certain potential therapeutic applications, such as the possibility of using them to suppress immune responses.

The first proteasome inhibitors synthesized by the company were simply peptide aldehydes *(29)*, which were analogs of the preferred substrates of the proteasome's chymotrypsin-like active site. Genetic studies in yeast had suggested that this site was the most important one in protein breakdown *(14,31)*, and we knew that hydrophobic peptides would be likely to penetrate cell membranes readily. The first inhibitors synthesized at the company were called MG compounds (for MyoGenics), such as MG132, which is still the proteasome inhibitor most widely used in basic research in cell biology because it is inexpensive, and its actions are readily reversible *(28,30)*. Most other inhibitors, including bortezomib, were derived from these initial molecules by peptide chemistry, in which a peptide with high affinity for the proteasome's chymotrypsin site was linked to different inhibitory pharmacophores. Julian Adams, who introduced the highly potent boronate as the inhibitory warhead, led these synthetic efforts. This pharmacophore had originally been developed to inhibit serine-proteases by scientists at DuPont and led to much more potent and selective inhibitors of the proteasome. Further medicinal chemistry efforts to modify the peptidic portion yielded bortezomib, a dipeptide-boronate, which was initially named MG341, but has since undergone multiple name changes as the company underwent various transitions. A major development leading to a change in the company's focus came from the discovery by Palombella et al. *(32)* (in a collaboration between Maniatis's lab and my own) of the involvement of the proteasome in activation of the key transcription factor, NF-κB, which plays a fundamental role in inflammation and cancer. Eventually, the company's role in muscle atrophy research became secondary, and its focus changed to the anti-inflammatory and antineoplastic actions of these inhibitors. The company therefore changed its name to ProScript, for Proteasomes and Transcription (hence, PS-341) and was taken over by a larger biotech company, Leukosite (hence, LDP-341) and then by Millennium Pharmaceuticals (MLN-341), who recently rechristened the drug bortezomib for commercial purposes.

It is noteworthy that these promising inhibitors were initially synthesized based on simple biochemical knowledge of the specificity of the proteasome's active sites, through directed medicinal chemistry, and by the use of classical enzyme and intracellular assays. They were not developed through a purely random screening of huge chemical libraries, as is the practice in most drug development efforts. Moreover, at the time, the nature of

Table 1
Distinctive Properties of the 26S Proteasome

Very large complex (2.5 MDa) composed of 44 polypeptides
Activity linked to ATP hydrolysis
Six proteolytic sites: two "chymotrypsin-like," and two
    "trypsin-like," and two caspase-like
Degrades proteins processively
Unfolds globular proteins
Degrades primarily proteins with polyubiquitin chain
Has isopeptidases that disassemble ubiquitin chains

the proteasome's architecture was unknown *(31)*; therefore, no structural information was available from X-ray crystallographic analysis to facilitate drug optimization. Nevertheless, exciting drug candidates emerged within 1 yr of the start of this company with less than a dozen talented scientists.

2. THE 26S AND 20S PROTEASOME

2.1. The 20S Core Particle

The degradation of most cellular proteins is catalyzed by the 26S proteasome, an extremely large (2.4-MDa), ATP-dependent proteolytic complex that differs in many respects from typical proteolytic enzymes *(14,31)* (Fig. 1 and Table 1). The great majority of proteases (which typically are 20–40-kDa enzymes) cleave the substrate once and then release the two fragments. By contrast, proteasomes (and other ATP-dependent proteases) are highly processive *(33)*, i.e., they cut polypeptides at multiple sites without the release of polypeptide intermediates. They degrade the proteins all the way down to small peptides ranging from 2 to 24 residues in length, with a median size of six to seven residues *(34)*. The 26S proteasome consists of a cylindrical proteolytic particle, the 20S (720-kDa) proteasome, in association with one or two 19S (890-kDa) regulatory complexes *(35)*, also termed PA700. These complexes associate with each other in an ATP-dependent process *(14,31)*. It remains unclear whether the symmetric (19S-20S-19S) complexes or the asymmetric, singly capped (19S-20S) complexes have different functional properties and are of equal importance in protein breakdown in vivo.

Free 20S proteasomes also exist in mammalian cells *(36,37)*, but when isolated by gentle approaches, they are inactive against peptide or protein substrates *(14,31)*. In the absence of the 19S particle, the 20S proteasomes are not ATP-dependent and are unable to degrade ubiquitin-conjugated proteins. Thus, they are unlikely to play a major role in intracellular proteolysis, which in vivo is largely an ATP-dependent process *(5,15,38)* and generally requires substrate modification by ubiquitination. Additional forms of the proteasome exist in vivo; for example, the cytokine interferon-γ induces a heptameric ring complex, PA28 (also termed Reg), which enhances peptide entry and exit in vivo *(39)*. Also, single-capped 26S particles may associate with the PA28 (11S) complex *(36)* to form hybrid 19S-20S-PA28 complexes *(40)*. These structures enhance the production of MHC class I-presented antigenic peptides by proteasomes *(41)* in most cells during inflammation and constitutively in immune tissues *(42,43)*.

The 20S proteasome is a hollow, cylindrical particle consisting of four stacked rings. Each outer ring contains seven distinct but homologous α-subunits; each inner ring contains seven distinct but homologous β-subunits *(5,14,31,44)*. Three of these β-subunits contain proteolytic active sites, which were first identified by X-ray diffraction as the sites of binding of a peptide aldehyde inhibitor *(45)*. These active sites face the inner chamber of the cylinder. Because the outer walls of the proteasome are very tightly packed, the only way for substrates to reach this central degradative chamber or for products to exit is by passage through the narrow gate channels in the α-rings *(45,46)*. This channel is too narrow to be traversed by tightly folded globular proteins; therefore, the breakdown of most proteins requires their unfolding prior to translocation into the core particle *(47)*.

This entry channel in the α-ring is tightly regulated. It has long been recognized that 20S proteasomes can be isolated in an active or an inactive (latent) form, which can be activated by various treatments (e.g., low concentrations of detergents, heat, dialysis against low ionic strengths). In the inactive 20S proteasomes, these entry channels are closed, as demonstrated by X-ray diffraction *(45)*, whereas the active forms all have open gates allowing substrate entry. Spontaneous gate opening and activation are inhibited by intracellular concentrations of potassium *(48*; K.M. Woo and A.L. Goldberg, in preparation), and one key function of the 19S (PA700 complex) is to facilitate substrate entry. Binding of ATP by this particle can trigger gate opening as part of the ATP-dependent translocation of substrates into the 20S particle *(48*; I. Bize and A.L. Goldberg, in preparation). The diameter of this gate in the α-ring also influences the sizes of products generated during proteolysis *(48)*. In fact, the interferon-γ-induced complex, PA28, increases the yield of peptides appropriate for antigen presentation in part by promoting gate opening *(39)* and allowing larger products to exit *(49)*. In addition, small hydrophobic peptides allosterically trigger gate opening, which may represent a mechanism by which peptide products exit *(50)*.

Because the particle's active sites are localized on its inner cavity, this architecture must have evolved to prevent the uncontrolled destruction of cellular proteins. Similarly, the 19S complexes, as well as substrate ubiquitination, may be viewed as mechanisms that ensure the entry only of substrates into the 20S proteolytic core particle in a highly selective, carefully regulated manner.

2.2. The 19S Regulatory Particle and the Role of ATP

Dramatic progress has been made recently in defining the composition of the 19S (PA700) regulatory particle and the functions of individual subunits *(11,31)*. The 19S particle can be separated into a base and a lid *(11,51)*. The lid contains at least nine polypeptides, including multiple isopeptidases that disassemble the poly-ubiquitin chain, allowing free ubiquitin to be reutilized in further rounds of proteolysis. The removal of the ubiquitin chain is an ATP-dependent process catalyzed by a specific subunit (rpn11), and this step is essential for ATP-dependent degradation of the substrate *(52,53)* by the 20S particle. The base, which associates with the 20S particle, contains eight polypeptides, including six homologous ATPases, which serve multiple functions. They interact directly with the α-rings of the 20S, allowing ATP-dependent opening of the channel, which is essential for polypeptide entry into the proteolytic chamber. In fact, one ATPase (Rpt2) subunit appears to be especially important in regulating this gating process *(48)*.

Table 2
Essential Roles of ATP in Protein Degradation
by 26S Proteasome[a]

Association of 19S regulatory complex with 20S proteasome
Unfolding of globular protein
Translocation of protein substrates into the 20S particle
Gate-opening into 20S particle (especially rpn2)
Binding of ubiquitin chains
Action of isopeptidase (rpn11)

[a]Based on studies with 26S complex or PAN-20S complex.

The ATPases also have chaperone-like functions that enable them to bind a polypeptide substrate, trigger gate opening, unfold a globular protein, and catalyze protein translocation into the 20S proteasome *(54)* (Table 2).

Much has been learned about the role of ATP hydrolysis by studying the analogous complexes from archaebacteria, which lack ubiquitin but contain simpler forms of the 20S proteasomes *(55)*. These particles function in protein breakdown together with the hexameric ring ATPase complex termed PAN, whose subunit is highly homologous to the ATPases in the base of the 19S complex *(56,57)*. PAN shares more than 40% identity with the six ATPases in the 19S complex and thus appears to be the evolutionary precursor to the 19S base, as well as regulated proteasome function before proteolysis became linked to ubiquitination in eukaryotes.

These ATPases are all members of the AAA family of multimeric ATPases *(58)*, which includes the ATP-dependent protease Lon and the regulatory components of the bacterial ATP-dependent proteases ClpAP, ClpXP, and HsIUV, which catalyze protein breakdown in bacteria and mitochondria *(59)*. Like these enzymes, PAN increases its rate of ATP consumption several fold when it binds an appropriate substrate *(54)*. This complex of ATPases has been shown to catalyze ATP-dependent unfolding of the globular model substrate GFPssrA *(60)*. This process occurs somehow on the surface of the ATPase ring *(61)*, but its mechanism is completely unclear. In addition, the ATPase complex is necessary for the ATP-dependent entrance of substrates, even denatured proteins, into the core proteasome. These substrates appear to be translocated through a central opening in the ATPase ring and then through the gate in the α-ring *(61)*. Some proteins enter exclusively in a C to N direction, whereas others are translocated in an N to C direction (Navon and Goldberg, in preparation). Recent studies have determined the actual amounts of ATP utilized during degradation of model proteins by this complex. Surprisingly, for the model unfolded substrate casein and the tightly folded protein GFPssrA, the same amount of ATP is hydrolyzed, about 350 ATP molecules/molecule of the protein, which is perhaps a third of what is consumed by the ribosome in synthesis of a polypeptide of this size *(54)*. The inhibitors of the proteasome available now all inhibit the active sites of the 20S particle, primarily the chymotrypsin-like site. However, the 26S particle contains many other subunits and enzymatic activities in its 19S component. Therefore, it seems very likely that this particle contains many other possible targets for selective inhibition and perhaps drug development in the future. At least in theory, agents affecting the 19S particle might even be anticipated to affect degradation of different substrates of the proteasome differentially.

2.3. The Proteasome's Unusual Proteolytic Mechanism

Proteasomes comprise a new class of proteolytic enzymes called threonine proteases, whose catalytic mechanism differs from that of other types of proteases (29,31). The active sites in proteasomes utilize the N-terminal threonines of certain β-subunits as the nucleophile that attacks peptide bonds. The proteasome thus is an N-terminal hydrolase, a family of enzymes that have similar three-dimensional structures and utilize the side chains of their N-terminal serine, threonine, or cysteine residues to cleave various amide bonds (62). Much of our understanding of this unique proteolytic mechanism has come through studies using proteasome inhibitors (29) and site-directed mutagenesis (8,63). The first strong evidence that the threonine hydroxyl is the catalytic nucleophile was the finding by X-ray diffraction that a peptide aldehyde inhibitor (ALLN) forms a hemiacetal bond with the hydroxyl group of the N-terminal threonines of the proteasome's β-subunits (45,64). Also, mutation of this threonine to alanine completely abolished the activity of the proteasome, whereas mutation to a serine retained significant activity against small peptides (8,65). This catalytic threonine residue is covalently modified by different irreversible proteasome inhibitors, lactacystin (66), vinyl sulfones (67), and epoxyketones (68).

The proteasome thus lacks the catalytic triad characteristic of serine and cysteine proteases (36). Instead, the free N-terminal amino group of catalytic threonine is likely to accept the proton from the side chain hydroxyl. To summarize the proteasome's catalytic mechanism: First, the hydroxyl group of the catalytic threonine directly attacks the scissile bond, resulting in the formation of the tetrahedral intermediate, which then collapses into an acyl enzyme with the release of the first reaction product. Deacylation of the catalytic threonine residue by water leads to the release of the second peptide product and the regeneration of the free N-terminal threonine on the proteasome's active site.

3. PHYSIOLOGIC FUNCTIONS OF THE PROTEASOME

Prior to the development of proteasome inhibitors, the functions of the ubiquitin-proteasome pathway and its different cellular roles were studied primarily by biochemical methods or by genetic analysis of yeast mutants defective in this process. The degradation of a model protein was typically studied using cell-free extracts (especially from mammalian reticulocytes or, more recently, frog oocytes). These approaches, unfortunately, are often technically difficult, and genetic analysis can be quite time-consuming. Also, many complex cellular processes involving the proteasome have to this day never been reconstituted in cell extracts and cannot be studied in yeast (e.g., antigen presentation or muscle atrophy). The availability since 1994 of specific inhibitors of the proteasome that enter intact cells and block or reduce its function (28) has allowed much more rapid analysis of the role of the proteasome in the breakdown of specific proteins and in complex cellular responses (28–30). Thus, if such inhibitors prevent a decrease in activity of an enzyme or cause an increase in the cellular content of a protein, then proteasome-mediated degradation is very likely to play a key role, especially if these inhibitors cause the protein to accumulate in a ubiquitin-conjugated, high-molecular-weight form. However, further biochemical analysis of the process is still necessary to identify the responsible ubiquitination enzymes and the critical regulatory factors (e.g., kinases that may trigger ubiquitination and proteasomal degradation).

3.1. Proteasomes Degrade Short-Lived Regulatory Proteins

The nonlysosomal ATP-dependent proteolytic system, which we now call the ubiquitin–proteasome pathway, was first discovered as the system responsible for the selective degradation in mammalian reticulocytes of proteins with highly abnormal conformations *(9)*. Such abnormal proteins may result from nonsense or missense mutations, intracellular denaturation, damage by oxygen radicals, or failure of polypeptides to fold correctly. Both prokaryotic and eukaryotic cells have evolved mechanisms to degrade such proteins selectively, whose accumulation could be highly toxic. This process is particularly important in various human inherited diseases, for example, in the various "unstable hemoglobinopathies" and cystic fibrosis, in which the mutant protein fails to accumulate because it is degraded very rapidly. It is also likely that a failure of this degradative process somehow plays a major role in the accumulation of abnormal polypeptides that form toxic aggregates in various neurodegenerative diseases *(69)*. Interestingly, treatment with proteasome inhibitors prevents the rapid degradation of abnormal proteins and causes the accumulation of aggregates of the abnormal proteins resembling the inclusions seen in such diseases *(69)*.

Another critical role of the ubiquitin–proteasome pathways is in the degradation of various short-lived regulatory proteins, including many transcription factors, oncogene products, tumor suppressors, cell-cycle regulatory proteins (e.g., the various cyclins and cyclin-dependent kinase-inhibitors), and rate-limiting enzymes (Table 3) *(10,11)*. These proteins have evolved short half-lives, because their rapid degradation is important for regulation of cell growth and metabolism. Such proteins turn over within minutes after synthesis or, at most, with half-lives of a few hours. Thus, their levels can rise or fall rapidly with changes in physiologic conditions *(5)*, and they can serve as timing devices (e.g., in the cell cycle). Many of these important functions of the ubiquitin–proteasome pathway were uncovered initially by biochemical or genetic approaches but have been firmly established in cultured mammalian cells by treatment with proteasome inhibitors (e.g., MG132 or lactacystin). These inhibitors block up to 90% of the degradation of abnormal and short-lived proteins *(26)*. Moreover, studies with these inhibitors have uncovered many additional such substrates of the proteasome and have tremendously advanced our understanding of the role of protein degradation in normal and disease states, as discussed below *(10,11)*. The ability of bortezomib to promote apoptosis is probably due to its stabilization of certain key short-lived regulatory proteins (e.g., p53 or p27) and perhaps also to the stabilization of abnormal polypeptides whose accumulation can be toxic.

For a detailed discussion of the proteasome's regulation of NF-κB, *see* Chapter 6.

3.2. Proteasomes Degrade the Bulk of Cell Proteins

Although significant numbers (perhaps 20%) of newly synthesized proteins are short lived, with half lives of less than 3 h, most cell proteins are much more stable, with half-lives of many hours or days. The degradation of such long-lived proteins had long been believed to occur within lysosomes, an incorrect conclusion still stated in many textbooks. However, the long-lived and short-lived cell proteins show a similar ATP depen-

Table 3
Important Regulatory Proteins Rapidly Degraded
by the 26S Proteasome

Oncogenic products and tumor suppressors

> p53 and MDM2
> c-fos
> c-jun
> c-Mos
> E2A proteins

Cell cycle regulatory proteins

> CDK inhibitors (p27, p21, and others)
> Cyclins (mitotic cyclins, G1 cyclins, and others)

Transcriptional regulators

> β-catenins
> IκB and NK-κB (p105)
> HIF1 (hypoxia-inducible factor 1)
> ATF2 (activating transcription factor 2)
> STAT proteins

Enzymes

> DNA topoisomerase
> Ornithine decarboxylase
> Receptor-associated protein kinases
> RNA polymerase II large subunit
> IRF2 (iron regulatory protein 2)

dence and a similar sensitivity to proteasome inhibitors *(26,70)*. Thus, 80–90% of long-lived proteins in cultured mammalian cells, under optimal nutritional conditions, are also degraded by the proteasome pathway. By contrast, inhibitors of the lysosome block only a small fraction (10–20%) of the total protein degradation, perhaps only the breakdown of endocytosed membrane-associated components *(26)*. (In fully differentiated cells, such as liver cells, however, the lysosomes, through autophagic vacuole formation, may account for a larger fraction of degradation, especially upon cell starvation or glucagon treatment.) Although proteasomal involvement in the breakdown of these long-lived components is clear, it still remains uncertain whether their degradation also requires ubiquitination of the substrate molecules, as is required for degradation of most short-lived cell proteins.

This involvement of the proteasome in the degradation of most cell proteins has had important implications for energy homeostasis in mammals and for evolution of the immune system. Cell proteins, especially proteins in skeletal muscle, also serve as a reservoir of metabolizable substrates, amino acids, that can be used for glucose production under poor nutritional states *(1,2)*. The activation of this degradative pathway in muscle during fasting or systemic disease helps mobilize essential amino acids from cell proteins for glucogenesis and is regulated by glucoregulatory hormones (e.g., insulin glucocorticoids). In muscles, the degradation of most cell proteins is normally quite slow unless it is activated by hormones (e.g., glucocorticoids) or cytokines (tumor necrosis factor, interleukin-1). In fact, whether a muscle cell grows or atrophies is determined largely by the overall rate of proteolysis in the tissue. For example, it is now well established that the major cause of the muscle wasting seen in fasting, in cancer cachexia following denervation, and in patients with sepsis is the excessive proteolysis caused by a general activation of the ubiquitin–proteasome pathway *(2)*. Atrophying muscles show a series of adaptations indicating an activation of this pathway, including increased expression of ubiquitin and many proteasome genes, an accumulation of ubiquitinated proteins, the induction of specific E3s *(23,24)*, and more rapid ubiquitin conjugation in cell-free extracts *(2)*. Also, studies with proteasome inhibitors have proved that enhanced degradation of normally long-lived muscle proteins is the primary mechanism leading to the rapid loss of muscle mass in cancer and other disease states. In fact, as discussed above, these insights were the original justification for mounting an effort to synthesize proteasome inhibitors for therapeutic purposes.

3.3. Proteasomes and MHC Class I Antigen Presentation

Eukaryotic cells contain two primary systems for degrading proteins in the nucleus and cytosol—the ubiquitin–proteasome pathway and the lysosomes in animal cells (or the vacuole in plants and yeast). In higher vertebrate cells, these two major proteolytic systems also function in the generation of antigenic peptides presented to the two functional arms of the immune system. The breakdown of extracellular proteins by the lysosome–endosome pathway is the source of antigenic peptides that are presented on MHC class II molecules and elicit antibody production. Similarly, some of the peptides generated during breakdown of intracellular proteins by the proteasome are transported into the endoplasmic reticulum and are delivered to the cell surface bound to MHC class I molecules for presentation to cytotoxic T-lymphocytes. This process allows the immune system to monitor continually for non-native proteins within cells that may arise during viral infection or cancer. If non-native (e.g., viral and oncogenic proteins) epitopes are presented on the cell surface, then the presenting cells are quickly killed by cytotoxic T-cells. Another important finding that linked proteasome function to immune surveillance was the discovery by many laboratories that specialized forms of the 20S and 26S particles, often termed immunoproteasomes, are induced upon exposure of cells to interferon-γ and certain other cytokines (ror review, see ref. *71*). With time, these alternative forms replace the normal species in most tissues. These immunoproteasomes are found constitutively in spleen, thymus, and presumably other immune cells. They differ from normal 20S particles in containing three alternative interferon-γ-induced β-subunits, termed LMP2, LMP7, and MECL1, which are incorporated in newly synthesized proteasomes. They encode the active sites, and their incorporation in place of the normal subunits enhances the particle's ability to cleave proteins after hydrophobic and basic residues and reduce cleavages after acidic amino acids *(72)*. These alterations do not influence the rate at which proteins are degraded, but rather change the nature of the peptides generated *(40,49)*. As a consequence, more peptides are produced with C-termini that are appropriate for binding to MHC class I molecules (which require ligands with hydrophobic and basic C-termini). Surprisingly, these alternative subunits in immunoproteasomes also influence the length of antigenic peptides generated *(49)*.

The involvement of the proteasome in the generation of antigenic peptides had been proposed but remained controversial until the proteasome inhibitors were introduced

(26,71). Peptide aldehyde inhibitors (MG132) and lactacystin, at concentrations that block the ATP-dependent degradation of cell proteins, were shown to prevent MHC class I presentation of an antigenic peptide (SIINFEKL) derived from a microinjected protein, ovalbumin. These inhibitors prevented the generation of the antigenic peptide but did not affect its transport into the endoplasmic reticulum (ER) or delivery to the cell surface. Moreover, the presentation of most antigenic peptides was also blocked by proteasome inhibitors. Thus, the great majority of MHC class I-presented peptides are generated by 26S proteasomes during the course of protein breakdown, in accord with our previous demonstration that protein ubiquitination is important in class I antigen presentation *(73)*.

Nearly all MHC class I peptides are 8–9 (or occasionally 10) residues long. This length is necessary for a peptide to fit within the groove in the class I molecule. By contrast, 70% of proteasome products are too small to function in this process, whereas perhaps 15% are too large unless trimmed by cellular enzymes *(34)*. Recent studies with proteasome inhibitors have led to the surprising discovery that proteasomes, although essential for the generation of the C-termini of most antigenic peptides, are not required for the production of their N-termini *(43,71)*. In other words, the proteasome, while degrading polypeptides, generates longer precursors of the presented peptides with N-terminal extensions *(43,49,71)*. The proteolytic trimming of these N-extended precursors is then catalyzed by cellular aminopeptidases to generate the presented eight- or nine-residue peptide. In fact, in leukocytes normally and in all cells in inflammatory states, the specialized forms of proteasomes induced by interferon-γ (termed immunoproteasomes) and the PA28 proteasome–activator complex both favor the production of such N-extended antigenic precursors, which require subsequent trimming before association with MHC class I molecules. In addition, interferon-γ signals induction of two aminopeptidases, leucine aminopeptidases in the cytosol *(74)* and a novel aminopeptidase, which we named ERAP1 *(75)* in the ER, that trim the N-extended peptides to the presented epitopes *(75,76)*. Thus, multiple proteolytic enzymes are involved in the production of antigenic peptides, and each of these steps is altered in inflammatory states by interferon-γ so as to enhance the efficiency of production of antigenic peptides *(43)*. Although proteasome inhibitors in vivo can block the generation of most MHC class I-presented peptides in patients or animals receiving therapeutic doses of these inhibitors, no immune deficiencies have been observed, presumably because the inhibition of proteasome function is only partial and of limited duration.

3.4. Proteasome Inhibitors and the Heat-Shock Response

It has long been known that in all cells an increase in the ambient temperature leads to the induction of a characteristic group of stress proteins, known as heat shock proteins. This adaptive response is induced not only by high temperatures, but also by a variety of stressful conditions that damage cell proteins, including exposure to heavy metals or oxygen radicals or incorporation of amino acid analogs *(69)*. The common feature of these various conditions is that they all cause the accumulation in cells of unfolded or denatured proteins. Accordingly, the expression or microinjection of an unfolded protein into intact cells causes the induction of heat shock proteins *(76,77)*. Therefore, the capacity of the ubiquitin–proteasome pathway to degrade such unfolded proteins rapidly is a major factor that indirectly suppresses the expression of heat shock proteins. However, if this degradative process is blocked with proteasome inhibitors, an accumulation of unfolded proteins should occur, and as a result, induction of the heat shock response *(72,78,79)*. The resulting changes in expression of heat shock genes leads to production of various molecular chaperones, which promote protein folding, and of ubiquitin and other components of the degradative machinery *(76)*. Thus, cells are better able to cope with the onslaught of unfolded proteins. A similar protective response, termed *the unfolded protein response*, occurs when abnormal proteins arise in the ER *(73)* and enhances the level of chaperones in the ER. When cells are exposed to proteasome inhibitors, both responses occur *(80)*. As a consequence, the cells show an enhanced capacity to refold such damaged proteins, to prevent their aggregation, and to degrade the abnormal polypeptides.

The treatment of cells with proteasome inhibitors leads to a coordinate induction of many, if not all, cytosolic heat shock proteins, as well as various molecular chaperones in the ER *(72,79)*. This effect involves increased transcription of these genes and is seen within 1–3 h of exposure of mammalian cells to various proteasome inhibitors. In mammalian cells, this induction of heat shock proteins was shown to be mediated by the activation of the heat shock transcription factors (HSFs). Thus, the ubiquitin–proteasome pathway seems to degrade a short-lived transcription factor(s) (e.g., an HSF) that is stabilized by these inhibitors, leading to the induction of heat shock proteins. It is well established that the induction of heat shock proteins is a protective response that enhances cellular resistance to high temperatures and other highly toxic agents (e.g., oxygen radicals). Accordingly, exposure to the proteasome inhibitors dramatically increased the cell's resistance in mammalian cells and yeast to many lethal insults, such as exposure to heat, high concentration of ethanol, or oxygen radicals *(72,79)*. The magnitude of this protective effect depends on the duration and the extent of the inhibition of proteolysis. This effect may contribute to some of the therapeutic actions of the proteasome inhibitor. However, it is noteworthy that the continual accumulation of abnormal proteins in the cytosol or ER (e.g., as occurs in cells at higher temperatures and cells treated with proteasome inhibitors) eventually can exceed the protective capacity of these responses and can trigger apoptosis by activating JNK-kinase *(81)*. Such a mechanism may also be occurring and may be important in the anticancer actions of bortezomib, especially in myeloma cells, which generate large amounts of aberrant, rapidly degraded immunoglobulins.

3.5. *Proteasomes Degrade Abnormal Secretory and Membrane Proteins*

Another unexpected discovery resulting from the use of proteasome inhibitors has been that cytosolic proteasomes are also responsible for the rapid degradation of many membrane or secretory proteins during their passage through the ER. The presence of this degradative process and its importance in quality control in the secretory pathway had been recognized for some time, but it had been attributed to an unidentified degradative system within the ER. However, recent studies with the proteasome inhibitors and genetic analysis of yeast mutants have led to the recognition that many such proteins, if they are not folded properly or if they fail to bind cofactors or form correct oligomeric structures, are translocated from the ER to the cytosol for ubiquitin-dependent proteasome-mediated proteolysis *(82,83)*. For example, the human cystic fibrosis transmembrane conductance regulator (CFTR) *(84,85)*, mutant forms of human α_1-antitrypsin *(86)*, unlipidated apolipoprotein B *(87)*, and MHC class I molecules in cytomegalovirus-infected cells *(88)* are rapidly degraded by the ubiquitin–proteasome pathway and stabilized by treatment with proteasome inhibitors. In addition to serving in quality control, this process is responsible for the tightly regulated degradation of ER-bound enzymes, such as 3-hydroxy-3-methylglutaryl coenzyme A (HMG CoA) reductase, the key enzyme in cholesterol biosynthesis.

The selective destruction of these misfolded membrane or mutant secretory proteins by the ubiquitin–proteasome pathway requires that they be translocated back into the cytoplasm. In some cases, proteasome inhibition leads to an accumulation of the nondegraded proteins in the cytosol, whereas in others, their extraction from the ER is also blocked. The Sec61 complex, which functions in the translocation of polypeptides into the ER, is also a key component of this retrograde transport system. Other components in the ER, including the ER chaperones BiP, calnexin, and a novel ER membrane protein Cue1p, are also required for this process *(89)*. Apparently, these substrates can be ubiquitinated while in the membrane, but their extraction from the membrane seems to require the function of the ATP-dependent molecular chaperone p93 (cdc48) *(90)*. However, it remains to be elucidated how this translocation out of the ER takes place and which other components are required for this process. It is noteworthy that the cell's capacity to carry out the process is enhanced by exposure of cells to proteasome inhibitors, but if this adaptation (termed the *unfolded protein response*) fails to prevent the continued accumulation of abnormal proteins, the apoptotic cell program is activated *(91)*.

For a detailed discussion of proteasome inhibition and apoptosis, *see* Chapter 10.

4. CONCLUSIONS

This chapter has described the scientific origins of the development of bortezomib and reviewed our knowledge of how the proteasome functions both as an isolated molecular machine and in vivo as the key site for degradation of cell proteins. Aside from their inherent scientific interest and exciting medical promise, these stories nicely illustrate several truths about medical research, namely that:

1. Improved therapies (especially in cancer) are tightly linked to advances in our understanding of basic biochemistry and cell biology.
2. The teamwork possible between industrial applied scientists and academic investigators in biotechnology companies can achieve practical ends impossible in university settings.
3. The paths to scientific progress are often unpredictable. I certainly never anticipated that in studying the mechanisms of muscle wasting or the selective degradation of abnormal proteins in *E. coli* that this work might somehow lead to the discovery of the proteasomal apparatus, or that this finding would, in turn, lead to insights about immune surveillance or even indirectly to novel therapies for cancer. In fact, had we ever suggested in a grant proposal that this research program might have such benefits, every granting agency or study section would have rejected such statements as fantasy, nonsense, or pure hogwash. It would be good if the lessons clearly illustrated by the development of proteasome inhibitors were appreciated by the governmental, private, and industrial offices that decide on research policies.

ACKNOWLEDGMENTS

These studies have been supported by grants from the National Institutes of Health (NIGHS), the Muscular Dystrophy Association, the National Space Biology Research

Institute, and the Hereditary Disease Foundation. The author is very grateful for the expert assistance of Sarah Trombley in preparing this manuscript.

REFERENCES

1. Mitch WE, et al. Mechanisms of muscle wasting. The role of the ubiquitin-proteasome pathway. *N Engl J Med* 1996;335:1897–1905.
2. Lecker SH, et al. Muscle protein breakdown and the critical role of the ubiquitin-proteasome pathway in normal and disease states. *J Nutr* 1999;129(1S suppl):227S–237S.
3. Goldberg AL. Protein turnover in skeletal muscle II: Effects of denervation and cortisone on protein catabolism in skeletal muscle. *J Biol Chem* 1969;244:3223–3229.
4. Goldberg AL, et al. Intracellular protein degradation in mammalian and bacterial cells. *Annu Rev Biochem* 1990.
5. Goldberg AL, et al. Intracellular protein degradation in mammalian and bacterial cells. *Annu Rev Biochem* 1976;45:747–803.
6. Goldberg AL. A role of aminoacyl-tRNA in the regulation of protein breakdown in *Escherichia coli*. *Proc Natl Acad Sci USA* 1971;68:362–366.
7. Goldberg AL. Degradation of abnormal proteins in *E. coli*. *Proc Natl Acad Sci USA* 1972;69:422–426.
8. Seemüller E, et al. Proteasome from *Thermoplasma acidophilum*—a threonine protease. *Science* 1995;268:579–582.
9. Etlinger JD, et al. A soluble ATP-dependent proteolytic system responsible for the degradation of abnormal proteins in reticulocytes. *Proc Natl Acad Sci USA* 1977;74:54–58.
10. Hershko A, et al. The ubiquitin system. *Annu Rev Biochem* 1998;67:425–479.
11. Glickman M, et al. The ubiquitin-proteasome proteolytic pathway: destruction for the sake of construction. *Physiol Rev* 2002;82:373–428.
12. Goldberg AL. The mechanism and functions of ATP-dependent proteases in bacterial and animal cells. *Eur J Biochem* 1992;203:9–23.
13. Wickner S, et al. Posttranslational quality control: folding, refolding, and degrading proteins. *Science* 1999;286:801–847.
14. Coux O, et al. Structure and functions of the 20S and 26S proteasomes. *Ann Rev Biochem* 1996;65:801–847.
15. DeMartino GN, et al. Identification and partial purification of an ATP-stimulated alkaline protease in rat liver. *J Biol Chem* 1979;254:3712–3715.
16. Hough R, et al. Purification of two high molecular weight proteases from rabbit reticulocyte lysate. *J Biol Chem* 1987;261:2400–2408.
17. Waxman L, et al. A soluble ATP-dependent system for protein degradation from murine erythroleukemia cells: evidence for a protease which requires ATP hydrolysis but not ubiquitin. *J Biol Chem* 1985;260:11994–12000.
18. Orlowski M. The multicatalytic proteinase complex, a major extralysosomal proteolytic system. *Biochemistry* 1990;29:10289–10297.
19. Arrigo A, et al. Identity of the 19S 'prosome' particle with the large multifunctional protease complex of mammalian cells (the proteasome). *Nature* 1988;331:192–194.
20. Matthews W, et al. Involvement of the proteasome in various degradative processes in mammalian cells. *Proc Natl Acad Sci USA* 1989;86:2597–2601.
21. Eytan E, et al. ATP-dependent incorporation of 20S protease into the 26S complex that degrades proteins conjugated to ubiquitin. *Proc Natl Acad Sci USA* 1989;86:7751–7755.
22. Driscoll J, et al. The proteasome (multicatalytic protease) is a component of the 1500kDa proteolytic complex which degrades ubiquitin-conjugated proteins. *J Biol Chem* 1990;265:4789–4792.
23. Bodine SC, et al. Identification of ubiquitin ligases required for skeletal muscle atrophy. *Science* 2001;294:1704–1708.
24. Gomes M, et al. Atrogin-1, a muscle-specific F-box protein highly expressed during muscle atrophy. *Proc Natl Acad Sci USA* 2001;98:14440–14445.
25. Tawa, NE, et al. Inhibitors of the proteasome reduce the accelerated proteolysis in atrophying rat skeletal muscles. *J Clin Invest* 1997;100:197–203.
26. Rock KL, et al. Inhibitors of the proteasome block the degradation of most cell proteins and the generation of peptides presented on MHC class 1 molecules. *Cell* 1994;78:761–771.

27. Silverman N, et al. NF-κB signaling pathways in mammalian and insect innate immunity. *Genes Dev* 2001;15:2321–2342.
28. Lee DH, et al. Proteasome inhibitors: valuable new tools for cell biologists. *Trends Cell Biol* 1998;8:397–403.
29. Kisselev AF, et al. Proteasome inhibitors: from research tools to drug candidates. *Chem Biol* 2001;8:739–758.
30. Lee DH, et al. The proteasome inhibitors and their uses. In: *Proteasomes: The World of Regulatory Proteolysis*. (Wolf DH and Hilt W, eds.). Georgetown, TX: Landes Bioscience, 1999.
31. Voges D, et al. The 26S proteasome: a molecular machine designed for controlled proteolysis. *Annu Rev Biochem* 1999;68:1015–1068.
32. Palombella VJ, et al. The ubiquitin-proteasome pathway is required for processing the NF-kappa-B1 precursor protein and the activation of NF-kappa-B. *Cell* 1994;78:773–785.
33. Nussbaum AK, et al. Cleavage motifs of the yeast 20S proteasome beta subunits deduced from digests of enolase 1. *Proc Natl Acade Sci USA* 1998;95:12504–12509.
34. Kisselev AF, et al. The sizes of peptides generated from protein by mammalian 26S and 20S proteasomes: implications for understanding the degradative mechanism and antigen presentation. *J Biol Chem* 1999;274:3363–3371.
35. Holzl H, et al. The regulatory complex of *Drosophila melanogaster* 26S proteasomes: subunit composition and localization of a deubiquitylating enzyme. *J Cell Biol* 2000;150:119–129.
36. Tanahashi N, et al. Hybrid proteasomes. Induction by interferon-gamma and contribution to ATP-dependent proteolysis. *J Biol Chem* 2000;275:14336–14345.
37. Yang Y, et al. In vivo assembly of the proteasomal complexes, implications for antigen processing. *J Biol Chem* 1995;270:27687–27694.
38. Gronostajski RM, et al. The ATP dependence of the degradation of short- and long-lived proteins in growing fibroblasts. *J Biol Chem* 1985;260:3344–3349.
39. Whitby FG, et al. Structural basis for the activation of 20S proteasomes by 11S regulators. *Nature* 2000;408:115–120.
40. Cascio P, et al. Properties of the hybrid form of the 26S proteasome containing both 19S and PA28 complexes. *EMBO J* 2002;21:2636–2645.
41. Rechsteiner M, et al. The proteasome activator 11 S REG (PA28) and class I antigen presentation. *Biochem J* 2000;345:1–15.
42. Goldberg AL, et al. Not just research tools—proteasome inhibitors offer therapeutic promise. *Nat Med* 2002;8:338–440.
43. Goldberg AL, et al. The importance of the proteasome and subsequent proteolytic steps in the generation of antigenic peptides. *Mol Immunol* 2002;1169:1–17.
44. Baumeister W, et al. The proteasome: paradigm of a self-compartmentalizing protease. *Cell* 1998;92:367–380.
45. Groll M, et al. Structure of 20S proteasome from yeast at 2.4 Å resolution. *Nature* 1997;386:463–471.
46. Groll M, et al. A gated channel into the proteasome core particle. *Nat Struc Biol* 2000;7:1062–1067.
47. Wenzel T, et al. Conformational constraints in protein degradation by the 20S proteasome. *Nat Struc Biol* 1995;2:199–204.
48. Kohler A, et al. The axial channel of the proteasome core particle is gated by the Rpt2 ATPase and controls both substrate entry and product release. *Mol Cell* 2001;7:1143–1152.
49. Cascio P, et al. 26S proteasomes and immunoproteasomes produce mainly N-extended versions of an antigenic peptide. *EMBO J* 2001;20:2357–2366.
50. Kisselev AF, et al. Binding of hydrophobic peptides to several non-catalytic sites promotes peptide hydrolysis by all active sites of 20S proteasomes. Evidence for peptide-induced channel opening in the alpha-rings. *J Biol Chem* 2002;277:22260–22270.
51. Glickman MH, et al. A subcomplex of the proteasome regulatory particle required for ubiquitin-conjugate degradation and related to the COP9-signalosome and eIF3. *Cell* 1998;94:615–623.
52. Hochstrasser M. New proteases in a ubiquitin stew. *Science* 2002;298:549–552.
53. Verma R, et al. Role of Rpn11 metalloprotease in deubiquitination and degradation by the 26S proteasome. *Science* 2002;298:611–615.
54. Benaroudj N, et al. ATP hydrolysis by the proteasome regulatory complex PAN serves multiple functions in protein degradation. *Mol Cell* 2003;11:69–78.
55. Zwickl P, et al. Proteasomes in prokaryotes. In: *Proteasomes: The World of Regulatory Proteolysis* (Wolf DH and Hilt W, eds.). Georgetown, TX: Landes Bioscience, 1999:8–20.

56. Zwickl P, et al. An archaebacterial ATPase, homologous to ATPases in the eukaryotic 26 S proteasome, activates protein breakdown by 20 S proteasomes. *J Biol Chem* 1999;274:26008–26014.
57. Wilson HL, et al. Biochemical and physical properties of the *Methanococcus jannaschii* 20S proteasome and PAN, a homolog of the ATPase (Rpt) subunits of the eucaryal 26S proteasome. *J Bacteriol* 2000;182:1680–1692.
58. Ogura T, et al. AAA+ superfamily ATPases: common structure-diverse function. *Genes Cells* 2001;6:575–597.
59. Gottesman S, et al. Regulatory subunits of energy-dependent proteases. *Cell* 1997;91:435–438.
60. Benaroudj N, et al. PAN, the proteasome activating nucleotidase from archaebacteria, is a molecular chaperone which unfolds protein substrate. *Nat Cell Biol* 2000;2:833–839.
61. Navon A, et al. Proteins are unfolded on the surface of the ATPase ring before transport into the proteasome. *Mol Cell* 2001;8:1339–1349.
62. Brannigan JA, et al. A protein catalytic framework with an N-terminal nucleophile is capable of self-activation. *Nature* 1995;378:416–419.63. Dick T , et al. Contribution of proteasomal beta-subunits to the cleavage of peptide substrates analyzed with yeast mutants. *J Biol Chem* 1998;273:25637–25646.
64. Löwe J, et al. Crystal structure of the 20S proteasome from the archaeon T. acidophilum at 3.4 Å resolution. *Science* 1995;268:533–539.
65. Kisselev AF, et al. Why does threonine, and not serine, function as the active site nucleophile in proteasomes? *J Biol Chem* 2000;275:14831–14837.
66. Fenteany G, et al. Inhibition of proteasome activities and subunit-specific amino-terminal threonine modification by lactacystin. *Science* 1995;268:726–731.
67. Bogyo M, et al. Covalent modification of the active site Thr of proteasome beta-subunits and the *E. coli* homologue HslV by a new class of inhibitors. *Proc Natl Acad Sci USA* 1997;94:6629–6634.
68. Meng L, et al. Epoxomicin, a potent and selective proteasome inhibitor, exhibits in vivo antiinflammatory activity. *Proc Natl Acad Sci USA* 1999;96:10403–10408.
69. Sherman M, et al. Cellular defenses against unfolded proteins: a cell biologist thinks about neurodegenerative diseases [Review]. *Neuron* 2001;29:15–32.
70. Gronostajski R, et al. The ATP-dependence of the degradation of short- and long-lived proteins in growing fibroblasts. *J Biol Chem* 1985;260:3344–3349.
71. Rock KL, et al. Degradation of cell proteins and generation of MHC class I-presented peptides. *Annu Rev Immunol* 1999;17:739–779.
72. Gaczynska M, et al. Gamma-interferon and expression of MHC genes regulate peptide hydrolysis by proteasomes. *Nature* 1993;365:264–267.
73. Michalek MT, et al. A role for the ubiquitin-dependent proteolytic pathway in MHC class I-restricted antigen presentation. *Nature* 1993;363:552–554.
74. Beninga J, et al. Interferon-gamma can stimulate post-proteasomal trimming of the N-termini of an antigenic peptide by inducing leucine aminopeptidase. *J Biol Chem* 1998;273:18734–18742.
75. Saric T, et al. ERAP1, an interferon-gamma-induced aminopeptidase in the endoplasmic reticulum, that trims precursors to MHC class I-presented peptides. *Nat Immunol* 2002;3:1169–1176.
76. York IA, et al. Endoplasmic reticulum aminopeptidase1 (ERAP1) generates antigenic peptides in interferon-γ-stimulated cells. *Nat Immunol* 2002;3:1177–1184.
77. Goff SA, et al. Production of abnormal proteins in *E. coli* stimulates transcription of lon and other heat-shock genes. *Cell* 1985;41:587–595.
78. Ananthan J, et al. Abnormal proteins serve as eukaryotic stress signals and trigger the activation of heat-shock genes. *Science* 1986;232:522–524
79. Lopes UG, et al. p53-dependent induction of apoptosis by proteasome inhibitors. *J Biol Chem* 1997;272:12893–12896.
80. Bush KT, et al Proteasome inhibition leads to a heat-shock response, induction of endoplasmic reticulum chaperones, and thermotolerance. *J Biol Chem* 1997;272:9086–9092.
81. Wang CY, et al. Control of inducible chemoresistance: enhanced anti-tumor therapy through increased apoptosis by inhibition of NF-kappaB. *Nat Med* 1999;5:412–417.
82. Sadoul R, et al. Involvement of the proteasome in the programmed cell death of NGF-deprived sympathetic neurons. *EMBO J* 1996;15:3845–3852.
83. Berenson JR, et al. The role of nuclear factor-kappaB in the biology and treatment of multiple myeloma. *Semin Oncol* 2001;28:626–633.
84. Jensen TJ, et al. Multiple proteolytic systems, including the proteasome, contribute to CFTR processing. *Cell* 1995;83:129–135.

85. Ward CL, et al. Degradation of CFTR by the ubiquitin-proteasome pathway. *Cell* 1995;83:121–127.
86. Qu D, et al. Degradation of a mutant secretory protein, alpha1-antitrypsin Z, in the endoplasmic reticulum requires proteasome activity. *J Biol Chem* 1996;271:22791–22795.
87. Fisher EA, et al. The degradation of apolipoprotein B100 is mediated by the ubiquitin-proteasome pathway and involves heat shock protein 70. *J Biol Chem* 1997:20427–20434.
88. Hughes EA, et al. Misfolded major histocompatibility complex class I heavy chains are translocated into the cytoplasm and degraded by the proteasome. *Proc Natl Acad Sci USA* 1997;94:1896–1901.
89. Sommer T, et al. Endoplasmic reticulum degradation: reverse protein flow of no return. *FASEB J* 1997;11:1227–1233.
90. Ye Y, et al. The AAA ATPase Cdc48/p97 and its partners transport proteins from the ER into the cytosol. *Nature* 2001;414:652–656.
91. Kaufman RJ. Orchestrating the unfolded protein response in health and disease. *J Clin Invest* 2002;110:1389–1398

3   Structures of the Yeast Proteasome Core Particle in Complex with Inhibitors

Michael Groll and Robert Huber

Contents

1. INTRODUCTION

Intracellular proteolysis is an essential process *(1)*. The ubiquitin–proteasome pathway represents a strictly controlled complex enzymatic machinery for nonlysosomal protein degradation in eukaryotic cells. Thus, it is particularly important for the turnover of many critical proteins controlling a vast array of biologic pathways, including proliferation, differentiation, and inflammation *(2–4)*. The system functions in two steps: first, a protein substrate is marked by covalent addition of a poly-ubiquitin chain; second, the poly-ubiquitinated substrate is degraded by a 2500-kDa proteolytic complex called the 26S proteasome.

The 26S proteasome is formed by a cylindrical-shaped multimeric complex referred to as the 20S proteasome (core particle [CP]), capped at each end by another multimeric component called the 19S complex (regulatory particle [RP]) or PA700. Proteolysis of the ubiquitinated substrates occurs within the CP. The X-ray structure of the 20S proteasome from the archaeon *Thermoplasma acidophilum (5)* showed for the first time the architecture of the CP at atomic resolution. The molecule is composed of four stacked rings, with each ring consisting of seven subunits following an $\alpha_{1-7}\beta_{1-7}\beta_{1-7}\alpha_{1-7}$ stoichiometry. Proteolysis occurs within the central chamber at the β-subunits with Thr1Oγ acting as the nucleophile. The general $\alpha_7\beta_7\beta_7\alpha_7$ architecture of the *Thermoplasma* proteasome is also found in eukaryotes. In yeast, the α- and β-subunits have diverged into seven different subunits each, which are present in unique locations in two copies per CP, so that the D7 symmetry of the archaebacterial particle is reduced to C2 symmetry *(6)*. The α- and β-nomenclature reflects the location of the α- and β-subunits in the 20S proteasome. Unique locations of individual subunits within the particle are defined by subunit-specific contact surfaces formed by unique sequence insertions and extensions.

From: *Cancer Drug Discovery and Development: Proteasome Inhibitors in Cancer Therapy*
Edited by: J. Adams © Humana Press Inc., Totowa, NJ

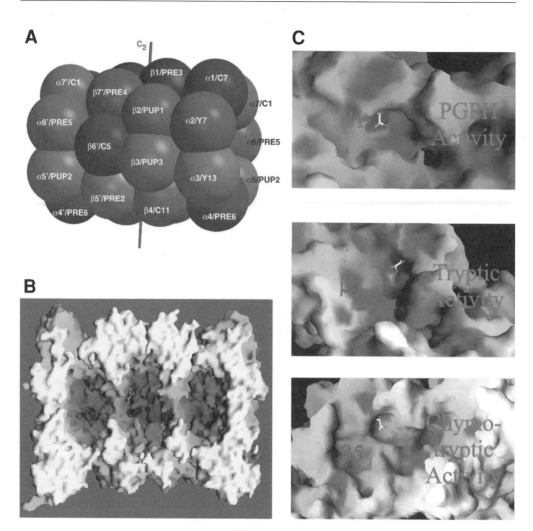

Fig. 1. (A) Topology of the 28 subunits of the yeast 20S proteasome drawn as spheres. **(B)** Surface view of the yeast 20S proteasome crystallized in the presence of calpain inhibitor 1, clipped along the cylindrical axis. The inhibitor molecules are shown as space-filling models in yellow. The sealed α-ports at both ends of the yeast proteasome and a few narrow side windows can be seen. **(C)** Surface representation of the three active sites in the yeast 20S proteasome. Each picture shows the nucleophilic Thr1 in sticks, the basic residues in blue, the acidic residues in red, and the hydrophobic residues in white. PGPH, peptidylglutamyl-peptide hydrolyzing.

As in archaebacterial CPs, the α-subunits are inactive. Four of the seven different β-subunits in yeast lack residues that have been shown to be essential in archaebacterial proteasomes for proteolytic activity, whereas the remaining three subunits, β1, β2, and β5, represent the active site (Fig. 1). By comparison with substrate specificities of known proteases, the three peptidase activities of the 20S proteasome, cleaving substrates after large hydrophobic, basic, or acidic residues, were designated as *chymotrypsin-like*, *trypsin-like*, and *peptidylglutamyl-peptide hydrolyzing* (PGPH) activities, respectively *(7)*. Recently, the latter has also been termed *postacidic* or *caspase-like* activity *(8)*.

2. PROTEASOME INHIBITORS

Inhibitors have been used to study the role of the proteasome in biological processes in vivo and in vitro. Initially, cell-penetrating peptide aldehydes, such as AC-LLNL-AL, MG115, MG132, and PSI, were developed. More recently, new compounds were synthesized with increased potency and selectivity for the proteasome *(9,10)*; based on the crystal structure of the yeast CP *(6)*, molecular modeling can now be used to engineer improved inhibitors *(11)*. In addition to the synthetic molecules especially developed as proteasome inhibitors, a variety of natural compounds have been described that inhibit the CP. Some of these natural products were discovered through their biologic effects on cells before it was recognized that their main target is the proteasome. Lactacystin *(12)*, eponemycin *(13)*, and epoxomicin *(14)* are such molecules. With a multifunctional enzyme like the proteasome, it is difficult to obtain clear results concerning the effects of its inhibitors. However, structure analyses of the yeast CP in complex with several inhibitors, as well as experiments performed with radiolabeled irreversible inhibitors, show that most proteasome inhibitors bind covalently in the active site.

N-Acetyl-Leu-Leu-norleucinal (Ac-LLnL-al, also called calpain inhibitor 1) has been widely used to study proteasome function in vivo, despite its lack of specificity *(15,16)*. This inhibitor binds reversibly to the N-terminal threonine of the active subunits and abolishes the chymotrypsin-like and, to a lesser extent, the trypsin-like and postacidic activities of the proteasome. The crystal structure of the CP in complex with Ac-LLnL-al shows the inhibitor covalently bound to Thr1Oγ of all active subunits, as a hemiacetal. It adopts a β-conformation and fills a gap between strands to which it is hydrogen bonded, generating an antiparallel β-sheet structure *(6)*. The norleucine side chain projects into the S1 pocket, which opens sidewise toward a tunnel leading to the particle surface, whereas the leucine side chain at P2 is not stabilized. The leucine side chain at P3 is in contact with the amino acids of the adjacent β-type subunit and is therefore fixed (Fig. 2A).

Lactacystin is a natural product from *Streptomyces* that was discovered as a result of its ability to induce neurite outgrowth in a murine neuroblastoma cell line. Incubation of cells in the presence of radioactive lactacystin resulted mainly in the labeling of the β5 subunit *(12)*, although lactacystin can be found to bind to all active β-type subunits of the CP in certain conditions *(17)*. Lactacystin effectively and irreversibly inhibits the chymotrypsin-like activity of the proteasome. It also blocks the trypsin-like and the postacidic activities with lower efficiencies. In aqueous solutions at pH 8, lactacystin is spontaneously hydrolyzed into *clasto*-lactacystin β-lactone, which is in fact the active compound inhibiting the CP *(18)*. The crystal structure of the complex between lactacystin and yeast proteasome shows the molecule covalently bound only to subunit β5 *(6)*, in accord with the observed chemical modification of subunit X/MB1 of the mammalian proteasome. Thus, lactacystin displays a host of hydrogen bonds with protein main chain atoms (Fig. 2A). The irreversible inhibition by lactacystin of the active site of the proteasome is due to the formation of an ester bond with the N-terminal threonine. In principle, this ester bond and almost every hydrogen-bonding interaction with lactacystin could be made in all active subunits. However, subunits β1 and β2 do not form a covalent complex in the crystal of the yeast proteasome, as there is a major difference in their S1 pocket in comparison with subunit β5. The dimethyl side chain of lactacystin mimics a valine or

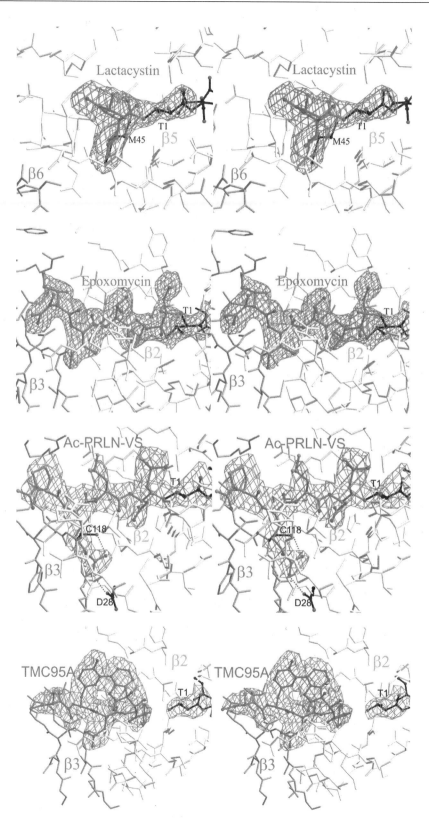

a leucine side chain. Met45, which is mainly responsible for the chymotryptic activity, closely interacts with the branched side chain of lactacystin and has a major role in selective inhibition. The S1 pocket of β5 consists additionally of several acidic amino acids contributed by subunit β6, which may allow binding of basic residues, consistent with the observation that lactacystin inhibits both the chymotrypsin-like and, to a lesser extent, the trypsin-like activity against chromogenic substrates *(6,12)*. These data gave impetus to the first structure-based design efforts to develop inhibitors *(19)*.

Recently, it was shown that the α',β'-epoxyketone peptide natural product epoxomicin potently and irreversibly inhibits the catalytic activity of the CP *(14)*. Unlike most other proteasome inhibitors, epoxomicin is highly specific for the proteasome and does not inhibit other proteases. The crystal structure of epoxomicin bound to the yeast CP reveals the molecular basis for selectivity of α',β'-epoxyketone inhibitors *(20)*. The complex showed an unexpected morpholino ring formation between the amino-terminal threonine and epoxomicin, providing the first insights into the unique specificity of epoxomicin for the proteasome (Fig. 2B). The morpholino derivative formation is most likely a two-step process. First, activation of the Thr1Oγ is believed to occur by its N-terminal amino group acting as a base either directly or via a neighboring water molecule. Subsequent nucleophilic attack of the Thr1Oγ on the carbonyl of the epoxyketone pharmacophore would produce a hemiacetal, as is observed in the proteasome:Ac-LLnL-al complex. The formation of the hemiacetal facilitates the second step in the formation of the morpholino adduct. In this cyclization, the N-terminus of Thr1 opens the epoxide ring by an intramo-

---

Fig. 2. *(Fig. 2 on opposite page)* Stereoview of yeast 20S proteasome subunits (colored in white and gray) in complex with the inhibitor (colored in green) **(A)** lactacystin, **(B)** epoxomicin, **(C)** MB1, and **(D)** TMC95A. The electron density maps (colored in blue) are contoured from 1σ on in similar orientations around Thr1 (colored in black) with $2F_O$-F_C coefficients after twofold averaging. Apart from the bound inhibitors, no structural changes were noted. Temperature fracture refinement indicates full occupancies of all inhibitor binding sites. The inhibitors have been omitted for phasing. **(A)** β5 covalently bound with the natural *Streptomyces* metabolite lactacystin. The S1 pockets from β1 and β2 differ from that of β5 and do not make covalent complexes with lactacystin. Met45 of subunit β5 (indicated in black) forms the bottom of the β5-S1 pocket and is in contact with the branched side chain of lactacystin, which stabilizes in particular the proteasome inhibitor complex and plays a dominant role for subunit specificity. **(B)** β2 covalently bound with the natural specific proteasome inhibitor epoxomicin. The electron density reveals the presence of a unique six-membered ring. This morpholino derivative results from adduct formation between epoxomicin and the proteasomal N-terminal threonyl 1Oγ and N (pink sticks) thus emphasizing the selectivity of epoxyketones for Ntn-hydrolases. **(C)** β2 covalently bound with the synthetic β2 specific vinyl sulfone inhibitor MB1. Favorable hydrogen bonds between Asp28 of β2 at the bottom of the S3 pocket and Cys118 of β3 within the walls of the S3 pocket are shown as orange dots. These residues make productive contacts with the amine groups of the P3 arginine of MB1 and are in particular responsible for the MB1 subunit specificity. β1 and β5 do not form stable complexes with MB1, because of their different S3 pockets. **(D)** β2 noncovalently bound to the natural specific proteasome inhibitor TMC-95A from *Apiospora montagnei*. TMC-95A binds near the proteolytic center in all active subunits in the extended substrate binding site not modifying the nucleophilic Thr1 and therefore forms the basis for non-covalent proteasome inhibitors.

lecular displacement, with consequent inversion of the C2 carbon *(20)*. The observed specificity of epoxomicin for the proteasome is explained by the requirement for both an N-terminal amino group and a side chain nucleophile for adduct formation with the epoxyketone pharmacophore.

The human immunodeficiency virus protease inhibitor ritonavir, used successfully in AIDS therapy, has recently been found to inhibit the chymotrypsin-like activity of the human CP *(21)*. No electron density for bound ritonavir was seen by analyzing the yeast proteasome-inhibitor complex crystallographically (Groll, unpublished data). However, a structural model in which ritonavir interacts with the yeast subunit β5 has been modeled *(22)*.

A new class of proteasome inhibitors comprises peptides that possess a vinyl sulfone moiety *(23)*. However, these inhibitors have similar limitations as the peptide aldehydes insofar as they have also been reported to bind and block intracellular cysteine proteases such as cathepsin S. The crystal structure of the proteasome:Ac-YLLN-vs complex shows covalent binding of the Thr1Oγ of all active subunits to the β-carbon atom of the vinyl sulfone group. Previous work using libraries of peptide-based covalent inhibitors has identified structural elements that can be used to control the substrate selectivity of synthetic inhibitors *(24)*. By comparison with proteasome-aldehyde inhibitors, it is possible to make the vinyl sulfones specific against the active subunits by altering the P3 and P4 position, as indicated by Ac-PRLN-vs *(25)*. The crystal structure analyses of the eukaryotic CP in complex with the vinyl sulfones suggest that favorable interactions between the P3 residue and the large S3 pocket generated at the interface of neighboring β-subunits are responsible for inhibitor selectivity (Fig. 2C). Furthermore, the P1 residue was bound in the S1 pocket of each of the active sites, regardless of seemingly unfavorable electrostatic interactions. Taking these data together, it is possible to design a model in which specificity can be controlled predominantly by interactions at the S3 site for substrates with favorable interactions at this site and poor interactions at other sites. However, strong interactions at P1 may overcome the need for a favorable P3 residue. This model for substrate binding may aid in the development of inhibitors of the proteasome with tunable selectivity for each of the active sites.

3. THE FUTURE OF PROTEASOME INHIBITORS AS THERAPY

As proteasomes play an important role in many irreversible intracellular processes such as mitosis, differentiation, signal transduction, and antigen processing *(26)*, inhibitors that specifically block proteasomal activities may be promising candidates for tumor or inflammation therapy. However, all the aforementioned proteasome inhibitors bind covalently to the active β-subunits and usually cause cell death by induction of apoptosis *(4)*. Reversible and time-limited inactivation of the different proteasome activities may reduce the cytotoxic effects of these compounds. It was recently shown that natural products from *Apiospora montagnei*, the TMC-95s (TMC-95A, -B, -C, and -D), block the proteolytic activity of the CP selectively and competitively in the low n*M* range *(27,28)*. The inhibitor is not related to any previously reported proteasome inhibitors and consists of modified amino acids forming a heterocyclic ring system. Crystal structure analysis of the yeast CP in complex with TMC-95A shows the inhibitor bound at all three active sites *(29)*. The structure indicates a noncovalent linkage of TMC-95A to the active β-subunits, not modifying their N-terminal threonines, in contrast to all previously structurally analyzed proteasome inhibitor complexes (Fig. 2D).

TMC-95A displays a host of hydrogen bonds with the protein, giving further stabilization to the compound in its bound state. In particular, all these interactions are performed with main chain atoms and strictly conserved residues of the CP, revealing a common mode of proteasome inhibition among different species. The arrangement of TMC-95A in the CP is similar to that of the already reported aldehyde and epoxyketone inhibitors *(20)*. The *n*-propylene group of TMC-95A protrudes into the S1 pocket, making weak hydrophobic contacts with Lys33, whereas the S2 subsite is shallow and does not contribute to the stabilization of TMC-95A, as already observed in the proteasome:Ac-LLnL-al adduct *(6)*. The side chain of the asparagine is inserted deeply into the S3 pocket and has been ascribed a major role in the differing median inhibitory concentration values among the different activities. The TMC-95 compounds specifically block the CP and do not inhibit other proteases like m-calpain, cathepsin L, and trypsin *(27)*. The nuclear magnetic resonance structure of unbound TMC-95A in solution *(28)*, when superimposed with the structure bound to the CP, as determined by X-ray crystallography, shows a similar conformation *(29)*.

Because of the crosslink between the tyrosine and the oxoindol side chain, the strained conformation of TMC-95s is stabilized suitably for optimal binding to the proteasome. Binding does not require major rearrangements of ligand and protein and is favored for entropic reasons compared with more flexible ligands. Analysis of the TMC-95A structure overlaid with that of the vinyl sulfone peptide inhibiting only β2 shows a remarkable overlap with both the backbone amides and the P1 and P3 residues, since TMC-95A interacts with the proteasome noncovalently *(25)*. By presenting its functional groups optionally, covalent attachment to the catalytic nucleophile is no longer required. Combining information from the crystal structures in complex with the CP inhibitors suggests the possibility of generating a scaffold based on the geometry of the bound TMC-95A that can present a variety of structures to the S1 and S3 pockets specific for each of the active sites of the CP. In particular, the P3 position offers itself for fine tuning of the selectivity of compounds for individual β-subunits and designing reversible, selective, and subunit-specific inhibitors of the CPs *(30)*.

REFERENCES

1. Hershko A, et al. The ubiquitin system. *Annu Rev Biochem* 1998;67:425–479.
2. Bochtler M, et al. The proteasome. *Annu Rev Biophys Biomol Struct* 1999;28:295–317.
3. Coux O, et al. Structure and functions of the 20S and 26S proteasomes. *Annu Rev Biochem* 1996;65:801–847.
4. Kloetzel PM. The proteasome system: a neglected tool for improvement of novel therapeutic strategies? *Gene Ther* 1998;5:1297–1298.
5. Löwe J, et al. Crystal structure of the 20S proteasome from the archaeon T. acidophilum at 3.4 Å resolution. *Science* 1995;268:533–539.
6. Groll M, et al. Structure of 20S proteasome from yeast at 2.4 Å resolution. *Nature* 1997;386:463–471.
7. Orlowski M. The multicatalytic proteinase complex, a major extralysosomal proteolytic system. *Biochemistry* 1990;29:10289–10297.
8. Kisselev AF, et al. The sizes of peptides generated from protein by mammalian 26 and 20 S proteasomes. Implications for understanding the degradative mechanism and antigen presentation. *J Biol Chem* 1999;274:3363–3371.
9. Adams J, et al. Potent and selective inhibitors of the proteasome: dipeptidyl boronic acids. *Bioorg Med Chem Lett* 1998;8:333–338.

10. Elofsson M, et al. Towards subunit-specific proteasome inhibitors: synthesis and evaluation of peptide alpha',beta'-epoxyketones. *Chem Biol* 1999;6:811–822.

11. Loidl G, et al. Bivalency as a principle for proteasome inhibition. *Proc Natl Acad Sci USA* 1999;96;5418–5422.

12. Fenteany G, et al. Inhibition of proteasome activities and subunit-specific amino-terminal threonine modification by lactacystin. *Science* 1995;268:726–731.

13. Meng L, et al. Eponemycin exerts its antitumor effect through the inhibition of proteasome function. *Cancer Res* 1999;59:2798–2801.

14. Meng L, et al. Epoxomicin, a potent and selective proteasome inhibitor, exhibits in vivo antiinflammatory activity. *Proc Natl Acad Sci USA* 1999;96:10403–10408.

15. Vinitsky A, et al. Inhibition of the proteolytic activity of the multicatalytic proteinase complex (proteasome) by substrate-related peptidyl aldehydes. *J Biol Chem* 1994;269:29860–29866.

16. Rock KL, et al. Inhibitors of the proteasome block the degradation of most cell proteins and the generation of peptides presented on MHC class I molecules. *Cell* 1994;78:761–771.

17. Craiu A, et al. Lactacystin and clasto-lactacystin beta-lactone modify multiple proteasome beta-subunits and inhibit intracellular protein degradation and major histocompatibility complex class I antigen presentation. *J Biol Chem* 1997;272:13437–13445.

18. Dick LR, et al. Mechanistic studies on the inactivation of the proteasome by lactacystin in cultured cells. *J Biol Chem* 1997;272:182–188.

19. Loidl G, et al. Bifunctional inhibitors of the trypsin-like activity of eukaryotic proteasomes. *Chem Biol* 1999;6:197–204.

20. Groll M, et al. Crystal structure of epoxomicin:20S proteasome reveals a molecular basis for selectivity of alpha',beta'-epoxyketone proteasome inhibitors. *J Am Chem Soc* 2000;122:1237–1238.

21. Andre P, et al. An inhibitor of HIV-1 protease modulates proteasome activity, antigen presentation, and T cell responses. *Proc Natl Acad Sci USA* 1998;95:13120–13124.

22. Schmidtke G, et al. How an inhibitor of the HIV-I protease modulates proteasome activity. *J Biol Chem* 1999;274:35734–35740.

23. Bogyo M, et al. Covalent modification of the active site threonine of proteasomal beta subunits and the *Escherichia coli* homolog HslV by a new class of inhibitors. *Proc Natl Acad Sci USA* 1997;94:6629–6634.

24. Nazif T, et al. Global analysis of proteasomal substrate specificity using positional-scanning libraries of covalent inhibitors. *Proc Natl Acad Sci USA* 2001;98:2967–2972.

25. Groll M, et al. Probing structural determinants distal to the site of hydrolysis that control substrate specificity of the 20S proteasome. *Chem Biol* 2002;9:1–20.

26. Groettrup M, et al. Peptide antigen production by the proteasome: complexity provides efficiency. *Immunol Today* 1996;17:429–435.

27. Koguchi Y, et al. TMC-95A, B, C, and D, novel proteasome inhibitors produced by *Apiospora montagnei* Sacc. TC 1093. Taxonomy, production, isolation, and biological activities. *J Antibiot (Tokyo)* 2000;53:105–109.

28. Kohno J, et al. Structures of TMC-95A-D: novel proteasome inhibitors from *Apiospora montagnei* sacc. TC 1093. *J Org Chem* 2000;65:990–995.

29. Groll M, et al. Crystal structure of the 20 S proteasome:TMC-95A complex: a non-covalent proteasome inhibitor. *J Mol Biol* 2001;311:543–548.

30. Kaiser M, et al. The core structure of TMC-95A is a promising lead for reversible proteasome inhibition. *Angew Chem Int Ed* 2002;41:780–783.

4 Natural Product and Synthetic Proteasome Inhibitors

Kyung Bo Kim and Craig M. Crews

CONTENTS

ABSTRACT

The ubiquitin–proteasome pathway has emerged as a major player in regulation several important signaling processes such as cell proliferation and inflammation. As a result, proteasome inhibitors are being intensely pursued as both molecular probes of proteasome biology and as therapeutic agents. Thus far, many proteasome inhibitors have been synthesized or isolated from natural sources, some of which are in clinical trial for cancer therapy. In this chapter, we discuss recent developments of both natural and synthetic proteasome inhibitors. Particular attention is focused on comparisons of the kinetic and/or biologic data for various proteasome inhibitors. Finally, we describe the design of novel proteasome inhibitors that target specific subunits of the proteasome.

KEY WORDS

ubiquitin; proteasome inhibitor; peptide aldehydes; peptide amides; vinyl sulfones; epoxy ketones; epoxomicin; lactacystin; boronic acids; polyphenols; macrocyclic inhibitors; PGPH-specific inhibitors; subunit-specific inhibitors

1. INTRODUCTION

Over the last decade, the proteasome–ubiquitin pathway has emerged as a central player in the regulation of diverse cellular processes. In addition, defects in various components of this pathway have been implicated in several human diseases (1). As a result, proteasome inhibitors from natural sources as well as those developed synthetically have been intensely pursued both as molecular probes of the proteasome biology and as potential therapeutic agents.

From: *Cancer Drug Discovery and Development: Proteasome Inhibitors in Cancer Therapy*
Edited by: J. Adams © Humana Press Inc., Totowa, NJ

There are a number of excellent reviews on proteasome inhibitors, mostly focusing on the chemical nature of inhibitors *(2–4)* In this chapter, we discuss the chemistry of both natural and synthetic proteasome inhibitors, updating recent studies on this class of compounds. Particular attention is focused on comparisons of the kinetic and/or biologic (median inhibitory concentration [IC_{50}]) data for various proteasome inhibitors.

2. SYNTHETIC INHIBITORS

Before recognition of the proteasome–ubiquitin pathway as a central player in many signaling pathways such as cell cycle control and inflammatory action, proteasome studies during the 1980s and early 1990s focused largely on the purification and characterization of this novel proteolytic machinery. Given the multiple proteolytic activities of the proteasome, which are referred to as the chymotrypsin-like (CT-L), trypsin-like (T-L), and peptidylglutamyl-peptide hydrolyzing (PGPH; or caspase-like) activities *(5,6)*, it is not surprising that inhibitors of better studied proteases, possessing analogous proteolytic activities to the proteasome, were the first proteasome inhibitor family shown to inhibit the activities of the 20S proteasome. The identification of compounds possessing dual inhibitory activities paved the way for the development of inhibitors with higher selectivity and potency for the 20S proteasome. Here, we broadly categorize the synthetic proteasome inhibitors into two groups, reversible and irreversible, referring to the ability to modify covalently the hydroxyl group of the catalytic amino terminal Thr within the proteasome active site.

2.1. Reversible Inhibitors

2.1.1. Peptide Aldehydes

During the 1980s, proteasome inhibitors were largely developed for use as molecular tools in the purification of proteasomes and for the characterization of the different proteolytic activities of the 20S proteasome. Because the proteasome displays similar proteolytic activities with several cysteine and serine proteases, not surprisingly, peptide aldehydes, which had long been used as inhibitors for both serine and cysteine proteases, were quickly identified as proteasome inhibitors (Fig. 1). For example, in the early 1980s, leupeptin, a standard serine (trypsin, plasmin) and cysteine (papain, cathepsin B) protease inhibitor, was shown to inhibit the 20S proteasome *(7)*. Of note, leupeptin has an Arg at the P1 position and, not unexpectedly, blocks the T-L activity of the 20S proteasome that cleaves a peptide bond after basic residues, analogous to trypsin.

Unlike leupeptin, calpain inhibitors I and II, which contain a large hydrophobic amino acid residue at the P1 position, were shown to inhibit selectively the CT-L activity of the 20S proteasome *(8,9)*. Later, combined with X-ray analysis data, extensive studies on direct inhibition of proteasome activities with these peptide aldehydes revealed that different proteasome β-subunits could be assigned to corresponding activities *(10,11)*.

The rediscovery of the serine and cysteine peptide aldehyde inhibitors as proteasome inhibitors has prompted the development of peptide aldehyde inhibitors with increased potency and selectivity for CT-L activity (Table 1). Some of these inhibitors have been widely used in studying the role of the proteasome in various cellular processes. For example, MG115 and MG132, tripeptide aldehydes developed by Rock and colleagues *(12)*, are both potent and CT-L-selective inhibitors that are widely used in proteasome

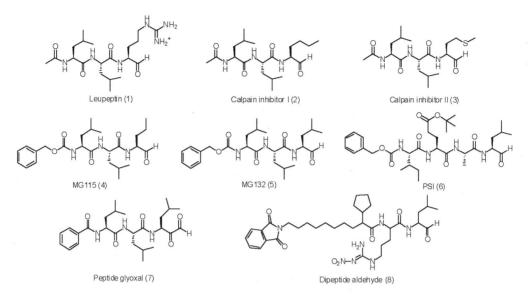

Leupeptin (1)
Calpain inhibitor I (2)
Calpain inhibitor II (3)
MG 115 (4)
MG 132 (5)
PSI (6)
Peptide glyoxal (7)
Dipeptide aldehyde (8)

Fig. 1. Peptide-based aldehyde inhibitors.

biology. Another good example is PSI, a tetrapeptide aldehyde developed by Wilk and colleagues *(13)*, a perhaps more potent and selective CT-L inhibitor but less widely used. Similarly, a myriad of peptide aldehyde inhibitors have been synthesized to improve the potency and selectivity, but none of them has been as successful as MG115 and MG132 so far. It should be noted that Orlowski and colleagues have attempted to develop peptide aldehydes to inhibit other activities of the 20S proteasome. For example, Z-GPFL-CHO has been reported to inhibit a minor activity of the proteasome, the branched-chain amino acid-preferring (BrAAP) activity of the proteasome *(14)*. Meanwhile, researchers have also attempted to improve the reactivity of aldehyde pharmacophore by adding an additional ketone moiety at the α-position, yielding a glyoxal *(15)*.

From extensive X-ray diffraction analysis and kinetic studies, the mode of inhibition of peptide aldehydes has been well characterized. Upon binding to the active site of the 20S proteasome, a peptide aldehyde forms a reversible hemiacetal adduct between the aldehyde group of the inhibitor and the hydroxyl group of the amino terminal Thr, analogous to the tetrahedral intermediate of a protease reaction *(10,11)*. Although peptide aldehydes of this class, in general, are cell-permeable potent inhibitors of the 20S proteasome and are still widely used in the study of the role of proteasome in many cellular processes, the crossreactivity with other cysteine and serine proteases is still a major concern for their use as potential therapeutics or as molecular probes in dissecting complex signaling pathways. Therefore, continuing efforts are being made to develop more specific and potent inhibitors toward the proteasome.

2.1.2. AMIDES

Proteasome inhibitors with electrophilic head groups such as aldehydes are thought to retain the inherent drawbacks of traditional serine and cysteine protease inhibitors, in that they are too reactive, unstable, non-target-specific, and possess poor membrane permeability. Therefore, researchers have attempted to replace the electrophilic pharmacophore

Table 1
Synthetic Peptide Aldehyde Inhibitors

Compound	$(k_{obs}/[I])$ (M/s)			In vivo activity	Crossreactivity	Ref.
	CT-L	T-L	PGPH			
MG132 (5)	K_i = 4.0 nM	K_i = 2760 nM	K_i = 900 nM	0.4 μM[a]	Calpain, cathepsins	4, 21, 59
PSI (6)	IC_{50} = 250 nM	25% inhibition at 65 μM	Stimulation (260%) at 65 μM	ND	Calpain, cathepsins	8
Glyoxal (7)	K_i = 3.7 μM	ND	ND	ND	ND	13
CEP1612 (8)	IC_{50} = 2 μM	No inhibition up to 1 μM	ND	IC_{50} = 1–2 μM[b]	Calpain I 100 μM Cathepsin B (IC_{50} = 90 μM)	59
Bifunctional aldehyde (35)	IC_{50} > 100 μM	IC_{50} = 0.5 μM	IC_{50} > 100 μM	ND	ND	57
PEG$_n$ (CO-RVR-H)$_2$ (34)	IC_{50} > 100 μM	IC_{50} = 0.071 μM	IC_{50} > 100 μM	ND	ND	56

CT-L, chymotrypsin-like; IC_{50}, median inhibitory concentration; ND, not determined; PGPH, peptidylglutamyl-peptide hydrolyzing; T-L, trypsin-like.
[a]80% growth inhibition of EL4 cells.
[b]For intracellular proteolysis of proteasome substrate and MHC1 processing.

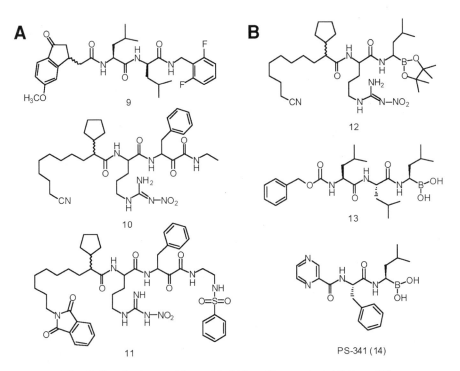

Fig. 2. Synthetic peptide amide (**A**) and boronate inhibitors (**B**).

with a less reactive but potentially hydratable head group, expecting less crossreactivity with other proteases (Table 2). For example, CV Therapeutics has introduced benzamide derivatives *(16,17)*, hoping to avoid the inherent drawbacks of the traditional serine and cysteine protease inhibitors. They identified a series of dipeptidyl indanylamide derivatives that are potent, competitive inhibitors of the CT-L activity of the 20S proteasome, from approximately 400 indanylamides prepared by a standard Fmoc solid-phase synthesis. These compounds have been shown to possess antiproliferative activity against RAW cells and, apparently, no calpain I inhibition activity, although no detailed kinetic and biologic data were provided. However, it should be noted that no inhibition study with other common proteases has been described for this class of compounds.

Meanwhile, Cephalon has developed other nonaldehyde reversible proteasome inhibitors (Fig. 2A), the family of dipeptide α-ketoamide inhibitors that are selective for the CT-L activity of the 20S proteasome *(18,19)*. Later, based on the backbone of these α-ketoamide inhibitors, Cephalon further developed P'-extended α-ketoamide inhibitors *(20)*, hoping to probe the importance of P'-sites on the inhibition of CT-L activity of proteasome. Like indanylamide inhibitors of the 20S proteasome, this class of P'-extended α-ketoamide inhibitors display selective inhibition of the CT-L activity of 20S proteasome. For example, compound **11** was unable to inhibit the T-L activity of the 20S proteasome at concentrations up to 1 μ*M*. Moreover, compound **11** has been shown to be more than 150-fold selective for the CT-L activity of proteasome in comparison with calpain I, although no inhibition studies toward other proteases have been reported.

Table 2

Synthetic Reversible Inhibitors: Peptide Amides and Boronates

Compound	$(k_{obs}/[I]$ (M/s)			In vivo activity	Crossreactivity	Ref.
	CT-L	T-L	PGPH			
Benzamide (9)	IC_{50} = 0.14 µM	IC_{50} > 20 µM	IC_{50} > 20 µM	IC_{50} = 8 µM[a]	No calpain I	16
α-ketoamide (10)	IC_{50} = 13–22 nM	No inhibition up to 1 µM	ND	ND	100-fold selective vs chymotrypsin	19
P'-extended α-ketoamide (11)	K_i = 1.1 nM	No inhibition up to 1 µM	ND	ND	150 times selective over calpain I	20
Dipeptidyl boronic ester (12)	IC_{50} = 8 nM	No inhibition up to 1 µM	ND	ND	100-fold selective vs chymotrypsin	19
Bortezomib (14)	53,000 IC_{50} = 0.62 nM	150	3200	0.02 µM[b]	None found	22, 61
Cbz-LLL-boronic acid (13)	K_i = 0.03 nM	ND	ND	0.04 µM[b]	ND	22, 61

For abbreviations, see Table 1 footnote.
[a] Antiproliferative activity against RAW cells.
[b] 80% growth inhibition of EL4 cells.

52

2.1.3. BORONIC ESTERS AND ACIDS

In addition to the amide derivatives described above, peptide boronates have been prepared as novel reversible inhibitors of the proteasome (Fig. 2B), yielding bortezomib (Velcade, formerly known as PS-341).

Before its use as a valuable proteasome inhibitory pharmacophore, the boronic functional group had been extensively employed as serine protease inhibitors, most notably as thrombin inhibitors. For example, researchers at DuPont Merck Pharm were able to develop extremely potent thrombin inhibitors with median inhibitory concentration (IC_{50}) values as low as 0.04 nM (21). Meanwhile, Cephalon developed a peptide boronic ester derived inhibitor (12) of the CT-L activity of the proteasome (19), demonstrating that these serine protease inhibitory moieties are capable of inhibiting the proteasome. Later, through systematic optimization studies, Adams and colleagues (22,23) developed potent and selective tri- and dipeptidyl boronic acid proteasome inhibitors, including bortezomib.

The activity of peptidyl boronic acids as serine protease inhibitors is presumably because an empty *p*-orbital on a boron atom is positioned to accept the oxygen lone pair of the active site serine residue to form a stable pseudo-tetrahedral complex. Moreover, this unique interaction between boron and oxygen is also thought to provide the selectivity for serine proteases over cysteine proteases, owing to the very weak nature of bonding between boron and thiol of cysteine proteases. Indeed, Cbz-Leu-Leu-Leu-boronic acid **13**, developed by Adams et al., showed high selectivity for the proteasome ($K_i = 0.03$ nM) over cathepsin B ($K_i = 6.1$ µM), representing a 200,000-fold selectivity for the proteasome (22). Based on this remarkable selectivity and potency of tripeptidyl boronic acids, they further developed the truncated dipeptidyl boronic acids with no apparent loss of activity. The best characterized compound of this family is the dipeptidyl boronic acid bortezomib. Surprisingly, bortezomib displayed extremely high selectivity for the proteasome over not just cysteine proteases but other serine proteases as well (Table 2). The biologic effects of bortezomib are extensively detailed elsewhere in this book. In vitro and mouse xenograft studies of bortezomib have shown antitumor activity in a variety of tumor types, including myeloma, chronic lymphocytic leukemia, prostate cancer, pancreatic cancer, and colon cancer, among others (22–24).

2.2. Irreversible Inhibitors

2.2.1. EPOXY KETONES

In order to develop a novel irreversible proteasome inhibitor, Spaltenstein et al. (25) first introduced an α',β'-epoxyketone pharmacophore in tripeptide backbones. By this approach, they were able to develop a potent peptide epoxyketone proteasome inhibitor **15** (Fig. 3). However, it should be emphasized that the importance of the peptide epoxyketones as specific proteasome inhibitors had not been realized until the mode of action studies of natural product epoxomicin and eponemycin discussed in Subheading 3.2. below.

2.2.2. VINYL SULFONES

Like a α', β'-epoxyketone functionality, a Michael acceptor vinyl sulfone has been exploited as a novel irreversible proteasome inhibitor. Originally, peptide vinyl sulfones were first introduced as mechanism-based cysteine protease inhibitors by Palmer and

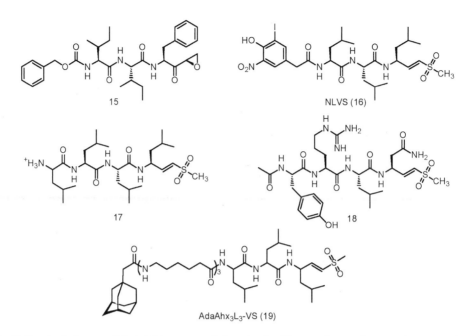

Fig. 3. Synthetic irreversible inhibitors containing vinyl sulfone and epoxyketone pharmacophores.

colleagues *(26,27)*. It was thought that the vinyl sulfones were sufficiently inert that they would act as a Michael acceptor only at the active site of cysteine proteases, where they are capable of forming hydrogen bonds with amino acid residues, thereby becoming more electrophilic and, eventually, forming a covalent bond with the active-site thiol, while being resistant to free thiols and serine proteases. Even though the vinyl sulfones are widely known as specific inhibitors of cysteine proteases, Bogyo et al. *(28,29)* have incorporated the vinyl sulfone pharmacophore into several novel proteasome inhibitors (Fig. 3). Later, the peptide vinyl sulfones were extensively used as active site-directed affinity probes to study the nature of substrate/inhibitor binding of the proteasome *(29)*. More recently, Kessler et al. *(30)* have developed a long hydrocarbon-containing peptide vinyl sulfone that labels all three active sites equally well, thereby providing an additional tool for ubiquitin–proteasome pathway studies. Nevertheless, the lack of specificity is a major concern for this class of inhibitors (Table 3), since the peptide vinyl sulfones inhibit both the proteasome and cysteine proteases.

3. NATURAL PRODUCT INHIBITORS

The synthetic inhibitors mentioned above have been rationally designed, synthesized, and optimized to improve the potency and specificity toward the proteasome, but nature has also provided selective and potent proteasome inhibitors (Table 4).

3.1. Lactacystin

Lactacystin **(20)** is a *Streptomyces lactacystinaeus* metabolite that was discovered because of its ability to induce neutrite outgrowth in the murine neuroblastoma cell line Neuro-2a *(31,32)*. Subsequently, others showed that lactacystin also inhibited cell cycle progression *(33,34)*. The biologic activity and unique structure promptly drew attention

Table 3
Synthetic Irreversible Inhibitors: Vinyl Sulfones and Epoxyketones

Compound	$(k_{obs}/[I])$ (M/s)			In vivo activity	Crossreactivity	Ref.
	CT-L	T-L	PGPH			
NLVS (16)	5000	3.4	4.0	8 μM^a	Cathepsin S and B	29
H₂N-LLLL-VS (17)	240	1500	29	ND	ND	29
Ac-PRLN-VS	No inhibition	2149	No inhibition	ND	ND	60
Ac-YRLN-VS (18)	No inhibition	1530	No inhibition	ND	ND	60
AdaAhx₃L₃VS (19)	8200	700	1024	ND	ND	30
YU101 (33)	166,000	7.1	21	0.25 μM^a	ND	45
YU102 (37)	5	No inhibition	254	ND	ND	57

For abbreviations, see Table 1 footnote.
^{a}80% growth inhibition of EL4 cells.

55

Table 4
Natural Product Inhibitors

Compound	$(k_{obs}/[I]$ (M/s) CT-L	T-L	PGPH	In vivo activity	Crossreactivity	Ref.
Lactacystin (20)	1500	110	17	$4\ \mu M^a$	Cathepsin A, TPPII	29
Clasto-lactacystin β-lactone (21)	7400	68	47	ND	Cathepsin A, TPPII	45
Epoxomicin (22)	20,000	300	40	$0.03\ \mu M^a$	None found	57
Dihydroeponemycin	114	17	217	$2\ \mu M^b$	Cathepsin (weak)	47, 57
TMC-95A/B (28)	$IC_{50} = 5.4\ nM$	$IC_{50} = 200\ nM$	$IC_{50} = 60\ nM$	ND	No calpain, no cathepsin L, and no trypsin	50
Gliotoxin (29)	72% inhibition at 40 μM	39% inhibition at 40 μM	6% inhibition at 40 μM	ND	At 100 μM, 12% chymotrypsin, 20% calpain, no trypsin inhibition: also FTase inhibitor ($IC_{50} = 1.1\ \mu M$)	55
Phepropeptin B (32)	$IC_{50} = 11\ \mu g/mL$	No inhibition	$IC_{50} > 100\ \mu g/mL$	ND	No chymotrypsin	53
EGCG (31)	$IC_{50} = 86\ nM$	No inhibition at 10 μM	Comparable to CT-L inhibition	ND	No calpain No caspase-3 inhibition	56

For abbreviations, see Table 1 footnote.
[a] 80% growth inhibition of EL4 cells.
[b] Antiproliferative activity against EL4 cells.

56

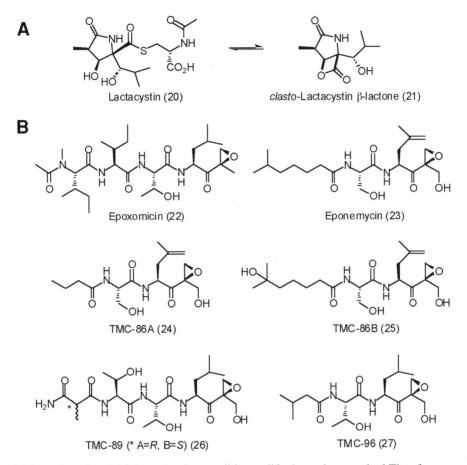

Fig. 4. Natural product inhibitors that irreversibly modify the amino terminal Thr of proteasome β–subunits.

to many elegant syntheses of lactacystin over the years *(35)*. Meanwhile, mode-of-action studies by Schreiber et al. revealed that lactacystin targets the 20S proteasome by a covalent modification of the amino-terminal threonine of β-subunits *(36)*. Researchers also showed that the active component of lactacystin is the *clasto*-lactacystin β-lactone (Fig. 4A), which is a rearrangement product of lactacystin in the aqueous condition *(37,38)*. Despite initial reports of high proteasome specificity and wide use in biologic studies, there have been reports that lactacystin also inhibits other cellular proteases *(39,40)*. Although lactacystin remains one of most used proteasome inhibitors in many biologic studies, partly because of the relatively specific inhibition of the proteasome over peptide aldehyde inhibitors, the development of lactacystin-based therapeutic agents has been hampered by its complex synthesis.

3.2. Epoxomicin (22) and the Family of Peptide Epoxyketone Natural Products

In a search for antitumor agents displaying specific activity against B16 murine melanoma, Hanada et al. *(41)* isolated peptidyl epoxyketone epoxomicin **(22)** from an unidentified actinomycete strain, Q996-17. Recently, Crews and colleagues reported its first total synthesis *(42)* and showed that epoxomicin targets the 20S proteasome *(43)*. More-

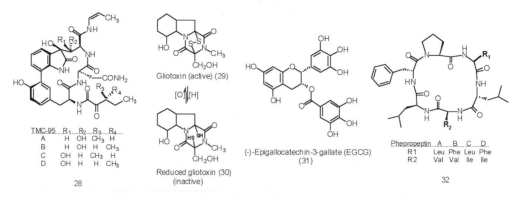

Fig. 5. Natural product inhibitors with unusual structures.

over, unlike other classes of proteasome inhibitors that show nontarget specificity, epoxomicin was shown to be highly specific for the 20S proteasome. The crystal structure of the yeast 20S proteasome complexed with epoxomicin revealed that the unique specificity of epoxomicin is partly because of to the formation of an unusual six-membered morpholino ring between the amino-terminal catalytic Thr-1 of the 20S proteasome and the a', b'-epoxyketone pharmacophore of epoxomicin *(44)*. Developed during the course of the total synthesis of epoxomicin, the facile synthetic strategy of linear peptide a', b'-epoxyketones has also prompted the development of more potent peptide a', b'-epoxyketones, such as YU101 *(45)*. Epoxomicin is a member of a growing family of linear peptide a', b'-epoxyketone natural products. Another example includes eponemycin **(23)**, an anti-angiogenic linear peptide a',b'-epoxyketone isolated from *Streptomyces hygroscopicus* P247-271 on the basis of its activity against B16 melanoma *(46)*. Eponemycin has been shown to target the 20S proteasome as well *(47)*. More recently, other linear peptide a', b'-epoxyketone natural products have been isolated on the basis of proteasome inhibition screening from microbial metabolites *(48,49)*.

3.3. Macrocyclic Compounds

Although lactacystin and epoxomicin are the best known natural product proteasome inhibitors, other natural products with novel structures have been isolated directly in the course of proteasome inhibitor screening procedures (Fig. 5). For example, a series of TMC-95s **(28)** were isolated from the fermentation broth of *Apiospora montagnei Sacc.* TC 1093 *(50,51)*, based on their proteasome-inhibition activities. Despite their unusual macrocyclic features, they possess potent inhibitory activity toward the CT-L activity of the 20S proteasome. Even so, they do not inhibit other proteases like m-calpain, cathepsin L, and trypsin. The crystal structure analysis of the yeast 20S proteasome:TMC-95 complex revealed that multiple hydrogen-bond networks between the main-chain atoms of the proteasome and TMC-95 are major contributors to the high-affinity binding with the proteasome *(52)*. More recently, Sekizawa et al. *(53)* isolated cyclic hexapeptides from *Streptomyces* sp. MK600-cF7 in the course of proteasome inhibitor screening. However, compared with the TMC-95 series, cyclic hexapeptides **(32)** are shown to possess a much weaker inhibition activity.

3.4. Gliotoxin

Another interesting natural product proteasome inhibitor is gliotoxin (**30**), a member of the fungal epipolythiodioxopiperazine toxins that are characterized by a heterocyclic core containing a disulfide bridge(s). In the mid-1990s, gliotoxin was shown to be a potent inhibitor of nuclear factor-κB (NF-κB) activation in T- and B-cells *(54)*. Recently, Kroll and colleagues showed that gliotoxin noncompetitively targets the CT-L activity of the 20S proteasome and that the disulfide bridge is essential for its inhibitory action, showing loss of activity by the reduced gliotoxin *(55)*.

3.5. Polyphenols

It has been known that green tea has strong cancer-preventive properties, and the major components of green tea are polyphenols. Recently, epigallocatechin-3-gallate (EGCG) (**31**) was shown to be a potent inhibitor toward the CT-L activity of the 20S proteasome *(56)*. Based on the limited atomic orbital analysis, structure-activity relationship studies, and high-performance liquid chromatography analysis of reaction products with the purified proteasome, it appears that the ester linkage between epigallocatechin and the gallate moiety is vital for the proteasome inhibition, thus suggesting a nucleophilic attack on the ester bond by the N-terminal Thr of proteasome. Given their unique polyphenol structures, it will be interesting to see how they bind to the active site of the 20S proteasome.

4. NEW GENERATIONS OF PROTEASOME INHIBITORS

The emergence of the ubiquitin–proteasome pathway as a potential therapeutic target for the treatment of several physiologic disorders has prompted many synthetic efforts. As a result, these efforts have yielded many peptide backbone-based cell-permeable proteasome-specific inhibitors, best exemplified by bortezomib. Meanwhile, proteasome-inhibition-driven systematic natural product screening has also offered a number of novel proteasome inhibitors with unusual structures, such as the TMC-95 series (Fig. 5). However, most of the natural product screening and synthetic efforts have been using the CT-L activity-driven assay system and, hence, most of the compounds described above are the CT-L activity-directed compounds (Fig. 6). Although CT-L activity inhibitors have been shown to be largely responsible for the proteolytic function of the proteasome in vivo and in vitro *(57)*, the role of other activities remains to be determined, mostly because of the lack of proper molecular probes. Therefore, a new generation of compounds that specifically inhibit the PGPH or T-L activities may be required to explore the function of individual subunits and to gain insights into the possibility for potential therapeutic intervention.

To date, few attempts have been made to develop such inhibitors. For example, Loidl et al. *(58,59)* developed bivalent (**34**) and bifunctional (**35**) T-L activity-specific aldehyde inhibitors using structure-based design. Bogyo and Nazif *(60)* also developed T-L activity-specific vinyl sulfone inhibitors by using a positional scanning strategy. Meanwhile, our lab has recently developed a series of PGPH-specific peptide α', β'-epoxyketones by optimizing the amino acids at the P1–P4 positions *(57)*. Moreover, we

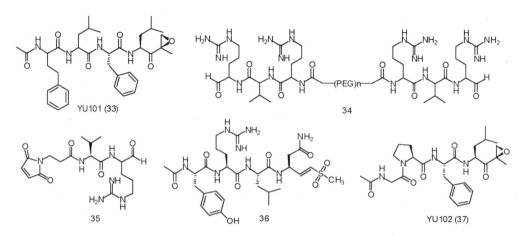

Fig. 6. Synthetic inhibitors that target specific activities of proteasome.

have successfully applied these compounds in cell-based protein degradation assays in living cells to probe the role of different catalytic subunits, revealing that selective PGPH inhibition was not sufficient to inhibit total protein degradation. However, it remains to be determined whether they can be developed into potential therapeutic agents, largely because of the unknown physiologic importance of the PGPH or T-L activities.

5. CONCLUSIONS

A better understanding of the ubiquitin–proteasome pathway and its role in many critical cellular processes has accelerated the development of proteasome inhibitors, yielding a boronate inhibitor and a lactacystin-derived inhibitor, both of which are currently in clinical trials. At the same time, new natural product screens for proteasome inhibitors are generating novel inhibitors with unusual backbones. These new inhibitors will undoubtedly provide valuable tools for the exploration of inhibitor proteasome interactions as well as aid in the design of proteasome inhibitors with novel structures. However, to achieve more specificity and thus increase the safety of therapeutic agents targeting the ubiquitin–proteasome pathway, the intervention of upstream proteasome degradation is desirable, i.e., ubiquitination by E3 ligase. Although such reagents are not yet available, the growing interest in and information about the ubiquitin-proteasome pathway may aid the design of potential therapeutic agents targeting the ubiquitin process.

ACKNOWLEDGMENT

The authors gratefully acknowledge support from the NIH (RO1-GM62120).

REFERENCES

1. Schwartz AL, et al. The ubiquitin-proteasome pathway and pathogenesis of human diseases. *Annu Rev Med* 1999;50:57–74.
2. Lee DH, et al. Proteasome inhibitors: valuable new tools for cell biologists. *Trends Cell Biol* 1998;8:397–403.
3. Myung J, et al. The ubiquitin-proteasome pathway and proteasome inhibitors. *Med Res Rev* 2001;21:245–273.
4. Kisselev AF, et al. Proteasome inhibitors: from research tools to drug candidates. *Chem Biol* 2001;8:739–758.

5. Cardozo C. Catalytic components of the bovine pituitary multicatalytic proteinase complex (proteasome). *Enzyme Protein* 1993;47:296–305.
6. Orlowski M. The multicatalytic proteinase complex (proteasome) and intracellular protein degradation: diverse functions of an intracellular particle. *J Lab Clin Med* 1993;121:187–189.
7. Wilk S, et al. Evidence that pituitary cation-sensitive neutral endopeptidase is a multicatalytic protease complex. *J Neurochem* 1983;40:842–849.
8. Figueiredo-Pereira ME, et al. A new inhibitor of the chymotrypsin-like activity of the multicatalytic proteinase complex (20S proteasome) induces accumulation of ubiquitin-protein conjugates in a neuronal cell. *J Neurochem* 1994;63:1578–1581.
9. Orlowski M. The multicatalytic proteinase complex, a major extralysosomal proteolytic system. *Biochemistry* 1990;29:10289–10297.
10. Groll M, et al. Structure of 20S proteasome from yeast at 2.4 Å resolution. *Nature* 1997;386:463–471.
11. Löwe J, et al. Crystal structure of the 20S proteasome from the archaeon *T. acidophilum* at 3.4 Å resolution. *Science* 1995;268:533–539.
12. Rock KL, et al. Inhibitors of the proteasome block the degradation of most cell proteins and the generation of peptides presented on MHC class I molecules. *Cell* 1994;78:761–771.
13. Wilk S, et al. Synthetic inhibitors of the multicatalytic proteinase complex (proteasome). *Enzyme Protein* 1993;47:306–313.
14. Vinitsky A, et al. Inhibition of the proteolytic activity of the multicatalytic proteinase complex (proteasome) by substrate-related peptidyl aldehydes. *J Biol Chem* 1994;269:29860–29866.
15. Lynas JF, et al. Inhibitors of the chymotrypsin-like activity of proteasome based on di- and tri-peptidyl alpha-keto aldehydes (glyoxals). *Bioorg Med Chem Lett* 1998;8:373–378.
16. Lum RT, et al. Selective inhibition of the chymotrypsin-like activity of the 20S proteasome by 5-methoxy-1-indanone dipeptide benzamides. *Bioorg Med Chem Lett* 1998;8:209–214.
17. Lum RT, et al. A new structural class of proteasome inhibitors that prevent NF-kappa B activation. *Biochem Pharmacol* 1998;55:1391–1397.
18. Iqbal M, et al. Potent inhibitors of proteasome. *J Med Chem* 1995;38:2276–2277.
19. Iqbal M, et al. Potent α-ketocarbonyl and boronic ester derived inhibitors of proteasome. *Bioorg Med Chem Lett* 1996;6:287–290.
20. Chatterjee S et al. P'-extended alpha-ketoamide inhibitors of proteasome. *Bioorg Med Chem Lett* 1999;9:2603–2606.
21. Fevig JM, et al. Rational design of boropeptide thrombin inhibitors: beta, beta-dialkyl-phenethylglycine P2 analogs of DuP 714 with greater selectivity over complement factor I and an improved safety profile. *Bioorg Med Chem Lett* 1998;8:301–306.
22. Adams J, et al. Potent and selective inhibitors of the proteasome: dipeptidyl boronic acids. *Bioorg Med Chem Lett* 1998;8:333–338.
23. Adams J. Development of the proteasome inhibitor PS-341. *Oncologist* 2002;7:9–16.
24. Adams J, et al. Proteasome inhibitors: a novel class of potent and effective antitumor agents. *Cancer Res* 1999;59:2615–2622.
25. Spaltenstein A, et al. Design and synthesis of novel protease inhibitors. Tripeptide α',β'-epoxyketones as nanomolar inactivators of the proteasome. *Tet Lett* 1996;37:1343–1346.
26. Bromme D, et al. Peptidyl vinyl sulphones: a new class of potent and selective cysteine protease inhibitors: S2P2 specificity of human cathepsin O2 in comparison with cathepsins S and L. *Biochem J* 1996;315:85–89.
27. Palmer JT, et al. Vinyl sulfones as mechanism-based cysteine protease inhibitors. *J Med Chem* 1995;38:3193–3196.
28. Bogyo M, et al. Covalent modification of the active site threonine of proteasomal beta subunits and the *Escherichia coli* homolog HslV by a new class of inhibitors. *Proc Natl Acad Sci USA* 1997;94:6629–6634.
29. Bogyo M, et al. Substrate binding and sequence preference of the proteasome revealed by active-site-directed affinity probes. *Chem Biol* 1998;5:307–320.
30. Kessler BM, et al. Extended peptide-based inhibitors efficiently target the proteasome and reveal overlapping specificities of the catalytic beta-subunits. *Chem Biol* 2001;8:913–929.
31. Omura S, et al. Lactacystin, a novel microbial metabolite, induces neuritogenesis of neuroblastoma cells [letter]. *J Antibiot (Tokyo)* 1991;44:113–116.
32. Omura S, et al. Structure of lactacystin, a new microbial metabolite which induces differentiation of neuroblastoma cells [Letter]. *J Antibiot (Tokyo)* 1991;44:117–118.

33. Fenteany G, et al. A beta-lactone related to lactacystin induces neurite outgrowth in a neuroblastoma cell line and inhibits cell cycle progression in an osteosarcoma cell line. *Proc Natl Acad Sci USA* 1994;91:3358–3362.

34. Katagiri M, et al. The neuritogenesis inducer lactacystin arrests cell cycle at both G0/G1 and G2 phases in neuro 2a cells [Letter]. *J Antibiot (Tokyo)* 1995;48:344–346.

35. Corey EJ, et al. Total synthesis and biological activity of lactacystin, omuralide and analogs. *Chem Pharm Bull* 1999;47:1–10.

36. Fenteany G, et al. Inhibition of proteasome activities and subunit-specific amino-terminal threonine modification by lactacystin. *Science* 1995;268:726–731.

37. Dick LR, et al. Mechanistic studies on the inactivation of the proteasome by lactacystin: a central role for clasto-lactacystin beta-lactone. *J Biol Chem* 1996;271:7273–7276.

38. Dick LR, et al. Mechanistic studies on the inactivation of the proteasome by lactacystin in cultured cells. *J Biol Chem* 1997;272:182–188.

39. Ostrowska H, et al. Lactacystin, a specific inhibitor of the proteasome, inhibits human platelet lysosomal cathepsin A-like enzyme. *Biochem Biophys Res Commun* 1997;234:729–732.

40. Ostrowska H, et al. Separation of cathepsin A-like enzyme and the proteasome: evidence that lactacystin/ beta-lactone is not a specific inhibitor of the proteasome. *Int J Biochem Cell Biol* 2000;32:747–757.

41. Hanada M, et al. Epoxomicin, a new antitumor agent of microbial origin. *J Antibiot* 1992;45:1746–1752.

42. Sin N, et al. Total synthesis of the potent proteasome inhibitor epoxomicin: a useful tool for understanding proteasome biology. *Bioorg Med Chem Lett* 1999;9:2283–2288.

43. Meng L, et al. Epoxomicin, a potent and selective proteasome inhibitor, exhibits in vivo anti-inflammatory activity. *Proc Natl Acad Sci USA* 1999;96:10403–10408.

44. Groll M, et al. Crystal structure of epoxomicin:20S proteasome reveals molecular basis for selectivity of α',β'-epoxyketone proteasome inhibitors. *J Am Chem Soc* 2000;122:1237–1238.

45. Elofsson M, et al. Towards subunit specific proteasome inhibitors: synthesis and evaluation of peptide α',β'-epoxyketones. *Chem Biol* 1999;6:811–822.

46. Sugawara K et al. Eponemycin, a new antibiotic active against B16 melanoma. I. Production, isolation, structure and biological activity. *J Antibiot* 1990;43:8–18.

47. Meng L, et al. Eponemycin exerts its antitumor effect through inhibition of proteasome function. *Cancer Res* 1999;59:2798–2801.

48. Koguchi Y, et al. TMC-89A and B, new proteasome inhibitors from *Streptomyces* sp. TC 1087. *J Antibiot (Tokyo)* 2000;53:967–972.

49. Koguchi Y, et al. TMC-86A, B and TMC-96, new proteasome inhibitors from *Streptomyces* sp. TC 1084 and *Saccharothrix* sp. TC 1094. II. Physico-chemical properties and structure determination. *J Antibiot (Tokyo)* 2000;53:63–65.

50. Koguchi Y, et al. TMC-95A, B, C, and D, novel proteasome inhibitors produced by *Apiospora montagnei Sacc.* TC 1093. Taxonomy, production, isolation, and biological activities. *J Antibiot (Tokyo)* 2000;53:105–109.

51. Kohno J, et al. Structures of TMC-95A-D: novel proteasome inhibitors from *Apiospora montagnei sacc.* TC 1093. *J Org Chem* 2000;65:990–995.

52. Groll M, Koguchi Y, Huber R, Kohno J. Crystal structure of the 20 S proteasome:TMC-95A complex: a non-covalent proteasome inhibitor. *J Mol Biol* 2001;311:543–548.

53. Sekizawa R, et al. Isolation and structural determination of phepropeptins A, B, C, and D, new proteasome inhibitors, produced by *Streptomyces* sp. *J Antibiot (Tokyo)* 2001;54:874–881.

54. Pahl HL, et al. The immunosuppressive fungal metabolite gliotoxin specifically inhibits transcription factor NF-kappaB. *J Exp Med* 1996;183:1829–1840.

55. Kroll M, et al. The secondary fungal metabolite gliotoxin targets proteolytic activities of the proteasome. *Chem Biol* 1999;6:689–698.

56. Nam S, et al. Ester bond-containing tea polyphenols potently inhibit proteasome activity in vitro and in vivo. *J Biol Chem* 2001;276:13322–13330.

57. Myung J, et al. Lack of proteasome active site allostery as revealed by subunit-specific inhibitors. *Mol Cell* 2001;7:411–420.

58. Loidl G, et al. Bivalency as a principle for proteasome inhibition. *Proc Natl Acad Sci USA* 1999;96:5418–5422.

59. Loidl G, et al. Bifunctional inhibitors of the trypsin-like activity of eukaryotic proteasomes. *Chem Biol* 1999;6:197–204.

60. Nazif T, et al. Global analysis of proteasomal substrate specificity using positional- scanning libraries of covalent inhibitors. *Proc Natl Acad Sci USA* 2001;98:2967–2972.

61. Harding CV, et al. Novel dipeptide aldehydes are proteasome inhibitors and block the MHC-I antigen-processing pathway. *J Immunol* 1995;155:1767–1775.

5 Other Proteasome Inhibitors

Carlos García-Echeverría

ABSTRACT

The involvement of the 20S proteasome in the degradation of critical intracellular regulatory proteins has suggested the potential use of proteasome inhibitors as novel therapeutic agents being applicable in many different disease indications. Early synthetic inhibitors of the 20S proeteasome were relatively nonspecific compounds but proved to be invaluable probes for improving our understanding of the ubiquitin/proteasome-dependent degradation pathway in vitro. New classes of inhibitors that target this proteolytic enzyme have emerged in the last few years by combining traditional drug discovery approaches with new methods to find and optimize lead structures. This chapter reviews recent salient medicinal chemistry achievements in the design, synthesis, and biologic characterization of a variety of inhibitors of the 20S proteasome. These compounds are capable of modulating the subunit-specific proteolytic activities of the 20S proteosome in ways not previously possible. Examples have been selected to illustrate the impact of structural-based design and natural product screening in this area of research.

KEY WORDS

Antitumor agents; structure-based design; enzyme inhibitors; peptidomimetics; boronic acids; proteolytic enzymes; aldehydes; a-ketoaldehydes; a-ketoamides; vinyl sulfones; non-covalent inhibitors; bifunctional; epoxyketone; HIV-1; drug discovery; ubiquitin; targeted therapy

From: *Cancer Drug Discovery and Development: Proteasome Inhibitors in Cancer Therapy*
Edited by: J. Adams © Humana Press Inc., Totowa, NJ

1. INTRODUCTION

Synthetic proteasome inhibitors have become valuable molecular probes for improving our understanding of biologic processes associated with the proteasome–ubiquitin pathway. These tool compounds are capable of modulating the subunit-specific proteolytic activities of the proteasome in ways not previously possible. Nonetheless, the transition from research tools to drug candidates has proved rather difficult. Most of the potent and selective synthetic proteasome inhibitors reported until now are peptide-like molecules (for recent reviews, see refs. *1–3*). Although peptides can display a diverse range of biologic properties both in vitro and in vivo, their use as drugs is compromised by proteolytic degradation, poor pharmacologic profiles, and low oral bioavailability. To overcome these problems, structure-based design efforts have been focused on reducing the size and peptide character of 20S proteasome inhibitors. However, this approach has met with limited success. Interestingly, only one 20S proteasome inhibitor—a peptide boronate, bortezomib (Velcade; formerly known as PS-341)—is currently in clinical trials against various cancers *(4,5)*. This chapter highlights key medicinal chemistry achievements in the design and synthesis of peptide-based 20S proteasome inhibitors containing diverse pharmacophores. The limits and potentials of other proteasome inhibitors not covered in previous chapters are also discussed here.

2. PEPTIDE ALDEHYDES, GLYOXALS, AND α-KETOAMIDES

Peptide aldehydes were one of the first class of proteasome inhibitors to be reported and have been widely used as tool compounds (e.g., MG132, Z-Leu-Leu-Leu-CHO) to study the role of proteasome in a variety of cellular processes. One of the major problems encountered with this class of derivatives was selectivity, and considerable effort had to be expended in overcoming this hurdle *(6–14)*. One representative example of this medicinal chemistry effort is CEP-1612 (see **1** in Fig. 1). This compound is a potent and reversible inhibitor of the chymotrypsin-like activity of the 20S proteasome median inhibitory concentration [IC_{50}] = 2 nM and does not block the trypsin-like activity of this enzyme at concentrations up to 1 μM *(10)*. Inhibition of calpain I and cathepsin B requires at least 45-fold higher concentrations. CEP-1612 induces apoptosis in a panel of human tumor cell lines. Apoptosis is p53-independent and is associated with accumulation of the cyclin-dependent kinase inhibitors p21 and p27 *(15)*.

Aldehyde head groups have also been used in bifunctional *(16)* and bivalent compounds *(17,18)* to develop subunit-specific inhibitors. Bifunctional peptides contain a maleimido moiety to react with the side chain of cysteine-118 in the S3 binding pocket of the trypsin-like active site and a *C*-terminal aldehyde group for hemiacetal formation with the catalytic threonine residue. These bifunctional derivatives are selective inhibitors of the trypsin-like activity of the yeast proteasome (*see* **2**, in Fig. 1; IC_{50} = 0.5 mM for trypsin-like activity; IC_{50} > 100 μM for chymotrypsin-like and peptidylglutamyl-peptide hydrolyzing ([PGPH] activities) *(16)*. High potency against the same subunit was also obtained by linking the N-terminus of two peptide aldehydes with a polyoxyethylene spacer that is appropiate for simultaneous binding at two active sites (*see* **3** in Fig. 1) *(17,18)*. The bivalent inhibitor is two orders of magitude more potent than the parent peptide aldehyde ($IC_{50}^{trypsin-like}$ = 0.071 μM for **3** vs $IC_{50}^{trypsin-like}$ = 6.4 μM for Ac-Arg-Val-Arg-CHO). Although these two approaches are good examples of structure-based

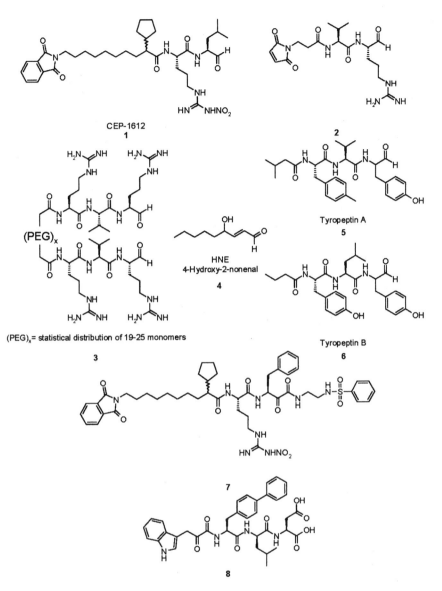

Fig. 1. Peptide aldehydes, glyoxals, and α-ketoamides.

design and provide subunit-specific inhibitors, the reactivity of the maleimido group toward thiols and the high molecular weight of the bivalent inhibitors might limit the utility of these compounds to only cell-free systems.

In addition to synthetic peptide aldehydes, non-peptidic and natural compounds containing this moiety have been shown to inhibit proteasome activity. 4-Hydroxy-2-nonenal (HNE; *see* **4** in Fig. 1) is a major end product of lipid peroxidation that can decrease the trypsin-like and PGPH activities of proteasome *(19,20)*. The mechanism of inactivation of the proteasome by HNE remains unclear, but this compound can react with the side chains of histidine, cysteine, and lysine residues, forming Michael addition-type products (histidine and cysteine) or pyrroles (lysine). Tyropeptins A and B (**5** and **6**, respec-

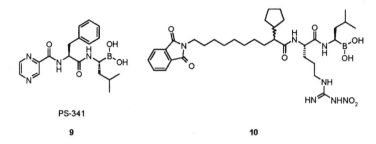

PS-341

9   **10**

Fig. 2. Peptide boronic acids.

tively; *see* Fig. 1), which were isolated from the culture broth of *Kitasatospora* sp. MK993-dF2 *(21,22)*, inhibit the chymotrypsin-like activity and trypsin-like activities of the 20S proteasome with IC_{50} values of 0.1/1.5 and 0.2/4.0 µg/mL, respectively, whereas no inhibition of the PGPH activity is observed at a concentration of 100 µg/mL. α-Chymotrypsin, cathepsin L, and m-calpain are also inhibited by these natural peptides ($IC_{50} \leq 1.0$ mg/mL).

Additional modifications of the carbonyl head group have been reported by different groups. Di- and tripeptide glyoxals (α-ketoaldehydes) were synthesized as putative inhibitors of the chymotryptic-like activity of proteasome, e.g., Cbz-Leu-Leu-Tyr-COCHO ($K_i = 3.1$ n*M*) and Bz-Leu-Leu-Leu-COCHO ($K_i = 3.7$ n*M*) *(23)*. Compound **7** (*see* Fig. 1), which is an analog of CEP-1612 (compound **1**) *(10)*, was identified as the most potent chymotrypsin-like activity inhibitor ($K_i = 1.1$ n*M*) of a series of P'-extended α-keto amide derivatives. This inhibitor was found to be >150-fold less active against calpain 1 and the trypsin-like activity of the proteasome *(24)*.

The α-ketoamide moiety has also been introduced at the N-terminus of peptides. For example, compound **8** (Fig. 1) inhibited in vitro the 20S proteasome with an IC_{50} value of 1 µg/mL *(25)*.

3. PEPTIDE BORONIC ACIDS

Another class of peptide-based inhibitors exploits a boronic-based electrophile at the *C*-terminus. It is presumed that the boron atom forms a reversible tetrahedral adduct with the side chain of the active-site threonine residue. The most well-characterized compound of this class is bortezomib (*see* **9** in Fig. 2) *(26–28)*, which is extensively covered in previous chapters. Besides this compound and its analogs, not many other peptide boronates have been described. In some examples, the *C*-terminal aldehyde moiety has been replaced with the boronic acid functional group. This is the case for **10** (*see* Fig. 2), which exploits the structure of the previously described CEP-1612 (*see* **1** in Fig. 1) *(10)*. Compound **10** significantly inhibits B16 tumor growth in female C57BL mice after ip administration (10 mg/kg/d) *(29)*.

4. PEPTIDE VINYL SULFONES

Peptide vinyl sulfones, which were originally designed to target cysteine proteases *(30)*, inhibit covalently the three hydrolytic activities of the proteasome *(31)*. Although not confirmed yet by structural data, the hydroxyl group of the catalytic threonine residue may react with the double bond of the vinyl sulfone, forming an irreversible covalent

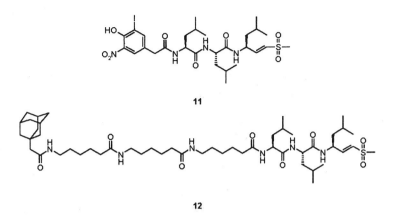

Fig. 3. Peptide vinyl sulfones.

adduct. Tri- and tetrapeptide vinyl sulfones (*see* **11** in Fig. 3; chymotrypsin-like activity, $IC_{50} = 0.1–0.5$ μ*M*; trypsin-like activity, $IC_{50} = 50–100$ μ*M*; and PGPH activity, $IC_{50} = 50–100$ μ*M*) were originally used to study substrate binding and specificity of the proteasome *(32)*. In this approach, some of these compounds were labeled with ^{125}I to trace binding to individual subunits by two-dimensional gels. A more detailed analysis of proteasomal substrate specificity was performed using an acetyl-capped tetrapeptide vinyl sulfone library and positional–scanning libraries in which tripeptide vinyl sulfones were varied through the P2 and P3 positions *(33)*. The resulting specificity profiles indicated that the P2–P4 substrate positions are critical for directing substrates to individual subunits of the proteasome. Cell-permeable peptide vinyl sulfones with proteasome inhibitory activity have been obtained by incorporating a number of aminohexanoic acid spacers into the (leucinyl)$_3$-vinyl-(methyl)-sulfone core and subsequent N-terminal capping (*see* **12** in Fig. 3) *(34)*.

5. 2-AMINOBENZYLSTATINE DERIVATIVES

A series of peptidomimetics containing the 2-aminobenzylstatine core structure *(35–37)* was identified by high-throughput screening to have in vitro inhibitory activity against the human 20S proteasome *(38)*. A representative example of this class of non-covalent 20S proteasome inhibitors is compound **13** (Fig. 4), which was originally synthesized to target the HIV-1 protease *(36)*. This compound inhibits the chymotrypsin-like activity of the 20S proteasome with an IC_{50} value of 0.9 μ*M* and shows selectivity over the trypsin-like and PGPH activities ($IC_{50} > 20$ μ*M*) *(38)*. Using the crystal structure of the yeast proteasome *(39,40)*, a structural model of compound **13** bound to the chymotrypsin-like activity site of the human 20S proteasome was developed to understand the structural basis of its inhibitory activity and to guide the medicinal chemistry optimization process *(41)*.

A large number of complementary hydrophobic and hydrogen bond interactions between the inhibitor and the S1/S3 pockets of the enzyme are observed in this model (Fig. 5). These interactions could account for the ability of this class of compounds to inhibit the chymotrypsin-like activity site of the human 20S proteasome without forming a covalent bond with the catalytic threonine residue. A structure-based optimization approach in conjunction with a modular chemistry strategy was used to improve the

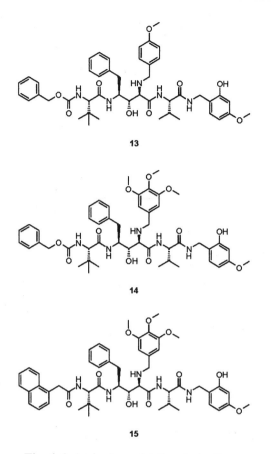

Fig. 4. 2-Aminobenzylstatine derivatives.

proteasome chymotrypsin-like inhibitory activity of compound **13**. A major increase in potency was obtained by targeting the S3 pocket. According to the model, the benzylamino group of the statine moiety is involved in two hydrogen bond interactions with Asp-153 and Ser-151 (Fig. 5). Examination of the model suggested that two other residues of the S3 pocket, Ser 157 and Tyr 135, could be targeted for additional hydrogen bond interactions (Fig. 6). Consistent with this hypothesis, a substantial increase in potency was observed with compound **14** (*see* Fig. 4; IC$_{50}$ = 0.05 μ*M*, chymotrypsin-like activity), which can form the targeted hydrogen bond interactions with the preceding residues *(42)*. Parallel to this effort, the possibility of enhancing potency by creating additional van der Waals interactions was explored by modifying the N-terminus of the inhibitor. The replacement of the benzyloxycarbonyl group by naphthalen-1-yl-acetic acid (*see* **15** in Fig. 4) improved sevenfold the potency of **14** (IC$_{50}$ = 0.007 μ*M* for **15** vs IC$_{50}$ = 0.05 μ*M* for **14**) *(42)*. This N-terminal change was designed to increase the strength of the interactions of the *N*-terminal group with a small cavity near the S3 pocket *(41)*. The modifications introduced in compound **13** did not affect the specificity profile of this class of inhibitors. Compound **15**, which is one of the most potent non-covalent inhibitors of the human 20S proteasome described to date, has a modest activity against the trypsin-like and PGPH activities of the 20S proteasome (IC$_{50}$ > 20 μ*M*).

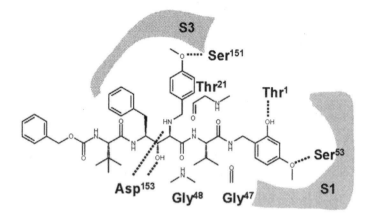

Fig. 5. Representation of the predicted hydrogen-bond interactions of compound 13 with the chymotrypsin-like active site of the human 20S proteasome.

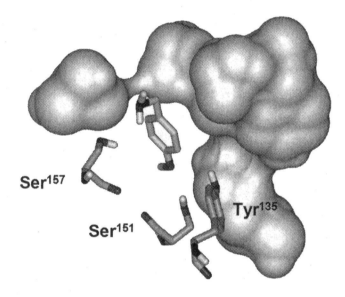

Fig. 6. The benzylamino group of the statine moiety embedded in the S3 pocket of the chymotrypsin-like site of the human 20S proteasome.

6. 5-METHOXY-1-INDANONE DIPEPTIDE BENZAMIDES

The 5-methoxy-1-indanone moiety was explored as an alternative to the traditional electrophilic *head groups* used to target the chymotrypsin-like activity of the 20S proteasome *(43)*. The most potent compounds identified by screening peptide libraries containing this new head group were **16** (CVT-659; Fig. 7) and **17** (Fig. 7). These compounds are selective for the chymotrypsin-like activity of the 20S proteasome (IC$_{50}$ = 0.14 and 0.20 μM for **16** and **17**, respectively), but only **16** displayed antiproliferative activity (IC$_{50}$ = 8 μM) against RAW cells (murine macrophage cell line). In addition to inducing tumor cell growth arrest, this class of derivatives has also been shown to inhibit

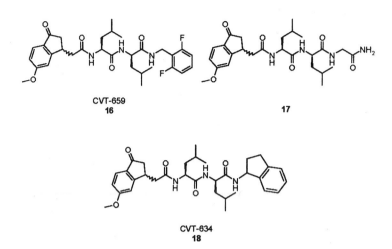

Fig. 7. 5-Methoxy-1-indanone dipeptide benzamides.

nuclear factor-κB (NF-κB) activation. Thus, **18** (CVT-634; Fig. 7) prevented activation of NF-κB *in vitro* and lipopolysaccharide-induced tumor necrosis factor synthesis in RAW cells (IC_{50} = 7 mg/mL) *(44)*. Serum tumor necrosis factor levels were significantly lower in female Swiss Webster mice pretreated with **18**, (ip) than in those mice that were treated only with lipopolysaccharide.

7. DRUGS THAT CAN MODULATE PROTEASOME ACTIVITIY

Several drugs have been reported to inhibit proteasome activitiy in different assays. The in vitro potency of these compounds is in general modest, and one can expect that these drugs do not have any effect on proteasome activity in vivo at the concentrations attained in the fluids of treated patients.

In addition to its HIV-1 antiviral activity, ritonavir (*see* **19** in Fig. 8) inhibits in vitro the chymotrypsin-like activity of the 20S proteasome and causes an increase in ubiquitin conjugates in murine B-cells when the compound is added at 100 μ*M (45,46)*. Apart from ritonavir, saquinavir also inhibits the chymotrypsin-like activity of the 20S proteasome, although much less efficiently. Under identical experimental conditions, indinavir and nelfinavir do not inhibit proteasome activity *(46)*. (For an additional example of an HIV-1 inhibitor that blocks 20s proteaseome activity, *see* Subheading 5.)

The prodrug (β-lactone ring) form of the hydroxymethyl-glutaryl (HMG)-coenzyme A reductase inhibitor lovastatin (*see* **20** in Fig. 8) *(47)* inhibits proteasome activity in cell extracts in a dose-dependent manner with half-maximal inhibition occurring at 40 μ*M (48)*. Treatment of MDA-MB-157 cells with the lactonized prodrug resulted in inhibition of cell proliferation as well as a pronounced induction and increased half-life of p21 and p27 (0.13 vs 1.5 h for both p21 and p27). The proteasome inhibitory activity of lovastatin seems to be ascribed to the β-lactone moiety.

Modest in vitro inhibition of proteasome activity has also been reported for the DNA-intercalating agent aclacinomycin A (**21**; IC_{50} = 50 μ*M*, chymotrypsin-like activity) *(49)* and the immmunosuppressive agent cyclosporin A *(50)*. The aglycone and sugar moieties of aclacinomycin A, which was the first nonpeptidic inhibitor described showing discrete

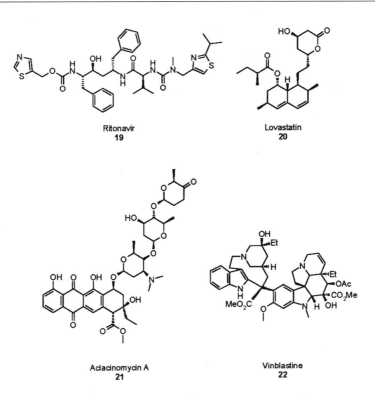

Fig. 8. Drugs that can modulate proteasome activity.

selectivity for the chymotrypsin-like activity of the 20S proteasome, are essential for inhibition.

Vinblastine (*see* **22** in Fig. 8), a *Vinca* alkaloid used as an antimitotic agent, inhibits proteasomal activity both in vitro and in vivo *(51)*. The three major peptidase activities of the 20S and 26S proteasome are reversibly inhibited by the drug at 3–110 μM, and accumulation of ubiquitin-protein conjugates (e.g., polyubiquitinated IκBα) was detected when HL60 cells were incubated for 6 h with vinblastine at 0.5–10 μM.

ACKNOWLEDGMENTS

I thank my colleagues Drs. P. Imbach, V. Guagnano, P. Furet, and M. Lang for helpful suggestions. Figures 5 and 6 were kindly provided by Dr. P. Furet.

REFERENCES

1. García-Echeverría C. Recent advances in the identification and development of 20S proteasome inhibitors. *Mini Rev Med Chem* 2002;2:247–259.
2. Myung J, et al. The ubiquitin-proteasome pathway and proteasome inhibitors. *Med Res Rev* 2001;21:245–273.
3. Kisselev AF, et al. Proteasome inhibitors: from research tools to drug candidates. *Chem Biol* 2001;8:739–758.
4. Adams J. Proteasome inhibition: a novel approach to cancer therapy. *Trends Mol Med* 2002;8:S49–S54.
5. Adams J. Proteasome inhibition in cancer: development of PS-341. *Semin Oncol* 2001;28:613–619.
6. Mundy GR, inventor; Osteoscreen Inc, assignee. Treatment of myeloma bone disease with proteasomal and NF-κB activity inhibitors. WO 0061167, 2000.
7. Anma T, et al, inventors; Takeda Chemical Industries, Ltd, assignee. Preparation of dipeptides and proteasome inhibitors. JP 11292833, 1999.

8. McCormack TA, et al. Kinetic studies of the branched chain amino acid preferring peptidase activity of the 20S proteasome: development of a continuous assay and inhibition by tripeptide aldehydes and clasto-lactacystin beta-lactone. *Biochemistry* 1998;37:7792–7800.

9. Stein RL, et al, inventors; ProScript, Inc, assignee. Preparation of peptide aldehyde derivatives as inhibitors of the 26S proteolytic complex and the 20S proteasome. US 5693617, 1997.

10. Iqbal M, et al. Potent inhibitors of proteasome. *J Med Chem* 1995;38:2276–2277.

11. Figueiredo-Pereira ME, et al. A new inhibitor of the chymotrypsin-like activity of the multicatalytic proteinase complex (20S proteasome) induces accumulation of ubiquitin-protein conjugates in a neuronal cell. *J Neurochem* 1994;63:1578–1581.

12. Figueiredo-Pereira ME, et al. Comparison of the effect of calpain inhibitors on two extralysosomal proteinases: the multicatalytic proteinase complex and m-calpain. *J Neurochem* 1994;62:1989–1994.

13. Rock KL, et al. Inhibitors of the proteasome block the degradation of most cell proteins and the generation of peptides presented on MHC class I molecules. *Cell* 1994;78:761–771.

14. Wilk S, et al. Evidence that pituitary cation-sensitive neutral endopeptidase is a multicatalytic protease complex. *J Neurochem* 1983;40:842–849.

15. An B, et al. Novel dipeptidyl proteasome inhibitors overcome Bcl-2 protective function and selectively accumulate the cyclin-dependent kinase inhibitor p27 and induce apoptosis in transformed, but not normal, human fibroblasts. *Cell Death Differ* 1998;5:1062–1075.

16. Loidl G, et al. Bifunctional inhibitors of the trypsin-like activity of eukaryotic proteasomes. *Chem Biol* 1999;6:197–204.

17. Loidl G, et al. Synthesis of bivalent inhibitors of eucaryotic proteasomes. *J Pept Sci* 2000;6:36–46.

18. Loidl G, et al. Bivalent inhibitors of the yeast proteasome. *Proc Eur Pept Symp* 1999;828–829.

19. Okada K, et al. 4-Hydroxy-2-nonenal-mediated impairment of intracellular proteolysis during oxidative stress. Identification of proteasomes as target molecules. *J Biol Chem* 1999;274:23787–23793.

20. Conconi M, et al. Proteasome inactivation upon aging and on oxidation effect of HSP 90. *Mol Biol Rep* 1997;24:45–50.

21. Momose I, et al. Tyropeptins A and B, new proteasome inhibitors produced by *Kitastospora* sp. MK993-dF2 I. Taxonomy, isolation, physico-chemical properties and biological activities. *J Antibiot 2001;*54:997–1003.

22. Momose I, et al. Tyropeptins A and B, new proteasome inhibitors produced by *Kitasatospora* sp. MK993-dF2 II. Structure determination and synthesis. *J Antibiot* 2001;54:1004–1012.

23. Lynas JF, et al. Inhibitors of the chymotrypsin-like activity of proteasome based on di- and tri-peptidyl α-keto aldehydes (glyoxals). *Bioorg Med Chem Lett* 1998;l8:373–378.

24. Chatterjee S, et al. P'-extended alpha-ketoamide inhibitors of proteasome. *Bioorg Med Chem Lett* 1999;9:2603–2606.

25. Wang L, et al, inventors; CV Therapeutics Inc, assignee. α-Ketoamide inhibitors of 20S proteasome. WO 9937666, 1999.

26. Adams J, et al. Proteasome inhibitors: a novel class of potent and effective antitumor agents. *Cancer Res* 1999;59:2615–2622.

27. Adams J, et al. Potent and selective inhibitors of the proteasome: dipeptidyl boronic acids. *Bioorg Med Chem Lett* 1998;8:333–338.

28. Adams J, et al., inventors; ProScript, Inc, assignee. Boronic ester and acid compounds, synthesis and uses. WO 9613266, 1996.

29. Siman R, et al., inventors; Cephalon Inc, assignee. Multicatalytic protease inhibitors for use as antitumor agents. WO 9930707, 1999.

30. Palmer JT. Vinyl sulfones as mechanism-based cysteine protease inhibitors. *J Med Chem* 1995;38:3193–3196.

31. Bogyo M, et al. Covalent modification of the active site threonine of proteasomal β-subunits and the *Escherichia coli* homolog HslV by a new class of inhibitors. *Proc Natl Acad Sci USA* 1997;94:6629–6634.

32. Bogyo M, et al. Substrate binding and sequence preference of the proteasome revealed by active-site-directed affinity probes. *Chem Biol* 1998;5:307–320.

33. Nazif T, et al. Global analysis of proteasomal substrate specificity using positional-scanning libraries of covalent inhibitors. *Proc Natl Acad Sci USA 2001;*98:967–2972.

34. Kessler BM, et al. Extended peptide-based inhibitors efficiently target the proteasome and reveal overlapping specificities of the catalytic β-subunits. *Chem Biol* 2001;8:913–929.

35. Lehr P, et al. Inhibitors of human immunodeficiency virus type 1 protease containing 2-aminobenzyl-substituted 4-amino-3-hydroxy-5-phenylpentanoic acid: synthesis, activity, and oral bioavailability. *J Med Chem* 1996;39:2060–2067.

36. Billich A, et al. Potent and orally bioavailable HIV-1 proteinase inhibitors containing the 2-aminobenzylstatine moiety. *Antiv Chem Chemother* 1995;6:327–336.

37. Scholz D, et al. Inhibitors of the HIV-1 proteinase containing 2-heterosubstituted-4-amino-3-hydroxy-5-phenylpentanoic acid: synthesis, enzyme inhibition, and antiviral activity. *J Med Chem* 1994;37:3079–3089.

38. García-Echeverría C, et al. A new structural class of non-covalent and selective inhibitors of the chymotrypsin-like activity of the 20S proteasome. *Bioorg Med Chem Lett* 2000;11:1317–1319.

39. Groll M, et al. Structure of 20S proteasome from yeast at 2.4 Å resolution. *Nature* 1997;386:463–471.

40. Loewe J, et al. Crystal structure of the 20S proteasome from the archaeon *T. acidophilum* at 3.4 Å resolution. *Science* 1995;268:533–539.

41. Furet P, et al. Modeling of the binding mode of a non-covalent inhibitor of the 20S proteasome. Application to structure-based analogue design. *Bioorg Med Chem Lett* 2001;11:1321–1324.

42. Furet P, et al. Structure-based optimisation of 2-aminobenzylstatine derivatives: potent and selective inhibitors of the chymotrypsin-like activity of the human 20S proteasome. *Bioorg Med Chem Lett* 2002;12:1331–1334.

43. Lum RT, et al. Selective inhibition of the chymotrypsin-like activity of the 20S proteasome by 5-methoxy-1-indanone dipeptide benzamides. *Bioorg Med Chem Lett* 1998;8:209–214.

44. Lum RT, et al. A new structural class of proteasome inhibitors that prevent NF-κB activation. *Biochem Pharmacol* 1998;55:1391–1397.

45. Andre P, et al, inventors; INSERM, assignee. Novel use of HIV protease inhibiting compounds. WO 9963998, 1999.

46. Andre P, et al. An inhibitor of HIV-1 protease modulates proteasome activity, antigen presentation, and T cell responses. *Proc Natl Acad Sci USA* 1998;95:13120–13124.

47. Retterstol K, et al. Results of intensive long-term treatment of familial hypercholesterolemia. *Am J Cardiol* 1996;78:1369–1374.

48. Rao S, et al. Lovastatin-mediated G1 arrest is through inhibition of the proteasome, independent of hydroxymethyl glutaryl-CoA reductase. *Proc Natl Acad Sci USA* 1999;96:7797–7802.

49. Figueiredo-Pereira ME, et al. The antitumor drug aclacinomycin A, which inhibits the degradation of ubiquitinated proteins, shows selectivity for the chymotrypsin-like activity of the bovine pituitary 20S proteasome. *J Biol Chem* 1996;271:16455–16459; Erratum in: *J Biol Chem* 1996;271:23602.

50. Meyer S, et al. Cyclosporine A is an uncompetitive inhibitor of proteasome activity and prevents NF-κB activation. *FEBS Lett* 1997;413:354–358.

51. Piccinini M, et al. Proteasomes are a target of the anti-tumour drug vinblastine. *Biochem J* 2001;356:835–841.

6 The Proteasome in Cell-Cycle Regulation

Julian Adams

CONTENTS

ABSTRACT

The cyclin-dependent kinases (CDKs) are essential for cell-cycle progression. Cyclins and CDK inhibitors regulate the activity of CDKs, and, in turn, the proteasome regulates these proteins. Destruction of proteins that prevent transition into anaphase or S phase is controlled by two dedicated multiprotein complexes, the anaphase-promoting complex (APC) and Skp1-cullin-F-box protein ligase complex. These gatekeepers include ubiquitin E3 ligases that specify the proteins that will be targeted for degradation by the proteasome. Proteasome activity is required for progression through the cell cycle; and when proteasome activity is disrupted by any of a number of small molecule inhibitors, cell cycle arrest follows. The presence or absence of p53 affects proteasome inhibitor-induced cell cycle arrest: in p53+ cells, proteasome inhibitors cause arrest at the G_1/S boundary, while proteasome inhibition in p53– cells leads to G_2/M phase arrest. In some instances, proteasome inhibition also culminates in the cell death; however, proteasome inhibitor-induced apoptosis may be a consequence of effects on pathways not directly involved in cell-cycle progression, and may also be dependent on the specific proteasome inhibitor or cell line.

KEY WORDS

Cyclins; cyclin-dependent kinase inhibitors; bortezomib; proteasome; cell cycle; proteasome inhibitors.

1. THE CELL CYCLE

Eukaryotic cell division is dependent on two distinct processes: DNA replication in the S phase (synthesis phase) of the cell cycle, and cell division, including division of the duplicated DNA, during mitosis (M phase) to form two daughter cells *(1)*. The gap phase between M and S is called G_1, and the gap phase between S and M is called G_2. The G_1, S, and G_2 phases are collectively referred to as interphase. Following interphase the cell

From: *Cancer Drug Discovery and Development: Proteasome Inhibitors in Cancer Therapy*
Edited by: J. Adams © Humana Press Inc., Totowa, NJ

enters the M phase, which is divided into prophase, metaphase, anaphase, and telophase. Quiescent cells that have exited the cell cycle are described as being in the G_0 phase (1).

Ordered and unidirectional progression through the various stages of the cell cycle is at least partly dependent on ubiquitin–proteasome pathway-mediated proteolysis of regulatory factors that control entry of the cell into the S and M phases (1–4).

2. PROTEINS INVOLVED IN THE CELL CYCLE

The passage of a cell through the cell cycle is controlled by various regulatory proteins including cyclins, cyclin-dependent kinases (CDKs), and CDK inhibitors (CKIs). Central to progression through the cell cycle is the relationship between cyclins and CDKs: CDKs act as catalytic enzymes for cell-cycle progression and are regulated by the expression of cyclins (5). The activity of the cyclin:CDK complex may also be regulated by CKIs and other factors (5). Whereas CDK levels remain fairly constant at all times, the levels of the various cyclins rise and fall at specific stages of the cell cycle, through a process of synthesis and proteolysis (2).

2.1. Cyclins

At least 16 different cyclins have been identified in mammalian cells (1). Those associated with cell-cycle regulation include cyclins A, B, D, and E. Of these, cyclins A and B regulate progression through mitosis and are termed mitotic cyclins (although cyclin A has also been associated with entry into S phase) (1). The levels of cyclin F also fluctuate during the cell cycle, but the functions of this cyclin have yet to be fully determined, and its degradation is independent of the ubiquitin–proteasome pathway (6). Cyclins D and E regulate the transition from G_1 to S phase and are called G_1 cyclins.

2.1.1. MITOTIC CYCLINS

Cyclin A was one of the first cyclins to be identified. It can associate with both CDK2 (also a cyclin E partner) and CDK1 (also a cyclin B partner) in somatic cells (1,7). In higher eukaryotes it exists in two forms, an embryonic form (A1) and a somatic form (A2) (7). Cyclin A levels rise initially in the G_1 phase, and it associates with CDK2 to promote entry into S phase. In late S phase, cyclin A binds to CDK1 and is associated with completion of S phase and progression through G_2 phase into mitosis. Cyclin A negatively regulates some members of the E2F family of transcription factors and may also be actively involved in DNA synthesis (1). Levels of cyclin A are regulated by ubiquitination, and cyclin A must be degraded by the proteasome before the cell can exit M phase.

Cyclin B begins to be expressed in very late S phase and accumulates during G_2 and early M phases. Cyclin B forms a complex with CDK1, known as cdc2, in lower eukaryotes, and the cyclin B–CDK1 activity is necessary for progression from the G_2 phase into mitosis (8). Cyclin B–CDK1 activity is regulated by phosphorylation and dephosphorylation of specific amino acids of CDK1. However, the activated complex must be destroyed for progression from telophase into G_2 phase (2). The deactivation of the complex is dependent on ubiquitination of cyclin B and its subsequent proteasomal destruction (2,8).

Cyclin F levels fluctuate with a pattern similar to cyclin A, although it is highly unstable throughout much of the cell cycle (6). It appears to be associated with transition from G_2 to M phase (1). No CDK partner has been identified for cyclin F, and it is additionally unusual for its ability to bind to another cyclin (cyclin B) *(6)*. Cyclin F accumulates when the DNA damage checkpoint is activated, and it is degraded at a similar point in the cell cycle to cyclin A, when the spindle assembly checkpoint is activated *(6)*. The tight temporal expression and control of cyclin F indicates that it has an important role in the cell cycle, but the exact nature of this role has yet to be determined *(6)*.

2.1.2. G_1 CYCLINS

D cyclins (D1, D2, and D3) are synthesized during G_1 as a cell enters the cell cycle following G_0 phase *(1)*. Cyclin D activates CDK4 and CDK6, and the primary target for these activated kinases is the retinoblastoma tumor suppressor protein (pRb) *(1)*. Although cyclin D levels do not oscillate during the cell cycle in the way that some other cyclin levels do, degradation of cyclin D is mediated via the ubiquitin–proteasome pathway by the ubiquitin E3 ligase SCF *(9)*.

Cyclin E associates predominantly with CDK2, and the cyclin E–CDK2 complex controls exit from G_1 and entry into S phase *(1)*. Together with cyclin D, cyclin E regulates phosphorylation of pRb, thereby controlling exit from G_1 *(10)*. Levels of cyclin E increase during G_1 phase, peaking at the G_1–S transition, and degradation of cyclin E is mediated by the ubiquitin–proteasome pathway during S phase *(10,11)*. Free cyclin E is readily degraded by the ubiquitin–proteasome pathway, possibly via association with the F-box protein Skp2 *(12)*. Although cyclin E bound to CDK2 is protected from ubiquitination, CDK2 activity can reverse this protection by phosphorylating cyclin E itself, thus promoting disassembly of the cyclin E–CDK2 complex and promoting subsequent ubiquitination and degradation of free cyclin E *(11)*.

2.2. Cyclin-Dependent Kinases

CDKs, of which nine (CDK1–9) are present in mammalian cells, are primarily activated by association with cyclins *(1)*. The cyclin–CDK complexes that control progress through the cell cycle act by adding phosphate groups to a variety of protein substrates *(13)*. Unlike those of cyclins, CDK levels remain fairly stable throughout the cell cycle. CDK activity is regulated by cyclin binding, phosphorylation of the CDK, binding of CKIs *(13)*, and proteolytic degradation of cyclins and CKIs via the ubiquitin-proteasome pathway *(14)* (Fig. 1).

2.3. CDK Inhibitors

CKIs negatively regulate the activity of CDKs *(1)*. Two families of CKIs exist: the Cip/Kip family, which can act on most cyclin–CDK complexes, and the INK4 family, which acts specifically on CDK4 and CDK6.

2.3.1. THE CIP/KIP FAMILY

This family of CKIs consists of three members: p21*Cip1*, p27*Kip1*, and p57*Kip2*. The Cip/Kip family regulates the activities of cyclin A-, D-, and E-dependent kinases *(15)*. The first CKI of this family to be isolated was p21*Cip1* *(16,17)*. In addition to inhibiting cyclin–CDK activity, p21*Cip1* also inhibits the ability of proliferating cell nuclear antigen (PCNA) to function in DNA replication *(18)*. It has been demonstrated that one molecule of p21*Cip1* is enough to inhibit the activity of one cyclin–CDK molecule, and this inhibition occurs even when the p21*Cip1* molecule is phosphorylated *(19)*.

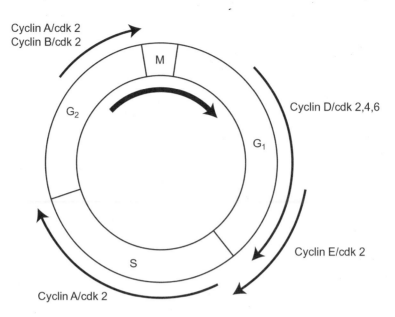

Fig. 1. The cycle/cyclin-dependent kinase (cdk) cycle. As the cell cycle progresses, the expression of the mitotic cyclins and their association with cyclin-dependent kinase changes. CDK activity requires association with a cyclin.

p27$Kip1$ appears to be the CKI primarily responsible for the control of the cell cycle at the G_1–S transition via inhibition of cyclin D–CDK4, cyclin E–CDK2, and cyclin A–CDK2 *(12,20)*.

It is present at high levels in cells in G_0 phase, but its levels decrease when cells enter into the cell cycle *(12)*. It is rapidly degraded during late G_1 via ubiquitination and subsequent proteasomal destruction *(20,21)*. Phosphorylation of p27$Kip1$ is mediated by cyclin E–CDK2, and this is required before proteasomal degradation can occur *(22)*.

The third member of the Cip/Kip family, p57$Kip2$, is essential for embryonic development in mice *(23)*, but its role in cell-cycle regulation is not well understood. Like p27$Kip1$, p57$Kip2$ is degraded via ubiquitination and subsequent proteasome-mediated proteolysis *(23)*.

2.3.2. THE INK4 CKIs

The INK4 family of CKIs includes four members: p16$INK4a$, p15$INK4b$, p18$INK4c$, and p19$INK4d$. All four INK4 proteins are closely related (approx 40% identical to each other), and all specifically prevent the association of cyclin D with CDK4 or CDK6 *(1)*. Of the four, only p19$INK4d$ is degraded via the ubiquitin–proteasome pathway; expression of the other three INK4 proteins is controlled by transcriptional regulation *(24)*.

2.4. Ubiquitin Ligases

Two E3 ubiquitin ligase enzymes catalyze degradation of cell-cycle proteins by the ubiquitin–proteasome proteolytic pathway—the anaphase-promoting complex (APC; also referred to as the cyclosome in some species) and the SCF complex (defined in Subheading 2.4.2.) *(12)*. The APC is active from late G_2 phase through mitosis to mid-G_1 phase; the SCF complex is primarily active through late G_1, S, and early G_2 phases *(12)*.

2.4.1. ANAPHASE-PROMOTING COMPLEX

The APC is a large complex composed of eight protein subunits in mammals *(25)*. It is required for the separation of sister chromatids at anaphase and for transition from M to G_1, mediated by the ubiquitination of anaphase inhibitors known as securins (Pds1 or Cut2) and of the mitotic cyclins A and B *(4,12,26)*.

2.4.2. SCF COMPLEX

The SCF complex is named after three of its main components: Skp1, Cdc53/cullin, and an F-box-containing protein *(9)*. SCF mediates ubiquitination of G_1 cyclins and CKIs by linking substrate proteins to the E2 ubiquitin-conjugating enzyme CDC34 *(2,27,28)* and is thus implicated in G_1–S progression *(12)*.

2.5. Retinoblastoma Tumor Suppressor Protein

Progression through the G_1 phase of the cell cycle and initiation of S phase requires inhibition of pRb, which otherwise halts G_1/S transition by sequestering cell-cycle-promoting transcription factors such as E2F *(24)*.

Phosphorylation of pRb occurs in mid to late G_1 phase and depends on formation of the cyclin D–CDK4 or cyclin D–CDK6 complexes. Once phosphorylated, pRb releases E2F and enables completion of G_1 phase and entry into S phase *(24)*.

2.6. Survivin

Survivin belongs to the inhibitor of apoptosis (IAP) protein family *(29)*, and has roles in both inhibition of apoptosis and cell-cycle regulation *(30)*. Levels of survivin peak during the G_2/M phase *(29)*. The ubiquitin–proteasome pathway is involved in the degradation of survivin in a cell-cycle-dependent manner *(30)*. Some members of the IAP family (XIAP, cIAP1, and cIAP2) have also demonstrated ubiquitin ligase activity of their own *(31–33)*.

2.7. p53 Tumor Suppressor

Levels of p53 tumor suppressor protein are normally very low in most cells, but they can increase when there is DNA damage, leading to cell cycle arrest in the G_1 phase. Normal turnover of p53, which has a very short half-life, is regulated by the ubiquitin-proteasome pathway *(34)*. Inhibition of the proteasome leads to accumulation of p53 in the nucleus, induction of the CKI p21*Cip1*, and cell cycle arrest in the G_1 phase *(35)*.

3. IMPACT OF PROTEASOME INHIBITION ON THE CELL CYCLE

Inhibition of the ubiquitin–proteasome pathway has been shown to block progression of the cell cycle at several points. In an study, 100 n*M* of bortezomib (Velcade; formerly known as PS-341) blocked mitogen-induced cell-cycle progression in a human pancreatic adenocarcinoma cell line (BxPC3). A total of 81.3% of cells were arrested in the G_1–G_0 phase, with only 6.7% of cells progressing to the S phase. Further experiments revealed a significant increase in the rate of apoptosis in cells exposed to 100 n*M* of bortezomib compared with control cells, as demonstrated by apoptotic fractions of the fluorescence-activated cell sorting sub-G_0 peak. Significant apoptosis was evident at 24 h, with further increases evident at 48 and 72 h. The effects of bortezomib appeared to be concentration-dependent, as a lower concentration of the drug (10 n*M*) was not associated with a significant increase in the rate of apoptosis. Furthermore, increased expression of p21$^{Cip1-Waf1}$, suggesting accumulation of p53, was evident after 3 h in cells exposed to bortezomib 100 nM, but not 10 nM (36). The effects of another proteasome inhibitor, MG115, on cell cycle progression in MR65 human non-small cell lung cancer cells were also concentration-dependent. Cell cultures treated with 54 μM of the proteasome inhibitor exhibited a complete block of G_1/S and G_2/M transitions. Lower concentrations of the drug decreased the exit rate from G_1 and M but did not completely block G_1/S or G_2/M transition. Progression through the S phase was evident with all concentrations of MG115, but was progressively retarded as the drug concentration increased (37).

The presence or absence of p53 appears to influence the point in the cell cycle at which proteasome inhibitor-induced cell cycle arrest occurs. In an in vitro study in diploid human fibroblasts, exposure to the proteasome inhibitor MG132 caused accumulation of p53, in turn leading to increased expression of p21^{Waf1} and cell cycle arrest at the G_1/S boundary. Conversely, cells deficient in p53 were found to arrest in the G_2/M phase of the cell cycle (38). Exposure of human PC3 prostate tumor cells, which are also deficient in functional p53 (39), to bortezomib 100 nM for 8 h also resulted in accumulation of cells in G_2/M. This was accompanied by a reduction in the number of cells in G_1 and a slight increase in the number of cells in S phase (40). Exposure of embryonic stem cells to MG132 10 μM was associated with greater accumulation of p53 null cells (E14 cells) at the G_2/M boundary (68 vs 30%) and a lower rate of apoptosis compared with cells expressing wild-type p53 (R72D27 cells) (41).

In another study, exposure of proliferating Rat-1 and PC12 cells to PSI-15 at 25 μM, or Rat-1 cells to MG115 at 30 μM, induced apoptosis. Accumulation of p53 was observed as early as 2 h after exposure to proteasome inhibitors in both cell types; increased expression of both p21 and Mdm-2 was also evident, suggesting that the p53 accumulating in response to proteasome inhibition was functional. Rat-1 and PC3 cells transfected with a plasmid-expressing mutant, nonfunctional p53 did not undergo apoptosis following exposure to MG115, indicating that functional p53 has a role in proteasome inhibitor-induced apoptosis (42).

There are conflicting data regarding the apoptotic effects of proteasome inhibition in actively dividing vs quiescent cells. Experiments with MG132 (5 μM for 24 h) in KIM-2 mammary epithelial cells suggest that proteasome inhibitor-induced apoptosis is more likely to occur in cells that have entered the cell cycle, as opposed to quiescent cells. Further analysis revealed retarded progression through G_2/M and that cell cycle arrest occurred either during or after the G_1/S transition (41). In another study, MG115 did not induce apoptosis in Rat-1 cells rendered quiescent by serum deprivation, but did induce apoptosis in differentiated, nonproliferating PC3 cells (42). A recent abstract reported that bortezomib induces apoptosis equally well in G_1-arrested and cycling colon tumor cells (43).

Proteasome inhibition has also been shown to induce apoptosis in spheroid cell cultures, which have a lower rate of proliferation than monolayer cultures. Bortezomib 5 nM induced apoptosis in monolayer, but not spheroid, cultures of SKOV3 cells; higher concentrations of the drug (50–500 nM), however, induced apoptosis to a similar extent in both cell cultures. Bortezomib 5 μM resulted in accumulation of p21 in SKOV3 cells plated in either monolayer or spheroid cultures, indicative of cell cycle arrest at the G_1/S boundary (44).

These conflicting data may result from differences in the susceptibility of different cell types to the apoptotic effects of proteasome inhibition or, indeed, to differing effects and/

or potency of the various proteasome inhibitors used. There is also evidence that proteasome inhibition interferes with cell viability via mechanisms other than disrupting transition between the various phases of the cell cycle. In one study, exposure to MG132 in HeLa cells in the S phase of the cell cycle resulted in re-replication of mid to late replicating genes and over-replication of DNA, indicating that proteasome-dependent mechanisms regulate the orderly progression of the S-phase *(45)*.

REFERENCES

1. Johnson DG, et al. Cyclins and cell cycle checkpoints. *Annu Rev Pharmacol Toxicol* 1999;39:295–312.
2. King RW, et al. How proteolysis drives the cell cycle. *Science* 1996;274:1652–1659.
3. Zwickl P, et al. The proteasome: a macromolecular assembly designed for controlled proteolysis. *Philos Trans R Soc Lond B Biol Sci* 1999;354:1501–1511.
4. Glickman MH, et al. The ubiquitin-proteasome proteolytic pathway: destruction for the sake of construction. *Physiol Rev* 2002;82:373–428.
5. Santella L, et al. Calcium, protease action, and the regulation of the cell cycle. *Cell Calcium* 1998;23:123–130.
6. Fung TK, et al. Cyclin F is degraded during G2-M by mechanisms fundamentally different from other cyclins. *J Biol Chem* 2002;277:35140–35149.
7. Yam CH, et al. Degradation of cyclin A does not require its phosphorylation by CDC2 and cyclin-dependent kinase 2. *J Biol Chem* 2000;275:3158–3167.
8. Nishiyama A, et al. A nonproteolytic function of the proteasome is required for the dissociation of Cdc2 and cyclin B at the end of M phase. *Genes Dev* 2000;14:2344–2357.
9. Koepp DM, et al. How the cyclin became a cyclin: regulated proteolysis in the cell cycle. *Cell* 1999;97:431–434.
10. Payton M, et al. Cyclin E2, the cycle continues. *Int J Biochem Cell Biol* 2002;34:315–320.
11. Clurman BE, et al. Turnover of cyclin E by the ubiquitin-proteasome pathway is regulated by cdk2 binding and cyclin phosphorylation. *Genes Dev* 1996;10:1979–1990.
12. Nakayama KI, et al. Regulation of the cell cycle at the G1-S transition by proteolysis of cyclin E and p27Kip1. *Biochem Biophys Res Commun* 2001;282:853–860.
13. Ekholm SV, et al. Regulation of G(1) cyclin-dependent kinases in the mammalian cell cycle. *Curr Opin Cell Biol* 2000;12:676–684.
14. Harper JW, et al. Cyclin-dependent kinases. *Chem Rev* 2001;101:2511–2526.
15. Sherr CJ, et al. CDK inhibitors: positive and negative regulators of G1-phase progression. *Genes Dev* 1999;13:1501–1512.
16. Xiong Y, et al. p21 is a universal inhibitor of cyclin kinases. *Nature* 1993;366:701–704.
17. Gu Y, et al. Inhibition of CDK2 activity in vivo by an associated 20K regulatory subunit. *Nature* 1993;366:707–710.
18. Li R, et al. Differential effects by the p21 CDK inhibitor on PCNA-dependent DNA replication and repair. *Nature* 1994;371:534–537.
19. Hengst L, et al. Complete inhibition of Cdk/cyclin by one molecule of p21(Cip1). *Genes Dev* 1998;12:3882–3888.
20. Piva R, et al. Proteasome-dependent degradation of p27/kip1 in gliomas. *J Neuropathol Exp Neurol* 1999;58:691–696.
21. Pagano M, et al. Role of the ubiquitin-proteasome pathway in regulating abundance of the cyclin-dependent kinase inhibitor p27. *Science* 1995;269:682–685.
22. Sheaff RJ, et al. Cyclin E-CDK2 is a regulator of p27Kip1. *Genes Dev* 1997;11:1464–1478.
23. Urano T, et al. p57(Kip2) is degraded through the proteasome in osteoblasts stimulated to proliferation by transforming growth factor beta 1. *J Biol Chem* 1999;274:12197–12200.
24. Thullberg M, et al. Ubiquitin/proteasome-mediated degradation of p19INK4d determines its periodic expression during the cell cycle. *Oncogene* 2000;19:2870–2876.
25. Yu H, et al. Identification of a cullin homology region in a subunit of the anaphase-promoting complex. *Science* 1998;279:1219–1222.
26. Weissman AM. Themes and variations on ubiquitylation. *Nat Rev Mol Cell Biol* 2001;2:169–178.
27. Bai C, et al. SKP1 connects cell cycle regulators to the ubiquitin proteolysis machinery through a novel motif, the F-box. *Cell* 1996;86:263–274.

28. Koepp DM, et al. Phosphorylation-dependent ubiquitination of cyclin E by the SCFFbw7 ubiquitin ligase. *Science* 2001;294:173–177.
29. Verdecia MA, et al. Structure of the human anti-apoptotic protein survivin reveals a dimeric arrangement. *Nat Struct Biol* 2000;7:602–608.
30. Zhao J, et al. The ubiquitin-proteasome pathway regulates survivin degradation in a cell cycle-dependent manner. *J Cell Sci* 2000;113 Pt 23:4363–4371.
31. Yang Y, et al. Ubiquitin protein ligase activity of IAPs and their degradation in proteasomes in response to apoptotic stimuli. *Science* 2000;288:874–877.
32. Huang H, et al. The inhibitor of apoptosis, cIAP2, functions as a ubiquitin-protein ligase and promotes in vitro monoubiquitination of caspases 3 and 7. *J Biol Chem* 2000;275:26661–26664.
33. Suzuki Y, et al. Ubiquitin-protein ligase activity of X-linked inhibitor of apoptosis protein promotes proteasomal degradation of caspase-3 and enhances its anti-apoptotic effect in Fas-induced cell death. *Proc Natl Acad Sci USA* 2001;98:8662–8667.
34. Maki CG, et al. In vivo ubiquitination and proteasome-mediated degradation of p53(1). *Cancer Res* 1996;56:2649–2654.
35. Chen F, et al. Role of p53 in cell cycle regulation and apoptosis following exposure to proteasome inhibitors. *Cell Growth Differ* 2000;11:239–246.
36. Shah SA, et al. 26S proteasome inhibition induces apoptosis and limits growth of human pancreatic cancer. *J Cell Biochem* 2001;82:110–122.
37. Machiels BM, et al. Detailed analysis of cell cycle kinetics upon proteasome inhibition. *Cytometry* 1997;28:243–252.
38. Chen F, et al. Role of p53 in cell cycle regulation and apoptosis following exposure to proteasome inhibitors. *Cell Growth Differ* 2000;11:239–246.
39. Tang DG, et al. Extended survivability of prostate cancer cells in the absence of trophic factors: increased proliferation, evasion of apoptosis, and the role of apoptosis proteins. *Cancer Res* 1998;58:3466–3479.
40. Adams J, et al. Proteasome inhibitors: a novel class of potent and effective antitumor agents. *Cancer Res* 1999;59:2615–2622.
41. MacLaren AP, et al. p53-dependent apoptosis induced by proteasome inhibition in mammary epithelial cells. *Cell Death Differ* 2001;8:210–218.
42. Lopes UG, et al. p53-dependent induction of apoptosis by proteasome inhibitors. *J Biol Chem* 1997;272:12893–12896.
43. Neumeier H, et al. Hypoxia increases potency of the proteasome inhibitor VELCADE™ (bortezomib) for injection: potential for a hypoxic cell cytotoxin in solid tumors. 2002;38(suppl 7):166.
44. Frankel A, et al. Lack of multicellular drug resistance observed in human ovarian and prostate carcinoma treated with the proteasome inhibitor PS-341. *Clin Cancer Res* 2000;6:3719–3728.
45. Yamaguchi R, et al. Proteasome inhibitors alter the orderly progression of DNA synthesis during S-phase in HeLa cells and lead to rereplication of DNA. *Exp Cell Res* 2000;261:271–283.

7 Proteasome Inhibition and Apoptosis

Simon A. Williams and David J. McConkey

1. INTRODUCTION

Programmed cell death is an energy-dependent process of cellular elimination that is necessary in all stages of life, including development, tissue homeostasis, and aging in multicellular organisms. Work by Wyllie, Kerr, and Currie identified the large phenotypic changes in the morphology of cells undergoing programmed cell death such as nuclear condensation and the dismantling of cellular material into membrane-enclosed packages; they termed these changes *apoptosis*. In 1972 they published a seminal paper that correctly predicted the physiologic and pathophysiologic relevance of their findings *(1)*, and Wyllie went on to explore some of the biochemical characteristics that are signs of apoptosis, describing the cleavage of DNA into discrete nucleosomal multimers (DNA ladders) *(2)*. In the 1970s Horvitz and colleagues described the loss of 131 cells during the development of the nematode *Caenorhabetitis elegans*. Mutagenesis studies subsequently implicated three genes in this process (*ced-3*, *ced-4*, and *egl-1*) that when inactivated caused the retention of the normally eliminated cells *(3,4)*. A fourth gene (*ced-9*) was identified that promoted cell survival, in that its loss resulted in the death of more cells than normal *(5)*. These proapoptotic gene products, EGL-1, CED-3, and CED-4, along with their antiapoptotic counterpart, CED-9, proved to be components of an evolutionarily conserved, biochemical cascade responsible for cellular elimination.

During the years since the work of Horvitz, mammalian homologs of the *C. elegans* genes have been identified. The caspases, for example, are homologous to CED-3 *(6)* and bcl-2 is similar to CED-9 *(7)*. Some of these, such as bcl-2, were immediately implicated in disease and initiated the explosion of discovery in the field of apoptosis. Figure 1 summarizes the central apoptotic cascade. During the decision stage, signals come from two main sources. The first sources, called extrinsic death stimuli, involve interactions

From: *Cancer Drug Discovery and Development: Proteasome Inhibitors in Cancer Therapy*
Edited by: J. Adams © Humana Press Inc., Totowa, NJ

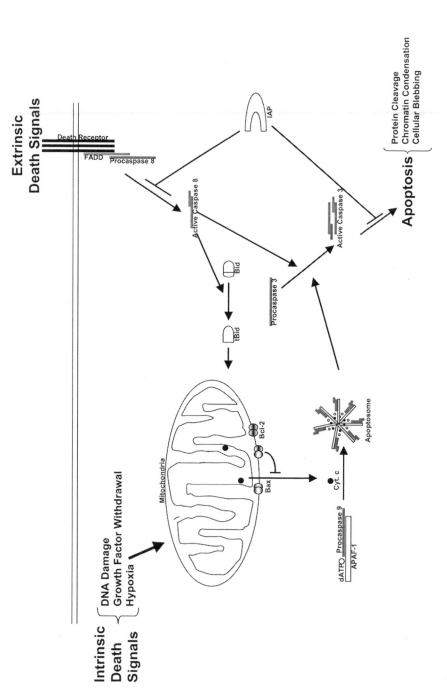

Fig. 1. The apoptotic cascade. Extrinsic or intrinsic signals ultimately result in the activation of caspases and the dismantling of the cellular architecture en route to death.

between a family of death receptors on the cell surface and their cognate ligands. Such interactions lead to receptor oligomerization and the activation of members of the caspase family of proteases (caspases 8 and 10). The other signal sources, called intrinsic death stimuli, act independently of death receptors, leading to the activation of caspase 9 and result from numerous cellular stressors such as DNA damage, growth factor withdrawal, or hypoxia. Both intrinsic and most extrinsic death stimuli converge on the mitochondria, and mitochondrial alterations mark the end of the decision stage. When the death signal is sufficient, factors such as cytochrome c are released from the mitochondria and initiate the execution stage. This step is essentially irreversible and centers on the actions of effector caspases, principally caspase 3. Effector caspases go on to amplify the death signal and dismantle the cellular architecture in much the same way as the *ced-3* gene product functions in the nematode, leading to the apoptotic phenotype described earlier. At the mitochondria, the Bcl-2 family of proteins regulates the release of death-signaling factors. They share structural features, and members of this family promote (i.e., Bad, Bak, Bax, tBid, and others) or suppress (i.e., Bcl-2, Bcl-X_L, A1, and others) progression of the signal to the execution stage. Many initiators and regulators of the death cascade have been characterized, painting the picture of an intricate and tightly regulated biochemical process of principal importance to the cell.

2. APOPTOSIS AND CANCER

Not until the discovery of Bcl-2 overexpression in B-cell follicular lymphoma did investigations on the role of programmed cell death in cancer begin to accelerate rapidly. These patients were found to display a high frequency of the 14;18 translocation. Subsequent molecular analyses revealed that the rearrangement promotes deregulated expression of the hitherto uncharacterized gene via juxtaposition of the immunoglobulin heavy chain enhancer *(8)*. Bcl-2 was found to prolong the life of leukemia cells and proved to be the first oncogene observed to confer an advantage that is independent of proliferation *(9,10)*.

Subsequently, apoptosis emerged as a process whose modulation is critical for disease progression and as a target for anticancer therapy. Inappropriate expression of key apoptotic cascade components has been observed in multiple forms of cancer and is frequently used as a diagnostic indicator. In prostate cancer, elevated Bcl-2 correlates with androgen-independent disease *(11)*. Multiple myeloma and an increasing number of solid tumor malignancies have exhibited elevated activity of the antiapoptotic transcription factor nuclear factor-κB (NF-κB) *(12,13)*. Bax, a proapoptotic Bcl-2 family member, was found to contain frameshift mutations in about half of the mismatch repair-deficient colon adenocarcinomas examined *(14)*. Measures of cancer cell death in nonclinical studies and clinical trials are considered important indicators of any potential chemotherapeutic agent's efficacy.

3. THE PROTEASOME AND APOPTOSIS

The ubiquitin–proteasome pathway is the major nonlysosomal system responsible for protein degradation in the cell and is discussed in detail elsewhere in this volume. The hawk moth *Manduca sexta* was the first system used to investigate the involvement of the ubiquitin–proteasome pathway in programmed cell death. As a result of a decrease in the levels of circulating 20-hydroxyecdysone during moth development, the intersegmental muscles undergo apoptosis *(15)*. Studies by Schwartz and colleagues have shown increases in ubiquitin mRNA levels, ubiquitination activity, and the ubiquitination state of proteins immediately before the onset of death. The levels of proteasome subunits were reported to increase as much as fivefold as a prelude to death, and ninefold increases in 26S proteasome function were also observed *(16)*.

4. EFFECTS OF PROTEASOME INHIBITION

The studies implicating proteasome activity in apoptotic progression in the moth suggested that proteasome inhibitors would block apoptosis. This was indeed found to be the case in primary cell cultures. For example, murine thymocytes exposed to γ-radiation, phorbol esters, dexamethasone *(17,18)*, or *etoposide (19,20)* undergo a death that is inhibited by lactacystin and various peptide aldehyde proteasome inhibitors *(21)*. Death induced by neural growth factor (NGF) withdrawal in rat sympathetic neurons was also suppressed by proteasome inhibition *(22)*. Primary thymocytes and rat sympathetic neurons both display less cleavage of poly-ADP ribose polymerase (PARP), a substrate of caspase 3, when proteasome inhibition suppressed death *(23)*. Thymocytes also displayed less caspase 3-like activity in this context along with retention of mitochondrial membrane potential and inhibited phosphotidyl serine exposure on their *surface (20)*.

Conversely, transformed cell lines consistently undergo apoptosis when treated with proteasome inhibitors. Lactacystin was the first reported proteasome inhibitor used in this kind of study. Human monoblast U937 cells lost viability upon treatment, suggesting a survival role for the proteasome in this context. The drug caused the formation of DNA ladders and other morphologic changes that are signs of apoptosis *(24)*. Lactacystin and peptidyl aldehydes have been used to induce death in a wide variety of other cell lines including the following: human T-cell leukemia MOLT-4, mouse lymphocytic leukemia L5178Y *(25)*, mouse RVC lymphoma *(26)*, HL60 *(27)*, DO.11.10 T-cell hybridoma *(28)*, Chinese hamster ovary *(29)*, HeLa *(30)*, Jurkat *(31,32)*, human Burkitt's lymphoma *(33)* and Ewing's sarcoma cells *(34)*, in addition to chronic lymphocytic leukemia (CLL) patients *(35–37)* and human lymphoblastic cells *(33)*. In our work with MG-132, cells from CLL patients that were resistant to glucocorticoids or nucleoside analogs proved to be selectively sensitive to proteasome inhibition as measured by DNA fragmentation, caspase activity, and caspase-substrate cleavage *(38)*.

The boronate dipeptide proteasome inhibitor bortezomib has also been shown to induce in apoptosis in vitro in a variety of cell lines *(39,40)*. Programmed cell death was induced in Jurkat cells, the human leukemia cell lines K562, HL60, and U937 *(41)*, and patient samples *(42)*, along with the multiple myeloma cell lines U266, RPMI8226, MM.1S, IM9, and ARH77 *(42)*. For regulatory reasons, please change to statement of the data rather than a conclusion *(43)*. The human and murine prostate lines PC-3 and TRAMP-C1, as well as MCF-7 human and EMT murine breast cell lines *(40)*, were induced to undergo apoptosis, observations that preceded the current and prospective clinical trials in these diseases. Colon (LOVO *[44]*, WiDR, HT29, KM12L4, and CCD841 *[45]*), squamous cell carcinoma (PAM212, PAM-LY2, B4B8, B7E3, UM-SCC-9, and UM-SCC-11B *[42,46]*), and pancreas cell lines (BxPC3 and MIA-PaCa-2 *[47]*) also undergo apoptosis in response to bortezomib treatment in vitro.

In vivo studies using xenographic mouse models have shown that bortezomib treatment consistently inhibits tumor growth as a single agent and improves the effects of most conventional cytotoxic agents. The earliest reports showed effects in PC-3 *(48)* and EMT-derived tumors, with a reduction in lung metastases noted with the latter system (40). Tumors derived from squamous cell carcinoma (46), colorectal (45), and lung cancer cells were all growth-inhibited. TRAMP-C1 tumors were growth-inhibited by bortezomib and sensitized to radiation. Tumors from BxPC3 cells were also growth-inhibited and induced to undergo apoptosis by bortezomib alone and in combination with the topoisomerase I inhibitor CPT-11 (49). This observation has also been made in LOVO tumors (45), and the same group used this system to demonstrate sensitization by bortezomib to radiation (44).

We have used bortezomib in vitro to induce apoptosis in several pancreas, prostate, and bladder cell lines (109–111) as well as in CLL patient samples (112). Our in vivo studies have demonstrated tumor growth suppression by bortezomib, with the best results occurring in combination with the nucleoside analog gemcitabine (47). Analysis of these tumors revealed elevated DNA fragmentation consistent with direct induction of tumor cell apoptosis. Angiogenic factors such as interleukin 8 (IL-8) and vascular endothelial growth factor (VEGF) are secreted by growing tumors in response to the stress of hypoxia and promote neovascularization. We have observed that bortezomib treatment reduces microvessel density and the levels of IL-8 and VEGF in prostate, bladder and pancreatic tumor models, suggesting that the drug may also function as an angiogenesis inhibitor (109–111).

The contrasting effects of proteasome inhibition on cell lines and primary cells have been attributed to their states of differentiation and proliferation. HL60 promyelocytic leukemia (PML) cells undergoing differentiation are less susceptible to the toxic effects of proteasome inhibition than their proliferating, undifferentiated counterparts (27). Rat-1 fibroblasts are more sensitive to proteasome inhibition while proliferating than not (50), and activated T-cells are also more sensitive than resting T-cells (28). The inhibitor of apoptosis protein (IAP) family of antiapoptotic proteins may also explain any differences. These bind to the active forms of caspases 3, 7, and 9 and inhibit their functions. There is evidence that these inhibitors also act as ubiquitin ligases that target caspases and themselves for degradation (51,52). Elevated IAP levels may therefore limit the killing effects of proteasome inhibition in primary cells.

5. MECHANISM OF PROTEASOME INHIBITOR-INDUCED APOPTOSIS

Of the many proteins stabilized as a result of proteasome inhibition, several candidates have emerged as mediators of the proapoptotic and antiangiogenic effects observed in tumor cells.

5.1. NF-κB

As mentioned earlier and in other chapters, NF-κB has been implicated in various forms of cancer and can be inhibited by proteasome inhibitors. This family of transcription factors was initially found to modulate aspects of the immune system but has subsequently been found to induce the expression of a wealth of genes involved with survival, proliferation, and angiogenesis (12,53). Typically, activation of NF-κB results from phosphorylation of the IκBα inhibitor by the IκB kinase (IKK) signalosome, followed by the ubiquitination and proteasomal degradation of IκBα, leaving the transcription factor free to translocate to the nucleus and transactivate target genes (54). Proteasome inhibition causes the accumulation of the phosphorylated inhibitor bound to its target transcription factor (55). Treatment causes the reduction of nuclear localized and DNA-bound NF-κB

(56). The inhibition of NF-κB causes cancer cells to be sensitized to apoptosis-inducing agents similar to the effects of expression of mutant IκB constructs that are not susceptible to degradation via the ubiquitin–proteasome pathway *(57)*. Our group and others have observed the inhibitory effects of proteasome inhibition on NF-κB in leukemic patient samples and solid tumor-derived cell lines *(46,109,112)*. Angiogenic factors such as VEGF and IL-8 were inhibited in vitro and in vivo by bortezomib, effects that are mimicked by dominant active IκB mutants *(58)*, and both factors have been identified as NF-κB targets by other groups *(59–62)*. The antiangiogenic effect of proteasome inhibitors and the resulting hypoxia-induced apoptosis and growth inhibition may prove to be among their most important contributions to these antitumor activities *(63)*.

5.2. p53

In normal cells, the tumor suppressor p53 is rapidly modified by the ubiquitin ligase, mdm-2, which exports this transcription factor from the nucleus and targets it for proteasomal degradation *(64)*. DNA strand breaks cause the activation of kinases such as DNA-PK *(65)* and ATM *(66)*, which inhibit p53 degradation; other stressors such as hypoxia can also stabilize the protein *(67)*. The phosphorylated form of p53 is released from mdm-2 *(68)* and takes on a tetrameric active state *(69)*. Once activated, p53 can bind to DNA and induce the expression of many genes *(70)*, some of which, such as p21/Waf-1/Cip-1 *(71)*, cause cell cycle arrest; others, including Gadd-45 *(72)*, engage in DNA repair. The proapoptotic genes upregulated by p53 are many and include APAF-1, SIAH-1, PTEN, Fas, DR5, Pmp22, Bax, Noxa, p53AIP1, and PUMA *(73)*. p53 induction of Fas is mediated by four p53-responsive elements in the promoter and the first intron of the gene. These elements are all bound by p53 and work cooperatively to induce Fas expression *(74)*. p53 can also inhibit the expression of Bcl-2 *(75)* and β-catenin *(76)*, genes responsible for survival, proliferation, and overall disease progression in various forms of cancer. Other evidence suggests a function of p53 that is independent of its DNA binding activities. The redistribution of Fas to the cell surface may be caused by p53 in a transcription-independent way *(77)*, and p53 has also been shown to directly interact with the mitochondria *(78,79)*.

As a target of the ubiquitin-proteasome pathway, wild-type p53 is stabilized by proteasome inhibition *(80)*. Previous studies generally reported correlations between p53 stabilization and cell death *(25,81)*, with some demonstrating more direct evidence for a causative role for functional p53 in apoptosis. As one example, Rat-1 cells treated with the peptide aldehydes proteasome-specific inhibitor (PSI) and MG-115 underwent death that was blocked by the introduction of a dominant-negative form of p53 *(50)*. In another study MG-132-induced apoptosis was blocked by SV40 T-antigen in the murine mammary cell line KIM-2 *(82)*. Even though p21 is a transcriptional target of p53, it is also degraded by the proteasome and so is not a valid measure of p53's transcriptional activity when protein levels are studied in cells treated with proteasome inhibitors *(30)*. However, some groups have reported elevated p21 mRNA, which suggests transcriptional activation indicative of p53 function *(80,83,84)*. Other groups have concluded that there is no causal association between p53 stabilization and death induced by treatment with proteasome inhibitors *(85–87)*. For example, reintroduction of wild-type p53 in PC-3 cells did not increase their sensitivity *(41)*, whereas in another study these cells displayed the same sensitivity to MG-132 as the p53-containing prostate cell line LNCaP *(88)*.

We have directly investigated how p53 contributes to proteasome inhibitor-induced apoptosis in the human prostate adenocarcinoma line, LNCaP-Pro5 *(89,113)*. Consistent with earlier studies, p53 was stabilized after bortezomib treatment, and stable transfectants expressing the E6 viral protein (which inhibits p53) displayed increased resistance to bortezomib-induced cell death. An RNase protection assay revealed that the mRNA levels of several p53 target proteins, including Fas, Bax, mdm-2, and p21, were elevated whereas the electrophoretic mobility shift assay showed that proteasome inhibitor-stabilized p53 binds to its consensus response element. Interestingly, we also observed that p53 remained bound to mdm-2 while exhibiting minimal levels of phosphorylation on serines 15 and 20, suggesting that these modifications may not be necessary for activity of the tumor suppressor *(113)*. The contribution of p53 to proteasome inhibitor-induced death is likely, if limited to certain cell types, and warrants further analysis of its structural and functional nature in this context.

5.3. Bcl-2 Family

Both pro- and antiapoptotic members of the Bcl-2 family of proteins regulate apoptosis at the point of the release of cytochrome c from the mitochondria (Fig. 1). The mechanisms of action of these proteins are unclear, but their observed ability to modulate the flow of cations and small molecules through lipid membranes in vitro may eventually prove to be of central physiologic relevance to their functions *(90)*. Additionally, Bcl-2 appears to bind to an array of proteins that are not immediately associated with the apoptotic cascade and so may elicit some component of its function through these interactions *(91)*. The balance between levels of pro- and antiapoptotic family members has a great impact on the susceptibility of a cell to an apoptotic signal, although knockout mouse studies suggest that certain aspects of regulation are independent of this kind of interplay *(92)*.

Many of these family members, including Bcl-2 *(93)*, Bax *(30,94)*, Bik *(31)*, and tBid *(95)*, have been identified as targets of the ubiquitin pathway. Typically, the proapoptotic proteins have a shorter half-life and so display a more distinct elevation as a result of proteasome inhibition when any changes are noted. In leukemia cells, for example, proteasome inhibition caused the mitochondrial accumulation of Bik and apoptosis *(31)*, whereas, in HeLa cells, tBid stabilization preceding cytochrome c release has been reported following treatment *(95)*. Bcl-2 has been described as being cleaved by caspases following proteasome inhibition in MO7e cells *(96)*, which may explain its observed downregulation in MIA-PaCa-2 pancreatic cells *(97)*. Lactacystin-induced cell death in Ewing's sarcoma cells is sensitive to bcl-2 overexpression *(98)*, as was also the case when human myeloid leukemic cells were treated with PSI *(99)*.

5.4. Caspases

As the effectors of the decision to undergo apoptosis, caspase activity is frequently used as a measure of activation of the process. With rare exceptions *(100,101)*, proteasome inhibitor treatment of cell lines results in caspase or caspase-like activation, as indicated by the use of fluorigenic substrates or inhibitors *(27)*. Generally, most studies suggest that proteasome inhibitors act upstream of cytochrome c-mediated activation of initiator caspase 9 and subsequent effector caspase activity *(37)*. There are reports, however, of caspase 8, the death receptor-activated initiator caspase, being activated by lactacystin in adult T-cell leukemia *(102)* and human glioma cells *(37,103,104)*. In the latter case there is also an increase in Fas ligand surface protein and mRNA levels that may be due to the stabilization of c-Myc *(37,104)*. Thus, proteasome inhibitors may also promote apoptosis by upregulating death receptor-ligand interactions.

5.5. Cell Cycle Regulators

The cell cycle is highly susceptible to perturbations in proteasomal function, because many regulators of progression must be degraded by the complex with precise timing. The inappropriate accumulation of these components may trigger the death program, particularly in cells that exhibit unrestricted division. In a recent study, we showed that bortezomib inhibited docetaxel-induced apoptosis in human pancreatic cancer cells in vitro, effects that were linked to accumulation of p21 and p27 and inhibition of cdk2 and cdc2 (114).

This observation may be important for the optimization of combination therapy that includes proteasome inhibition. The cyclin-dependent kinase (CDK) inhibitors p21 and p27 function by binding to cyclin/CDK complexes and are both stabilized by proteasome inhibition (106). Although many reports suggest an antiapoptotic result of p21 and p27 overexpression, proapoptotic effects have also been reported (107). Proteasome inhibitor-induced death of tumor cells has correlated with the stabilization of both p21 (87) and p27 (106,108), but the contribution of these proteins to any observed effect is unclear.

5.6. ER Stress

A third major molecular pathway that has recently been implicated in proteasome inhibitor–induced apoptosis is endoplasmic reticular stress (ER stress) (115,116). The proteasome plays a central role in quality control in protein synthesis and turnover, mediating the degradation of the misfolded or damaged proteins produced in the course of normal cell function (116). Proteasome inhibition leads to an accumulation of these polypeptides, and if cytoprotective mechanisms are overwhelmed, it can lead to induction of apoptosis (117–119). Cells with high secretory capacity appear to be particularly vulnerable to this pathway of cell death (120), which may explain why multiple myeloma cells are particularly susceptible (119). In our own studies we have been investigating the role of ER stress in the induction of apoptosis in human pancreatic cancer cells because they too display high secretory function. Our results confirm that bortezomib induces apoptosis in some human pancreatic cancer cell lines via ER stress but that others are highly resistant (S. Nawrocki et al., manuscript submitted). Thus, identification of the cytoprotective mechanisms(s) in place in the resistant cells could provide molecular targets that could be exploited within the context of bortezomib-based combination therapy.

Recent studies of the molecular mechanisms involved in proteasome inhibitor–induced ER stress have demonstrated that the activation of Jun N-terminal kinase (JNK) is required for the response (119,121). We have obtained direct evidence that uncontrolled protein synthesis promotes JNK activation and cell death in pancreatic cancer cells (S. Nawrocki et al., manuscript submitted). Agents that induce ER stress typically shut down protein synthesis to prevent further accumulation of proteins that would exacerbate cytotoxicity. This is accomplished via phosphorylation of a translation initiation factor (eIF2α) on S51 via activation of pancreas ER kinase (PERK) and/or PKR (115). However, in pancreatic cancer cells bortezomib fails to induce PERK activation, eIF2α phosphorylation, or translational suppression. Thus, in this unique example of ER stress, the accumulation of misfolded and damaged proteins is accompanied by ongoing protein synthesis. We found that the protein synthesis inhibitor, cycloheximide, blocks JNK activation and apoptosis, consistent with this model. Conversely, bortezomib overrides eIF2α phosphorylation and promotes cell death stimulated by other agents (thapsigargin,

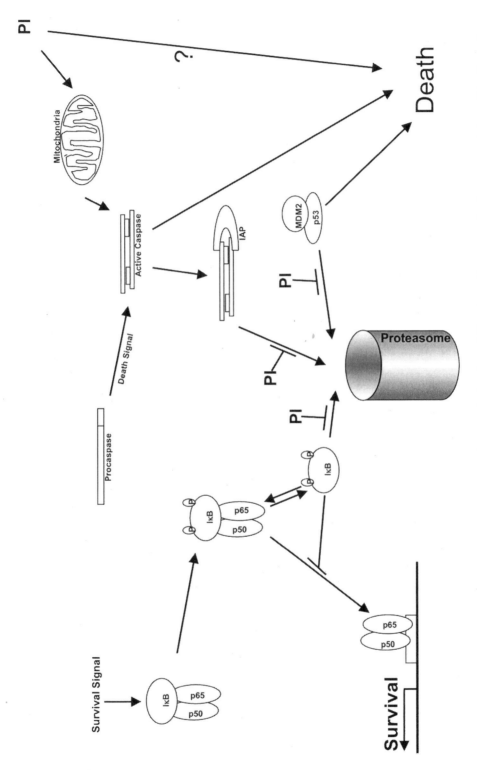

Fig. 2. The impact of proteasome inhibition on the apoptotic cascade. By the stabilization of known and unknown regulators of death, proteasome inhibition (**PI**) shifts the cell down the death pathway. IAP, inhibitor of apoptosis protein.

tunicamycin). We are currently exploring whether this effect of bortezomib can also be exploited in combination therapy.

6. SUMMARY AND CONCLUSIONS

Tissue homeostasis is the result of a balance between proliferation and the removal of cells. Part of the dysregulation process in cancer stems from genomic instability and includes the selection of characteristics that suppress a cell's tendency to initiate and complete the death signal. This is the reason for the importance of the apoptotic cascade in cancer progression and anticancer research.

The ubiquitin proteasome pathway is clearly involved modulating the apoptotic machinery. Figure 2 diagrams the points at which proteasome inhibition takes effect. The exact nature of the association and the reason for the opposing effects of proteasome inhibition observed between cell lines and primary cell cultures is unclear. It does appear, however, that the states of differentiation and proliferation weigh heavily on that decision. Such a difference in effect may be advantageous in the context of therapy in which toxic side effects place severe limits on a candidate agent. The stabilizing and activating of proapoptotic gene products such as Bcl-2 family members, p53, and the caspases contribute to the observed effects by shifting the overall state of the cell to an internal environment that will readily engage the apoptotic machinery. One should not ignore, however, the role of angiogenesis inhibition, with its indirect effect on the susceptibility of a tumor to apoptosis-inducing stress. The list of proteins relevant to the toxic effects of proteasome inhibitors on cancerous cells is far from complete and, although possessing great potential as a new class of chemotherapeutic agent, these drugs are also powerful analytical tools that will continue to further our understanding of apoptosis.

REFERENCES

1. Kerr JF, et al. Apoptosis: a basic biological phenomenon with wide-ranging implications in tissue kinetics. Br J Cancer 1972;26:239–257.
2. Wyllie AH, et al. Chromatin changes in apoptosis. Histochem J 1981;13:681–692.
3. Ellis HM, et al. Genetic control of programmed cell death in the nematode C. elegans. Cell 1986;44:817–829.
4. Conradt B, et al. The C. elegans protein EGL-1 is required for programmed cell death and interacts with the Bcl-2-like protein CED-9. Cell 1998;93:519–529.
5. Hengartner MO, et al. Caenorhabditis elegans gene ced-9 protects cells from programmed cell death. Nature 1992;356:494–499.
6. Xue D, et al. The Caenorhabditis elegans cell-death protein CED-3 is a cysteine protease with substrate specificities similar to those of the human CPP32 protease. Genes Dev 1996;10:1073–1083.
7. Xue D, et al. Caenorhabditis elegans CED-9 protein is a bifunctional cell-death inhibitor. Nature 1997;390:305–308.
8. Reed JC, et al. Oncogenic potential of bcl-2 demonstrated by gene transfer. Nature 1988;336:259–261.
9. McDonnell TJ, et al. bcl-2-immunoglobulin transgenic mice demonstrate extended B cell survival and follicular lymphoproliferation. Cell 1989;57:79–88.
10. Hockenbery D, et al. Bcl-2 is an inner mitochondrial membrane protein that blocks programmed cell death. Nature 1990;348:334–336.
11. Moul JW. Angiogenesis, p53, bcl-2 and Ki-67 in the progression of prostate cancer after radical prostatectomy. Eur Urol 1999;35:399–407.
12. Karin M, et al. NF-kappaB in cancer: from innocent bystander to major culprit. Nat Rev Cancer 2002;2:301–310.

13. Berenson JR, et al. The role of nuclear factor-kappaB in the biology and treatment of multiple myeloma. Semin Oncol 2001;28:626–633.

14. Rampino N, et al. Somatic frameshift mutations in the BAX gene in colon cancers of the microsatellite mutator phenotype. Science 1997;275:967–969.

15. Schwartz LM. Insect muscle as a model for programmed cell death. J Neurobiol 1992;23:1312–1326.

16. Jones ME, et al. Changes in the structure and function of the multicatalytic proteinase (proteasome) during programmed cell death in the intersegmental muscles of the hawkmoth, Manduca sexta. Dev Biol 1995;169:436–447.

17. Grimm LM, et al. Proteasomes play an essential role in thymocyte apoptosis. EMBO J 1996;15:3835–3844.

18. Grassilli E, et al. Inhibition of proteasome function prevents thymocyte apoptosis: involvement of ornithine decarboxylase. Biochem Biophys Res Commun 1998;250:293–297.

19. Stefanelli C, et al. Inhibition of etoposide-induced apoptosis with peptide aldehyde inhibitors of proteasome. Biochem J 1998;332:661–665.

20. Hirsch T, et al. Proteasome activation occurs at an early, premitochondrial step of thymocyte apoptosis. J Immunol 1998;161:35–40.

21. Dallaporta B, et al. Proteasome activation as a critical event of thymocyte apoptosis. Cell Death Differ 2000;7:368–373.

22. Sadoul R, et al. Involvement of the proteasome in the programmed cell death of NGF-deprived sympathetic neurons. EMBO J 1996;15:3845–3852.

23. Sadoul R, et al. Involvement of the proteasome in the programmed cell death of NGF-deprived sympathetic neurons. EMBO J 1996;15:3845–3852.

24. Imajoh-Ohmi S, et al. Lactacystin, a specific inhibitor of the proteasome, induces apoptosis in human monoblast U937 cells. Biochem Biophys Res Commun 1995;217:1070–1077.

25. Shinohara K, et al. Apoptosis induction resulting from proteasome inhibition. Biochem J 1996;317:385–388.

26. Tanimoto Y, et al. Peptidyl aldehyde inhibitors of proteasome induce apoptosis rapidly in mouse lymphoma RVC cells. J Biochem (Tokyo) 1997;121:542–549.

27. Drexler HC. Activation of the cell death program by inhibition of proteasome function. Proc Natl Acad Sci USA 1997;94:855–860.

28. Cui H, et al. Proteasome regulation of activation-induced T cell death. Proc Natl Acad Sci USA 1997;94:7515–7520.

29. Bertrand F, et al. A role for nuclear factor kappaB in the antiapoptotic function of insulin. J Biol Chem 1998;273:2931–2938.

30. Chang YC, et al. mdm2 and bax, downstream mediators of the p53 response, are degraded by the ubiquitin-proteasome pathway. Cell Growth Differ 1998;9:79–84.

31. Marshansky V, et al. Proteasomes modulate balance among proapoptotic and antiapoptotic Bcl-2 family members and compromise functioning of the electron transport chain in leukemic cells. J Immunol 2001;166:3130–3142.

32. You SA, et al. Potent antitumor agent proteasome inhibitors: a novel trigger for Bcl2 phosphorylation to induce apoptosis. Int J Oncol 1999;15:625–628.

33. Orlowski RZ, et al. Tumor growth inhibition induced in a murine model of human Burkitt's lymphoma by a proteasome inhibitor. Cancer Res 1998;58:4342–4348.

34. Soldatenkov VA, et al. Apoptosis of Ewing's sarcoma cells is accompanied by accumulation of ubiquitinated proteins. Cancer Res 1997;57:3881–3885.

35. Delic J, et al. The proteasome inhibitor lactacystin induces apoptosis and sensitizes chemo- and radioresistant human chronic lymphocytic leukaemia lymphocytes to TNF-alpha-initiated apoptosis. Br J Cancer 1998;77:1103–1107.

36. Masdehors P, et al. Increased sensitivity of CLL-derived lymphocytes to apoptotic death activation by the proteasome-specific inhibitor lactacystin. Br J Haematol 1999;105:752–757.

37. Almond JB, et al. Proteasome inhibitor-induced apoptosis of B-chronic lymphocytic leukaemia cells involves cytochrome c release and caspase activation, accompanied by formation of an approximately 700 kDa Apaf-1 containing apoptosome complex. Leukemia 2001;15:1388–1397.

38. Chandra J, et al. Proteasome inhibitors induce apoptosis in glucocorticoid-resistant chronic lymphocytic leukemic lymphocytes. Blood 1998;92:4220–4229.

39. Adams J, et al. Proteasome inhibitors: a novel class of potent and effective antitumor agents. Cancer Res 1999;59:2615–2622.

40. Teicher BA, et al. The proteasome inhibitor PS-341 in cancer therapy. Clin Cancer Res 1999;5:2638–2645.

41. An WG, et al. Protease inhibitor-induced apoptosis: accumulation of wt p53, p21WAF1/CIP1, and induction of apoptosis are independent markers of proteasome inhibition. Leukemia 2000;14:1276–1283.

42. Hideshima T, et al. The proteasome inhibitor PS-341 inhibits growth, induces apoptosis, and overcomes drug resistance in human multiple myeloma cells. Cancer Res 2001;61:3071–3076.

43. Adams J. Preclinical and clinical evaluation of proteasome inhibitor PS-341 for the treatment of cancer. Curr Opin Chem Biol 2002;6:493–500.

44. Russo SM, et al. Enhancement of radiosensitivity by proteasome inhibition: implications for a role of NF-kappaB. Int J Radiat Oncol Biol Phys 2001;50:183–193.

45. Cusack JC, Jr., et al. Enhanced chemosensitivity to CPT-11 with proteasome inhibitor PS-341: implications for systemic nuclear factor-kappaB inhibition. Cancer Res 2001;61:3535–3540.

46. Sunwoo JB, et al. Novel proteasome inhibitor PS-341 inhibits activation of nuclear factor-kappa B, cell survival, tumor growth, and angiogenesis in squamous cell carcinoma. Clin Cancer Res 2001;7:1419–1428.

47. Bold RJ, et al. Chemosensitization of pancreatic cancer by inhibition of the 26S proteasome. J Surg Res 2001;100:11–17.

48. Adams J, et al. Proteasome inhibitors: a novel class of potent and effective antitumor agents. Cancer Res 1999;59:2615–2622.

49. Shah SA, et al. 26S proteasome inhibition induces apoptosis and limits growth of human pancreatic cancer. J Cell Biochem 2001;82:110–122.

50. Lopes UG, et al. p53-dependent induction of apoptosis by proteasome inhibitors. J Biol Chem 1997;272:12893–12896.

51. Yang Y, et al. Ubiquitin protein ligase activity of IAPs and their degradation in proteasomes in response to apoptotic stimuli. Science 2000;288:874–877.

52. Suzuki Y, et al. Ubiquitin-protein ligase activity of X-linked inhibitor of apoptosis protein promotes proteasomal degradation of caspase-3 and enhances its anti-apoptotic effect in Fas-induced cell death. Proc Natl Acad Sci USA 2001;98:8662–8667.

53. Royds JA, et al. Response of tumour cells to hypoxia: role of p53 and NFkB. Mol Pathol 1998;51:55–61.

54. Palombella VJ, et al. The ubiquitin-proteasome pathway is required for processing the NF-kappa B1 precursor protein and the activation of NF-kappa B. Cell 1994;78:773–785.

55. Traenckner EB, et al. Appearance of apparently ubiquitin-conjugated I kappa B-alpha during its phosphorylation-induced degradation in intact cells. J Cell Sci Suppl 1995;19:79–84.

56. Traenckner EB, et al. A proteasome inhibitor prevents activation of NF-kappa B and stabilizes a newly phosphorylated form of I kappa B-alpha that is still bound to NF-kappa B. EMBO J 1994;13:5433–5441.

57. Jeremias I, et al. Inhibition of nuclear factor kappaB activation attenuates apoptosis resistance in lymphoid cells. Blood 1998;91:4624–4631.

58. Bellas RE, et al. Inhibition of NF-kappa B activity induces apoptosis in murine hepatocytes. Am J Pathol 1997;151:891–896.

59. Bancroft CC, et al. Effects of pharmacologic antagonists of epidermal growth factor receptor, PI3K and MEK signal kinases on NF-kappaB and AP-1 activation and IL-8 and VEGF expression in human head and neck squamous cell carcinoma lines. Int J Cancer 2002;99:538–548.

60. Huang S, et al. Blockade of nuclear factor-kappaB signaling inhibits angiogenesis and tumorigenicity of human ovarian cancer cells by suppressing expression of vascular endothelial growth factor and interleukin 8. Cancer Res 2000;60:5334–5339.

61. Huang S, et al. Blockade of NF-kappaB activity in human prostate cancer cells is associated with suppression of angiogenesis, invasion, and metastasis. Oncogene 2001;20:4188–4197.

62. Yoshida S, et al. Involvement of interleukin-8, vascular endothelial growth factor, and basic fibroblast growth factor in tumor necrosis factor alpha-dependent angiogenesis. Mol Cell Biol 1997;17:4015–4023.

63. Oikawa T, et al. The proteasome is involved in angiogenesis. Biochem Biophys Res Commun 1998;246:243-248.

64. Freedman DA, et al. Functions of the MDM2 oncoprotein. Cell Mol Life Sci 1999;55:96–107.

65. Shieh SY, et al. DNA damage-induced phosphorylation of p53 alleviates inhibition by MDM2. Cell 1997;91:325–334.

66. Siliciano JD, et al. DNA damage induces phosphorylation of the amino terminus of p53. Genes Dev 1997;11:3471–3481.

67. Koumenis C, et al. Regulation of p53 by hypoxia: dissociation of transcriptional repression and apoptosis from p53-dependent transactivation. Mol Cell Biol 2001;21:1297–1310.
68. Unger T, et al. Critical role for Ser20 of human p53 in the negative regulation of p53 by Mdm2. EMBO J 1999;18:1805–1814.
69. Sakaguchi K, et al. Phosphorylation of serine 392 stabilizes the tetramer formation of tumor suppressor protein p53. Biochemistry 1997;36:10117–10124.
70. Raycroft L, et al. Transcriptional activation by wild-type but not transforming mutants of the p53 anti-oncogene. Science 1990;249:1049–1051.
71. Gartel AL, et al. Transcriptional regulation of the p21 (WAF1/CIP1) gene. Exp Cell Res 1999;246:280–289.
72. Xiao G, et al. A DNA damage signal is required for p53 to activate gadd45. Cancer Res 2000;60:1711–1719.
73. Schuler M, et al. Mechanisms of p53-dependent apoptosis. Biochem Soc Trans 2001;29:684–688.
74. Muller M, et al. p53 activates the CD95 (APO-1/Fas) gene in response to DNA damage by anticancer drugs. J Exp Med 1998;188:2033–2045.
75. Miyashita T, et al. Identification of a p53-dependent negative response element in the bcl- 2 gene. Cancer Res 1994;54:3131–3135.
76. Sadot E, et al. Down-regulation of beta-catenin by activated p53. Mol Cell Biol 2001;21:6768–6781.
77. Bennett M, et al. Cell surface trafficking of Fas: a rapid mechanism of p53-mediated apoptosis. Science 1998;282:290–293.
78. Marchenko ND, et al. Death signal-induced localization of p53 protein to mitochondria. A potential role in apoptotic signaling. J Biol Chem 2000;275:16202–16212.
79. Sansome C, et al. Hypoxia death stimulus induces translocation of p53 protein to mitochondria. Detection by immunofluorescence on whole cells. FEBS Lett 2001;488:110–115.
80. Maki CG, et al. In vivo ubiquitination and proteasome-mediated degradation of p53 (1). Cancer Res 1996;56:2649–2654.
81. Kurland JF, et al. Protease inhibitors restore radiation-induced apoptosis to Bcl-2-expressing lymphoma cells. Int J Cancer 2001;96:327–333.
82. MacLaren AP, et al. p53-dependent apoptosis induced by proteasome inhibition in mammary epithelial cells. Cell Death Differ 2001;8:210–218.
83. Blagosklonny MV, et al. Proteasome-dependent regulation of p21WAF1/CIP1 expression. Biochem Biophys Res Commun 1996;227:564–569.
84. Chen F, et al. Role of p53 in cell cycle regulation and apoptosis following exposure to proteasome inhibitors. Cell Growth Differ 2000;11:239–246.
85. Kitagawa H, et al. Proteasome inhibitors induce mitochondria-independent apoptosis in human glioma cells. FEBS Lett 1999;443:181–186.
86. Wagenknecht B, et al. Proteasome inhibitors induce p53/p21-independent apoptosis in human glioma cells. Cell Physiol Biochem 1999;9:117–125.
87. Naujokat C, et al. Proteasome inhibitors induced caspase-dependent apoptosis and accumulation of p21WAF1/Cip1 in human immature leukemic cells. Eur J Haematol 2000;65:221–236.
88. Herrmann JL, et al. Prostate carcinoma cell death resulting from inhibition of proteasome activity is independent of functional Bcl-2 and p53. Oncogene 1998;17:2889–2899.
89. Pettaway CA, et al. Selection of highly metastatic variants of different human prostatic carcinomas using orthotopic implantation in nude mice. Clin Cancer Res 1996;2:1627–1636.
90. Schendel SL, et al. Channel formation by antiapoptotic protein Bcl-2. Proc Natl Acad Sci USA 1997;94:5113–5118.
91. Reed JC. Bcl-2 family proteins. Oncogene 1998;17:3225–3236.
92. Knudson CM, et al. Bcl-2 and Bax function independently to regulate cell death. Nat Genet 1997;16:358–363.
93. Dimmeler S, et al. Dephosphorylation targets Bcl-2 for ubiquitin-dependent degradation: a link between the apoptosome and the proteasome pathway. J Exp Med 1999;189:1815–1822.
94. Li B, et al. Bax degradation by the ubiquitin/proteasome-dependent pathway: involvement in tumor survival and progression. Proc Natl Acad Sci USA 2000;97:3850–3855.
95. Breitschopf K, et al. Ubiquitin-mediated degradation of the proapoptotic active form of bid. A functional consequence on apoptosis induction. J Biol Chem 2000;275:21648–21652.
96. Zhang XM, et al. Inhibition of ubiquitin-proteasome pathway activates a caspase-3-like protease and induces Bcl-2 cleavage in human M-07e leukaemic cells. Biochem J 1999;340:127–133.

97. Bold RJ, et al. Chemosensitization of pancreatic cancer by inhibition of the 26S proteasome. J Surg Res 2001;100:11–17.
98. Soldatenkov VA, et al. Apoptosis of Ewing's sarcoma cells is accompanied by accumulation of ubiquitinated proteins. Cancer Res 1997;57:3881–3885.
99. Soligo D, et al. The apoptogenic response of human myeloid leukaemia cell lines and of normal and malignant haematopoietic progenitor cells to the proteasome inhibitor PSI. Br J Haematol 2001;113:126–135.
100. Fujita E, et al. Enhancement of CPP32-like activity in the TNF-treated U937 cells by the proteasome inhibitors. Biochem Biophys Res Commun 1996;224:74–79.
101. Monney L, et al. Defects in the ubiquitin pathway induce caspase-independent apoptosis blocked by Bcl-2. J Biol Chem 1998;273:6121–6131.
102. Yamada Y, et al. Lactacystin activates FLICE (caspase 8) protease and induces apoptosis in Fas-resistant adult T-cell leukemia cell lines. Eur J Haematol 2000;64:315–322.
103. Wagenknecht B, et al. Proteasome inhibitor-induced apoptosis of glioma cells involves the processing of multiple caspases and cytochrome c release. J Neurochem 2000;75:2288–2297.
104. Tani E, et al. Proteasome inhibitors induce Fas-mediated apoptosis by c-Myc accumulation and subsequent induction of FasL message in human glioma cells. FEBS Lett 2001;504:53–58.
105. Wang TH, et al. Paclitaxel-induced cell death: where the cell cycle and apoptosis come together. Cancer 2000;88:2619–2628.
106. Pagano M, et al. Role of the ubiquitin-proteasome pathway in regulating abundance of the cyclin-dependent kinase inhibitor p27. Science 1995;269:682–685.
107. Roninson IB. Oncogenic functions of tumour suppressor p21 (Waf1/Cip1/Sdi1): association with cell senescence and tumour-promoting activities of stromal fibroblasts. Cancer Lett 2002;179:1–14.
108. Kudo Y, et al. p27Kip1 accumulation by inhibition of proteasome function induces apoptosis in oral squamous cell carcinoma cells. Clin Cancer Res 2000;6:916–923.
109. Nawrocki ST, et al. Effects of the proteasome inhibitor PS-341 on apoptosis and angiogenesis in orthotopic human pancreatic tumor xenografts. Mol Cancer Ther 2002;1:1243–1253.
110. William S, Pettaway C, Song R, Papandreou C, Logothetis C, and McConkey DJ. Differential effects of the proteasome inhibitor bortezomib on apoptosis and angiogenesis in human prostate tumor xenografts. Mol Cancer Ther 2003;2:835–843.
111. Kamat AM, et al. The proteasome inhibitor bortezomib synergizes with gemcitabine to block the growth of human 253JB-V bladder tumors in vivo. Mol Cancer Ther 2004;3:279–290.
112. Pahler JC, et al. Effects of the proteasome inhibitor, bortezomib, on apoptosis in isolated lymphocytes obtained from patients with chronic lymphocytic leukemia. Clin Cancer Res. 2003;9:4570–4577.
113. Williams SA, McConkey DJ. The proteasome inhibitor bortezomib stabilizes a novel active form of p53 in human LNCaP-Pro5 prostate cancer cells. Cancer Res 2003;63:7338–7344.
114. Nawrocki ST, et al. The proteasome inhibitor bortezomib enhances the activity of docetaxel in orthotopic human pancreatic tumor xenografts. Mol Cancer Ther 2004;3:59–70.
115. Kaufman RJ. Stress signaling from the lumen of the endoplasmic reticulum: coordination of gene transcriptional and translational controls. Genes Dev 1999;13:1211–1233.
116. Kaufman RJ. Orchestrating the unfolded protein response in health and disease. J Clin Invest 2002;110:1389–1398.
117. Hightower LE. Heat shock, stress proteins, chaperones, and proteotoxicity. Cell 1991;66:191–197.
118. Lee AH, et al. Proteasome inhibitors disrupt the unfolded protein response in myeloma cells. Proc Natl Acad Sci USA 2003;100:9946–9951.
119. Hideshima T, et al. Molecular mechanisms mediating antimyeloma activity of proteasome inhibitor PS-341. Blood 2003;101:1530–1534.
120. Ellgaard L, Helenius A. Quality control in the endoplasmic reticulum. Nat Rev Mol Cell Bio 2003;4:181–191.
121. Chauhan D, et al. JNK-dependent release of mitochondrial protein, Smac, during apoptosis in multiple myeloma (MM) cells. J Biol Chem 2003;278;17593–17596.

8 The Proteasome and the COMPARE Algorithm

Susan L. Holbeck and Edward A. Sausville

CONTENTS

ABSTRACT

A series of peptidic boronic acids that inhibit the activity of the proteasome were screened by the NCI for activity against a panel of 60 human tumor cell lines. Comparison to data from approx 80,000 other compounds demonstrated that these proteasome inhibitors exhibited a novel pattern of growth inhibition against these cell lines. The potency of these compounds in the cell line screen correlated well with activity against purified proteasomes, indicating that proteasome inhibition was likely causing the growth inhibition. Comparison of bortezomib (formerly known as PS-341) sensitivity to expression levels of thousand of molecular targets within the 60 cell line panel did not yield strong correlations with any single molecular target, consistent with the role of the proteasome in degradation of a multitude of proteins.

KEY WORDS

Proteasome; NCI COMPARE; correlation; molecular target.

1. INTRODUCTION

A potential role for proteasome inhibitors in cancer treatment has generated much interest. Proteasomal degradation regulates proteins that control the cell cycle, as well as those that are involved in signal transduction, control of transcription, and apoptosis. Polyubiquitinylation of proteins serves as a marker to target a protein to the 26S

From: *Cancer Drug Discovery and Development: Proteasome Inhibitors in Cancer Therapy*
Edited by: J. Adams © Humana Press Inc., Totowa, NJ

proteasome, where it is degraded in an ATP-dependent manner. The 20S central core of the proteasome has multiple proteolytic activities—chymotryptic, tryptic, and postglutamyl peptide hydrolytic *(1)*. This chapter reviews the role that the computational resources developed at the Developmental Therapeutics Program (DTP) of the National Cancer Institute (NCI) had in the initial characterization of one agent, bortezomib (Velcade®; formerly known as PS-341), which inhibits the chymotryptic activity of the proteasome *(2)*. Although we focus on this one agent, the use of these resources is applicable to the development of many other classes of compounds.

2. DEVELOPMENT OF THE COMPARE ALGORITHM

For more than a decade the DTP has conducted a screening program for potential anticancer drugs, testing more than 82,000 compounds for their ability to inhibit the growth of, or to kill, a panel of 60 human tumor cell lines *(3,4)*. These lines represent nine different tissues of origin. Each compound is tested over a 10,000-fold concentration range in a 2-d assay (described in detail at http://dtp.nci.nih.gov/branches/btb/ivclsp.html). Several endpoints are calculated—GI_{50} (50% growth inhibition, relative to no compound), TGI (total growth inhibition), and LC_{50} (50% lethality). Paull et al. *(5)* developed the Mean Graph, which displays the results of a particular endpoint for a given cell line relative to the mean of that endpoint across all the cell lines. This is a convenient way of displaying 60 cell line screening data. The Mean Graph simplifies the 60 dose–response curves into a format in which one can see at a glance which cell lines are more sensitive to a given compound. A Mean Graph for bortezomib (identified in the NCI-DTP database as NSC 681239) is shown in Fig. 1. From this display, it is readily apparent that certain cell lines (including the melanoma lines) are more sensitive, whereas others (e.g., the ovarian line SV-OV-3) are less responsive.

Paull et al. *(5)* noted that compounds with similar mechanisms of action tended to yield similar Mean Graphs across the 60 cell lines. The COMPARE algorithm was developed as a means of quantifying the relatedness of these Mean Graph patterns for compounds of interest. COMPARE evaluates the difference from the mean for each cell line at a compound/endpoint combination, and this Mean Graph pattern for a "seed" compound is compared quantitatively with all other Mean Graph patterns available. The algorithm calculates a Pearson correlation coefficient (PCC) for the relatedness of different Mean Graph patterns. A list of correlating compounds is generated, sorted by PCC. While not all compounds with high PCCs will be mechanistically related, this algorithm has been used successfully to suggest possible mechanisms of action for many novel compounds, including novel tubulin-interacting agents *(6–8)*, a new class of cyclin-dependent kinase inhibitors *(9)*, and novel antimetabolites *(10,11)*. As an example, many different structural classes of tubulin binders have been identified—some stabilize microtubules and others destabilize microtubules. Nevertheless, the 60 cell line panel responds to tubulin perturbation in a similar way, with paclitaxel (Taxol®) and colchicine showing a PCC of 0.7.

3. BORTEZOMIB IN THE NCI 60 CELL LINE SCREEN

If one has a novel compound, with either a known or unknown mechanism of action, one can run COMPARE with that compound as a "seed" and find compounds in the database that have the most similar behavior in the 60 cell line screen. In 1995, bortezomib and other related peptidic boronic acids were submitted to the NCI-DTP for 60 cell line

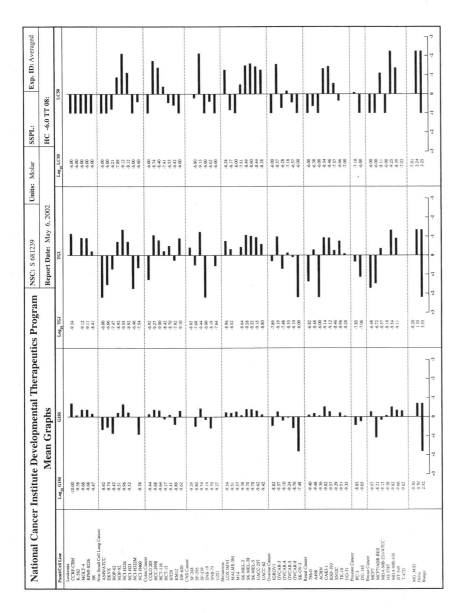

Fig. 1. A Mean Graph display of NCI 60 cell line screening data for bortezomib (NSC 681239). Dose-response data were used to calculate three endpoints for each cell line—GI$_{50}$ (the log$_{10}$ of the concentration that caused 50% growth inhibition), TGI (the log$_{10}$ of the concentration that caused total growth inhibition), and LC$_{50}$ (the log$_{10}$ of the concentration that caused 50% lethality). For each endpoint the mean across all the cell lines was calculated. The GI$_{50}$ data are graphed as the difference of the GI$_{50}$ for a particular cell line from the mean GI$_{50}$. Cell lines that are more sensitive are represented as bars deflecting to the right of the mean, and less sensitive cell lines project to the left of the mean. TGI and LC$_{50}$ Mean Graphs are generated in a similar fashion.

testing. The compounds showed quite potent activity in the screen. For bortezomib, the mean GI_{50} (4 nM) was lower than 99.8% of compounds that had been through the screen. In addition to its potent activity, COMPARE revealed that bortezomib and related compounds had a pattern of activity that was dissimilar to any seen before. However, the peptidic boronic acids correlated extremely well with one another (PCCs ranging up to 0.78), indicating that these related compounds were perturbing the cell lines in a similar manner to one another. The mean GI_{50} (across all 60 cell lines) correlated quite well with the IC_{50} (mean inhibitory concentration) of the compounds against purified proteasomes ($r^2 = 0.92$, ideal being 1.0), supporting the view that inhibition of the proteasome was responsible for the growth inhibition observed in the cell lines *(12)*. The mean TGI and LC_{50} also correlated well with the IC_{50} ($r^2 = 0.88$). Bortezomib showed a modest correlation (PCC of 0.48 at the LC_{50} endpoint) with another proteasome inhibitor, aclacinomycin A *(13)*, which also has DNA-binding activity. It did not correlate well with the activity of other (nonproteasome) protease inhibitors. Clustering of GI_{50} data for 2753 compounds of known mechanism of action (using either hierarchical or K-means clustering) groups bortezomib in a cluster containing only other peptidic boronic acids.

Interestingly, bortezomib was primarily cytostatic in the leukemia cell lines. At concentrations between 10^{-9} M and 10^{-4} M, cell growth was completely blocked in all the leukemia lines, with little loss of viable cells observed in the 2-d assay. In contrast, many of the cell lines derived from solid tumors showed virtually complete loss of viable cells at concentrations less than 10^{-8}–10^{-7} when treated with this agent (Fig. 2).

In the case of the proteasome inhibitors, as well as other classes of compounds, knowing what the target of the compound is does not reveal why it inhibits the growth of tumor cells. The proteasome degrades a very large number of proteins, including cell cycle-regulated proteins. Tumor growth could be disrupted by a global failure to degrade numerous proteins. Alternatively, there could be a small number of proteins whose degradation is crucial to tumor cell survival, and it would be the persistence of these proteins that would be toxic. A current clinical focus is the role of the proteasome in activation of nuclear factor-κB (NF–κB), by degradation of the inhibitor IκB *(14)*.

4. COMPARE AND MOLECULAR TARGETS

One can also use the COMPARE algorithm to attempt to identify molecular targets that may contribute to the action of a compound. For a number of years, the DTP has been coordinating the measurements of various molecular targets in the 60 cell line screen, *molecular targets* being defined in this context as any molecular entity (e.g., mRNA, protein levels, enzyme activity, mutation status, phosphorylation of a certain protein, and so on) that can be measured in the 60 cell line panel. Data are publicly available for 348 individually measured molecular targets (available at http://dtp.nci.nih.gov/mtargets/ mt_index.html), as well as data from microarray experiments *(15,16)*. With this information in hand, one can then ask whether the baseline levels of a molecular target can predict the sensitivity of a particular cell line to a given agent. Just as for compounds, molecular target data can be drawn as a Mean Graph. One defines the "average" expression of a target and displays individual cell line data as deviations from the mean. As COMPARE can assess the degree of similarity of the Mean Graph patterns of compounds, so can it determine whether these patterns are similar for a molecular target and a compound. Positive correlations occur when cells with higher levels of the molecular target tend to

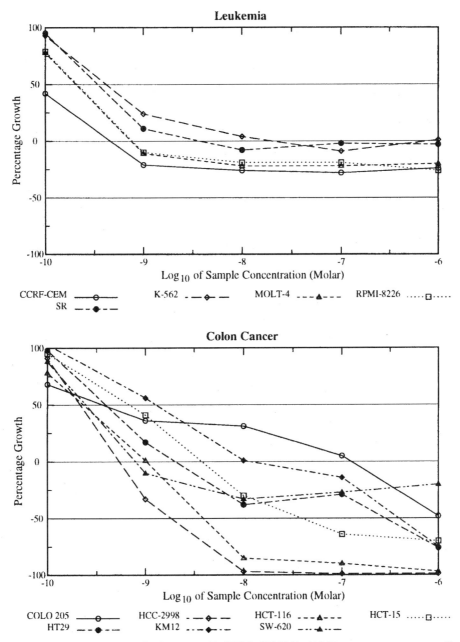

Fig. 2. Dose-response curves for bortezomib (NSC 681239). **(A)** Dose-response curves for the leukemia cell lines. These growth of these cell lines was completely inhibited at all the concentrations tested (from 10^{-10} to $10^{-6}\,M$), yet bortezomib (PS-341) was only modestly toxic to the leukemia cell lines at four of these doses. **(B)** Colon tumor cell lines tested in the same dose range. In contrast to the leukemia cell lines, most of the colon tumor cell lines showed significant lethality at the highest doses (10^{-7} and $10^{-6}\,M$).

exhibit greater sensitivity to a compound. When comparing compounds with other compounds, one is generally most interested in finding compounds that are most similar to the seed. When comparing compounds with molecular targets, it is often useful to look for negative as well positive correlations. Negative correlations are instances in which cells with lower levels of the target are more sensitive (or stated differently, those cells with higher levels tend to be more resistant).

Correlations between compound activity and molecular targets in the 60 cell line screen can provide hints as to various types of cellular processes that influence compound sensitivity. One may get clues as to molecules that influence uptake or efflux of compound. Measurement of the activity of P-glycoprotein (Pgp), a drug efflux pump, gives quite high negative correlations with compounds that are substrates for this pump—cells with higher levels of Pgp activity tend to be resistant to these compounds *(17–19)*. Conversely, one might also expect that if a compound requires a particular receptor or channel to enter the cell, then cell lines with higher levels of the receptor would have greater sensitivity to that compound.

Drugs may be activated or inactivated by cellular enzymes. COMPARE may help identify such enzymes. The enzyme DT-diaphorase activates a number of compounds, and known substrates of this enzyme show strong positive correlations in the 60 cell screen with DT-diaphorase activity *(20)*. By contrast, one would expect enzymes that degrade or inactivate a compound to show negative correlations.

Both Pgp and DT-diaphorase give very strong correlations with their substrates, indicating that these molecular targets are major determinants of cellular sensitivity to compounds on which they act. Both of these targets have a direct influence on the intracellular level of the active compound. In contrast, for many agents one might expect that multiple molecular targets might influence cellular response. In these cases, levels of a given molecular target would generate less impressive correlations; however, one might see modest correlations with multiple molecular targets in a given cellular pathway.

Several groups have identified novel inhibitors of specific pathways by screening compounds that correlated with levels of relevant molecular targets. Kubo et al. *(21)* identified a novel cyclin-dependent kinase inhibitor among compounds that correlated with their determination of alterations of the *p16INK4* gene. Wosikowski et al. *(22)* identified 14 compounds that inhibited the epidermal growth factor receptor (EGFR) or ErbB2 pathways by testing 20 compounds that correlated with RNA levels of the EGFR and ERBB2 genes. EGFR status was identified as a determinant of cell line sensitivity to a transforming growth factor-α (TGF-α) fusion protein toxin *(23)*. Higher levels of cellular metallothionein were demonstrated to correlate with resistance to several heavy metal-containing compounds *(24)*.

5. BORTEZOMIB AND DTP MOLECULAR TARGETS

COMPARE analysis of bortezomib against the DTP molecular targets and NCI60 Microarray databases did not reveal any striking correlations with a single molecular target. This is not surprising, given the large number of proteins involved in the function of the proteasome pathway, as well as the large number of substrates for proteasomal degradation. It seems unlikely that a single molecular target controls sensitivity of cells to this agent, rather, expression of multiple targets may together influence whether a cell responds to proteasome inhibition.

There were no significant correlations between expression of any of the proteasomal subunit genes and sensitivity to bortezomib. Of the genes encoding proteins involved in conjugation of ubiquitin to proteins, CUL1 [encoding cullin 1, a component of the Skp1, cullin, and F-box (SCF β-TrCP) complex that provides specificity to ubiquitin-conjugating enzymes] and CUL4A gave modest correlations with bortezomib sensitivity (PCCs of 0.38 and 0.43, respectively). Cells with higher levels of cullin mRNA expression tended to be more sensitive to bortezomib. Cullin 1 is associated with phosphorylated IκBα, an inhibitor of NF-κB that is regulated by proteasomal degradation *(25,26)*. Cullin 4A is reported to regulate DDB2, which is involved in repair of DNA damaged by ultraviolet light *(27)*. Of the genes encoding ubiquitin-specific proteases, which remove ubiquitin from proteins, USP4 showed a significant correlation (PCC of 0.53), with cells expressing higher levels of this gene showing greater sensitivity. Overexpression of the murine homolog of USP4 is tumorigenic *(28)*. Levels of several proteins subject to proteasomal degradation showed correlations with bortezomib sensitivity in the 60 cell line panel. Cell lines with lower levels of ErbB2 and EGFR proteins tended to be more sensitive (PCCs of –0.53 and –0.40, respectively).

6. CONCLUSIONS

Agents that inhibit the activity of the proteasome have a unique pattern of activity in the NCI's 60 human tumor cell line panel. Testing of multiple peptidic boronic acids in the 60 cell line screen demonstrated that those analogs that were more effective at inhibiting the activity of purified proteasomes also showed greater potency in their ability to inhibit the growth of tumor cells. Of this series of proteasome inhibitors, bortezomib was highly potent, in terms of both cell line activity and proteasome inhibition. The in vitro data from the cell line screen provided valuable information supporting bortezomib as a lead compound. Further testing using the NCI hollow fiber assay *(29)* demonstrated that bortezomib also had activity in vivo.

The NCI provides the 60 human tumor cell line screen as a free service available to academic researchers, as well as to companies of any size. Information on submitting a compound to the screen can be found at http://dtp.nci.nih.gov. Data obtained from the cell line screen can be used to guide selection of a lead compound. For compounds of unknown mechanism, use of the COMPARE algorithm may suggest possible mechanisms of action, which can be used to develop hypotheses that can be tested in laboratory experiments. Even if a compound shows no strong correlations to compounds of known mechanism, one may still be able to glean information on processes affected by the compound. Running COMPARE against the molecular targets and NCI60 Microarray databases may identify correlations with targets in a particular pathway or with targets that modulate the amount of active compound available within the cell. This may allow the generation of hypotheses that can be verified or refuted experimentally. If there are no data available on a molecular target of interest, researchers may collaborate with the NCI to evaluate this target in the 60 cell line panel. All the NCI-DTP data can be downloaded, or explored using DTP software freely available at http://dtp.nci.nih.gov/.

REFERENCES

1. Kopp F, et al. Subunit arrangement in the human 20S proteasome. *Proc Natl Acad Sci USA* 1997;94:2939–2944.

2. Lightcap ES, et al. Proteasome inhibition measurements: clinical application. *Clin Chem* 2000;46:673–683.
3. Alley MC, et al. Feasibility of drug screening with panels of human tumor cell lines using a microculture tetrazolium assay. *Cancer Res* 1988;48:589–601.
4. Monks A, et al. Feasibility of a high-flux anticancer drug screen using a diverse panel of cultured human tumor cell lines. *J Natl Cancer Inst* 1991;83:757–766.
5. Paull KD, et al. Display and analysis of patterns of differential activity of drugs against human tumor cell lines: development of mean graph and COMPARE algorithm. *J Natl Cancer Inst* 1989;81:1088–1092.
6. Paull KD, et al. Identification of novel antimitotic agents acting at the tubulin level by computer-assisted evaluation of differential cytotoxicity data. *Cancer Res* 1992;52:3892–900.
7. Bai RL, et al. Halichondrin B and homohalichondrin B, marine natural products binding in the vinca domain of tubulin. Discovery of tubulin-based mechanism of action by analysis of differential cytotoxicity data. *J Biol Chem* 1991;266:15882–158829.
8. Hamel E, et al. Antitumor 2,3-dihydro-2-(aryl)-4(1H)-quinazolinone derivatives. Interactions with tubulin. *Biochem Pharmacol* 1996;51:53–59.
9. Zaharevitz DW, et al. Discovery and initial characterization of the paullones, a novel class of small-molecule inhibitors of cyclin-dependent kinases. *Cancer Res* 1999;59:2566–2569.
10. Cleaveland ES, et al. Identification of a novel inhibitor (NSC 665564) of dihydroorotate dehydrogenase with a potency equivalent to brequinar. *Biochem Biophys Res Commun* 1996;223:654–659.
11. Cleaveland ES, et al. Site of action of two novel pyrimidine biosynthesis inhibitors accurately predicted by the compare program. *Biochem Pharmacol* 1995;49:947–954.
12. Adams J, et al. Proteasome inhibitors: a novel class of potent and effective antitumor agents. *Cancer Res* 1999;59:2615–2622.
13. Figueiredo-Pereira ME, et al. The antitumor drug aclacinomycin A, which inhibits the degradation of ubiquitinated proteins, shows selectivity for the chymotrypsin-like activity of the bovine pituitary 20 S proteasome. *J Biol Chem* 1996;271:16455–16459.
14. Sunwoo JB, et al. Novel proteasome inhibitor PS-341 inhibits activation of nuclear factor-kappa B, cell survival, tumor growth, and angiogenesis in squamous cell carcinoma. *Clin Cancer Res* 2001;7:1419–1428.
15. Scherf U, et al. A gene expression database for the molecular pharmacology of cancer. *Nat Genet* 2000;24:236–244.
16. Ross DT, et al. Systematic variation in gene expression patterns in human cancer cell lines. *Nat Genet* 2000;24:227–235.
17. Alvarez M, et al Using the National Cancer Institute anticancer drug screen to assess the effect of MRP expression on drug sensitivity profiles. *Mol Pharmacol* 1998;54:802–814.
18. Alvarez M, et al. Generation of a drug resistance profile by quantitation of mdr-1/P-glycoprotein in the cell lines of the National Cancer Institute Anticancer drug screen. *J Clin Invest* 1995;95:2205–2214.
19. Lee JS, et al. Rhodamine efflux patterns predict P-glycoprotein substrates in the National Cancer Institute drug screen. *Mol Pharmacol* 1994;46:627–638.
20. Fitzsimmons SA, et al. Reductase enzyme expression across the National Cancer Institute tumor cell line panel: correlation with sensitivity to mitomycin C and EO9. *J Natl Cancer Inst* 1996;88:259–269.
21. Kubo A, et al. The p16 status of tumor cell lines identifies small molecule inhibitors specific for cyclin-dependent kinase 4. *Clin Cancer Res* 1999;5:4279–4286.
22. Wosikowski K, et al. Identification of epidermal growth factor receptor and c-erbB2 pathway inhibitors by correlation with gene expression patterns. *J Natl Cancer Inst* 1997;89:1505–1515.
23. Chandler LA, et al. Targeting tumor cells via EGF receptors: selective toxicity of an HBEGF-toxin fusion protein. *Int J Cancer* 1998;78:106–111.
24. Woo ES, et al. Diversity of metallothionein content and subcellular localization in the National Cancer Institute tumor panel. *Cancer Chemother Pharmacol* 1997;41:61–68.
25. Suzuki H, et al. IkappaBalpha ubiquitination is catalyzed by an SCF-like complex containing Skp1, cullin-1, and two F-box/WD40-repeat proteins, betaTrCP1 and betaTrCP2. *Biochem Biophys Res Commun* 1999;256:127–132.
26. Suzuki H, et al. Identification of a novel 300-kDa factor termed IkappaB alphaE3-F1 that is required for ubiquitinylation of IkappaB alpha. *FEBS Lett* 1999;458:343–348.
27. Nag A, et al. The xeroderma pigmentosum group E gene product DDB2 is a specific target of cullin 4A in mammalian cells. *Mol Cell Biol* 2001;21:6738–6747.

28. Gilchrist CA, et al. Characterization of the ubiquitin-specific protease activity of the mouse/human Unp/
    Unph oncoprotein. *Biochim Biophys Acta* 2000;1481:297–309.
29. Hollingshead MG, et al. *In vivo* cultivation of tumor cells in hollow fibers. *Life Sci* 1995;57:131–141.

III   RATIONALE FOR PROTEASOME INHIBITORS IN CANCER

9 The Proteasome in Cancer Biology and Therapy

Frank Pajonk and William H. McBride

CONTENTS

1. INTRODUCTION

A perfect cancer treatment in a world of perfectly treatable cancers would target only the unique features of malignant cells and leave normal cells untouched. In the real world of real cancers, cancer-specific alterations of common pathways have been identified that can offer opportunities for the development of targeted drugs. A recent successful example is STI 571, which has been used to target the deregulated tyrosine-kinase bcr-abl in chronic myelogenous leukemia (CML) *(1)*. This is recognized as a key translocation in this disease. Unfortunately, most cancers have many mutations *(2)*, and several molecules may have to be targeted for success. Furthermore, recent data provide strong evidence that this process is not exclusively determined by mutations of the genome but is also driven by the tumor microenvironment and that, in principle, the process is reversible *(3)*.

A key regulator of many molecular pathways in eukaryotic cells is the ubiquitin/26S proteasome system *(4)*. It has the potential to take a unique position as a master controller that integrates multiple physiologic signals in a cell, and its interaction with pathways that are abnormal in cancer is an area of growing interest *(5)*. Cancers and rapidly growing embryonic cells generally have higher levels of proteasome activity than their normal well-differentiated counterparts *(6–9)*. The reason for this is unknown, but it may relate to the needs of rapidly proliferating cells, or to higher levels of oxidative stress, or to cytokines and growth factors. Proteasome structure and function appears to depend on the demands put on the cell and can be modulated by many factors. For example, the cytokines interferon-γ (IFN-γ) *(10)* and tumor necrosis factor-α (TNF-α) *(11)* affect proteasome structure as well as function, and we have evidence suggesting that autocrine interleukin-

From: *Cancer Drug Discovery and Development: Proteasome Inhibitors in Cancer Therapy*
Edited by: J. Adams © Humana Press Inc., Totowa, NJ

3 (IL-3) production by cancer cells increases proteasome activity (McBride et al., in press). Autocrine loops involving growth factors and their receptors, which are frequently overexpressed in cancer, may therefore drive alterations in proteasome structure and function. In addition, the proinflammatory tumor environment contains high levels of growth factors that might act through paracrine action to affect proteasomes. Also, hypoxia/reperfusion within the tumor microenvironment is known to affect the distribution and function of proteasomes (12). Differences in proteasomes between cancer and normal cells suggest that they may serve as a promising target for cancer therapy (13).

2. RESPONSE OF THE PROTEASOME TO HEAT, RADIATION, AND OXIDATIVE STRESS

The plasticity and heterogeneity expressed by cells with respect to proteasome structures and functions can be nicely seen in their response to oxidative stress. Cells use reactive oxygen and nitroxide species for many important physiologic processes. One result is damage to proteins that then have to be removed by proteolysis, since they are toxic. This is achieved mainly through degradation by non-ATP-dependent proteasomes. Oxidatively modified proteins increase with age and in certain pathologic conditions and this been ascribed to decreased proteasome function (14,15). One manifestation of protein accumulation is formation of aggresomes, the main components of which are misfolded proteins, ubiquitins, proteasomes, and heat shock proteins (especially hsp70 and hsp90). Cells appear to attempt to protect themselves from toxic intracellular protein overload by activating stress kinases (16,17) and increasing expression of cytosolic heat shock proteins, which is associated with acquisition of thermal tolerance (18). A number of disease states have as their hallmark accumulation of ubiquitinylated proteins, especially neurodegenerative diseases, such as Parkinson's (19), Alzheimer's (20), and Huntington's disease (21), as well as Angelman's syndrome (19,22).

The ubiquitin–proteasome system is itself sensitive to oxidative stress (14,23). Treatment with hydrogen peroxide has shown that the ATP-dependent 26S proteasome pathway is more sensitive than the ATP- and ubiquitin-independent 20S pathway (24–27). This suggests a division of labor between the 20S and 26S proteasomes in response to oxidative stress that allows the 26S proteasome to slow down degradation of ubiquitinylated proteins that might activate pathways leading to appropriate cellular responses without compromising the need to remove potentially cytotoxic nonfunctional proteins, which is performed independently. Our evidence indicates that N-acetyl-L-cysteine (28), tempol, and glutathione (Pervan, unpublished data) treatment inhibits proteasome function, suggesting that the proteasome may be a prime sensor of redox changes in the cell.

Proteasome function is also affected by hyperthermia treatment. Heating cultured myotubes increased the degradation of short- and long-lived proteins through the proteasome, with a maximal effect at 41°C (29). On the other hand, others have shown that heat shock impairs proteasome activity (18,30). Kuckelkorn and colleagues (31) suggest that 1 h at 44°C "locks" 20S proteasomes in their inactive state and does not allow de novo proteasome maturation or further activation of the 26S proteasome by ATP. They also showed that heat leads to a rapid intracellular redistribution of proteasomes. Our data, in contrast, show that heat exposure may preferentially inhibit 26S proteasome function in prostate cancer lines and that heat-induced impairment of proteasome function could be prevented by induction of immunoproteasomes using IFN-γ (Pajonk et al., in press). Variation in the responses of different cells to heat shock are well known, and some of this variation may be due to the presence and induction of varying levels of different types of heat shock proteins. The inhibition of proteasome function experienced by cells following heat exposure could also be responsible for the ability of hyperthermia to inhibit DNA repair processes when administered shortly before ionizing radiation *(32)*.

Recently, we showed that ionizing radiation had a rapid inhibitory effect on proteasome function in a variety of cell types, as assessed by degradation of specific fluorogenic substrates *(33,34)*. The inhibitory effect on proteasome activity that is achieved with exposure to ionizing radiation is not as complete as it is with drugs that directly target proteasomal enzymatic activity, but in many cell lines a 40–50% impairment in chymotrypsin-like activity was found within 15 min of exposure to doses as low as 5 cGy, and over a wide dose range up to 20 Gy. Because the proteasome is involved in DNA repair, cell-cycle arrest, and cell death, these findings have potential implications with respect to radiation-induced cellular responses, which in many respects mimic those of proteasome inhibitors.

Most of the radiation-induced impairment of proteasome function was associated with 26S activity, with minor effects on 20S activity, suggesting that the 19S regulatory subunit was the main target for radiation. Bulteau et al. *(35)* have shown similar rapid impairment of 26S proteasome function after exposure of human keratinocytes to ultraviolet (UV)-A and UV-B radiation. The inhibition following UV radiation became progressively greater with time, unlike that following ionizing radiation, which recovered to a large extent over a 24-h period of culture (Pajonk, unpublished data).

One possible explanation for impairment of proteasome function following exposure to radiation, heat, or oxidative stress is an increase in expression levels of endogenous inhibitors of proteasome activity. hsp90 *(36)* and PI31 *(37)* have been shown to inhibit proteasome function, as have other undefined factors found in low-molecular-weight cytosolic extracts (Pajonk, unpublished data). We have failed to detect any change in the level of endogenous inhibitors following irradiation, as measured in proteasome function assays with fluorogenic substrates. Also, although treatment of cells with geldanamycin, the hsp90 antagonist, increased proteasome function, the inhibitory effects of ionizing irradiation were still observed in the presence of the drug *(33)*, suggesting that hsp90 was not responsible. Bulteau et al. *(35)* provided evidence that extracts of UV-irradiated keratinocytes, including 4-hydroxy-2-nonenal modified proteins, inhibited degradation by the proteasome, but it is possible that the mechanism will vary with the type of radiation, and perhaps also the dose and (therefore) the extent of protein damage.

An alternative hypothesis for radiation-induced proteasome impairment is free radical damage to proteasome-associated molecules. Evidence for a direct effect of radiation was obtained using purified proteasomes, which impaired functional activity to an extent similar to that achieved by irradiation of whole cells *(33)*. The suggestion is that the 26S proteasome, or molecules tightly associated with the 26S proteasome, appear to serve as direct targets for ionizing radiation. This explains the rapidity of the inhibition.

We recently found that proteasomes that lack Lmp2 and Lmp7 appear to be more resistant to the inhibitory effects of irradiation than constitutive proteasomes (Pervan, unpublished data). This could allow differentials between different tumor and normal cell types with respect to radiation-induced responses. It might also have implications for radiation-induced immune suppression, because immune cells, which are involved in

MHC class I-mediated antigen processing and presentation, will be most affected. The concept that molecular substitutions in proteasome structure could redirect and fine-tune cellular responses is indirectly supported by the finding that hsp90 affects constitutive and not immunoproteasomes *(38)*.

3. CONSEQUENCES OF PROTEASOME INHIBITION

Modulation of proteasome activity has been shown to affect cellular processes as diverse as transcriptional activation *(39–41)*, cell-cycle progression *(42)*, cell survival *(43,44)*, DNA repair and chromosome stability *(45)*, receptor-mediated responses to external ligands *(46)*, and antigen presentation through the MHC class I-mediated pathway *(10)*. It therefore seems likely that the effects of radiation, hyperthermia, and oxidative stress on proteasomes is part of a mechanism by which cells make adaptive responses. The cellular consequences of radiation, for example, in cell-cycle arrest, apoptosis, and DNA repair are not dissimilar to those of proteasome inhibitors.

Specific inhibitors like lactacystein, MG-132, or bortezomib (Velcade®; formerly known as PS-341) prevent removal of cell-cycle regulators and thus block movement of cells through cell-cycle transition checkpoints and induce apoptosis. Apoptosis following exposure of cells to proteasome inhibitors has been demonstrated with many different tumor entities including Hodgkin's *(47)* and non-Hodgkin's lymphoma *(48)*, multiple myeloma *(49,50)*, leukemia *(51,52)*, prostate cancer *(52,53)*, glioblastoma *(52,54)*, pancreatic cancer *(55,56)*, gastric cancer *(57)*, cervical cancer (Pajonk et al., unpublished results), colorectal cancer *(58,59)*, ovarian cancer *(60)*, and lung cancer *(61)*. Numerous in vitro and in vivo studies have shown that such effects did not necessarily depend on classical molecular pathways like those dictated by p53 and bcl-2 *(53)*, but the exact mechanism is still not fully understood.

In vitro, proteasome inhibitors like MG-132, lactacystein, NLVS, and bortezomib induce apoptosis by a mechanism that involves activation of initiator caspases *(62)*. However, depending on the specificity of the inhibitors used, activation of effector caspases by proteasome inhibitors *(63)* cannot always be assumed. For example, drugs like MG-132 also inhibit calpains that are necessary for activation of caspase-3, at least in some cell types *(64)*. In solid cancer cells, apoptosis induced by proteasome inhibitors often resembles the caspase-independent apoptosis that has previously been described for other stimuli *(65)*, whereas cells of hematopoietic origin show full caspase-dependent apoptosis *(62)*.

Proteasome inhibitor-induced apoptosis might involve apoptosis-inducing factor (AIF) *(66)*, which is stabilized by proteasome inhibition and co-immunoprecipitates with ubiquitinated proteins (Pajonk et al., unpublished results). AIF is normally located in the inner membrane space of the mitochondria and is released into the cytoplasm upon mitochondrial damage. By a not fully understood mechanism, AIF activates a caspase-independent form of apoptosis, which results in large-scale fragmented DNA (50 kBp). One could propose a mechanism in which there is a permanent slow leakage of AIF into the cytoplasm, where it is rapidly degraded by the proteasome. In the presence of proteasome inhibitors, it would accumulate and initiate caspase-independent apoptosis. Another possible contributory mechanism that would be more general is based on the fact that many oncogenes and tumor repressor genes are regulated by the proteasome *(5)*.

Proteasome inhibition might partly reconstitute a normal oncogene or tumor suppressor gene expression profile and thus reassemble a benign phenotype with an increased apoptotic potential. Escape from proteasome inhibition-induced apoptosis also seems possible.

If proteasome degradation pathways are affected by radiation, one might expect levels of ubiquitinylated proteins to be altered. A general increase in expression of all ubiquitinylated proteins is not an expected consequence of radiation-induced proteasome inhibition, but alterations in specific molecular pools would be expected and do occur. Ubiquitinylated p53 levels increase following irradiation *(67)*. Levels of the cyclin kinase inhibitor p21, which is known to be degraded through the ubiquitin–proteasome system, are also elevated after irradiation, but not the ubiquitinylated form *(67)*, unlike the case following treatment with proteasome inhibitors. The difference may be that p21 can be unphosphorylated or dephosphorylated as a result of pathways activated by DNA damage, and this would inhibit ubiquitinylation *(68)*. Irradiation increased ubiquitin mRNA expression and ubiquitinylated nuclear proteins in human lymphocytes *(69)* and in Ewing's sarcoma cells *(70)*. It was suggested that this was associated with radiation-induced apoptosis.

One of the most studied effects of proteasome inhibition on a molecular pathway is inhibition of nuclear factor-κB (NF-κB) activation, which is a major mediator of gene transcription for oxidative stress, proinflammatory cytokines, and immune and cell survival responses (reviewed in refs. *71* and *72*). The ubiquitin–proteasome system is involved in three ways. First, NF-κB1 (p50) and NF-κB2 (p52) have to be processed from p105 and p100 precursor proteins, respectively, and this is achieved by partial degradation. Second, ubiquitinylation is required for activation of IκB kinase, which phosphorylates IκB. Third, the E3 ligase β-TrCP specifically ubiquitinylates phosphorylated IκBα, targeting it for degradation. Inhibition of proteasome function prevents the generation of new NF-κB molecules and stabilizes IκBα expression, preventing NF-κB nuclear localization *(33)*. Because NF-κB is involved in both inflammatory responses and as a survival factor for cancer cells, proteasome inhibitors are anti-inflammatory agents with potential antitumor activity, in particular for tumors that are addicted to the NF-κB pathway for survival.

Blocking NF-κB activation in tumors has many possible outcomes other than inducing apoptosis and decreasing inflammation. One interesting possibility is in prevention of metastasis. NF-κB is a key regulator of expression of matrix metalloproteases (MMPs), which digest extracellular matrix proteins and promote invasiveness of tumor cells by opening junctions between normal cells, allowing a tumor to spread into the resulting spaces. Blocking the NF-κB pathway using proteasome inhibitors prevents TNF-dependent MMP-1, MMP-3, intracellular adhesion molecule 1 (ICAM-1), and cyclo-oxygenase 2 (COX-2) expression *(73)* and is a possible mechanism for their antimetastatic effects *(74)*. In addition to proteasome inhibitors inhibiting MMP production, there is a report that metalloprotease inhibitors inhibit the proteasome *(75)*. This is further supported by the observation that proteasome inhibitors reduce tumor growth and angiogenesis in vivo *(76)* and stabilize tight junctions, preventing cell–cell dissociation *(77)*. In contrast, MMP-2 expression, which is controlled through the Akt pathway, was increased by proteasome inhibition, leading to increased cellular invasiveness *(78)*, showing the multiple levels of control that are being exerted on pathways by this structure and the need to take into consideration the cellular context in which they are used.

Radiation-induced impairment of proteasome function presents a paradox with respect to NF-κB activation. Proteasome inhibition would be expected to prevent NF-κB activation, but numerous studies have shown irradiation to activate this transcription factor *(79,80)* and promote proinflammatory responses. Radiation is known to increase expression of proinflammatory chemokines *(81)* and cytokines such as TNF-α *(82,83)*, IL-1α and -β *(84,85)*, IL-5 *(86)*, IL-6 *(87,88)*, granulocyte/macrophage colony-stimulating factor (GM-CSF) *(89)*, IFN-α *(90)*, basic fibroblast growth factor (bFGF) *(91)*, and vascular endothelial growth factor (VEGF) *(92,93)*, as well as proinflammatory cell adhesion molecules (ICAM-1 *[85,94,95]*, E-selectin *(96)*, and vascular cell adhesion molecule 1 [VCAM-1; *97*]), prostaglandins and leukotrienes *(98,99)*, and proteases *(85,100,101)*. The apparent paradox extends to the clinic. Although ionizing radiation has recognized proinflammatory effects, it has been used, especially in the first half of the last century, in the treatment of many benign inflammatory as well as hyperproliferative diseases, and in many European countries it is still a popular treatment modality for such conditions *(102)*. Such treatments, however, generally use considerably lower doses of radiation than are used in cancer therapy. We have recently shown that NF-κB may be activated only in response to high doses of radiation, in excess of 7 Gy *(33)*. The same was observed for radiation-induced ICAM-1 expression, which is considered a downstream readout of NF-κB activity (≥4 Gy; Pajonk, unpublished data). IκBα expression did not decrease at any dose, and in fact after 25 cGy, IκBα expression was increased, in keeping with what would be expected if irradiation induced proteasome inhibition. ICAM-1 expression was decreased after doses in the range 25–150 cGy. The suggestion is that radiation stabilizes expression of IκBα over a wide dose range and has an anti-inflammatory effect at low doses, but at high doses a pathway is activated that can overcome this inhibition.

4. PROTEASOMES AND RADIOSENSITIZATION

Whereas the permanent presence of nanomolar concentrations of proteasome inhibitors efficiently prevents tumor cell growth *(47)*, short-term treatment of cancer cells with these compounds sensitizes tumor cells to ionizing radiation *(47)*, suggesting the use of proteasome inhibitors in radiation therapy. The underlying mechanism is, again, not clear. At least in Hodgkin's lymphoma and prostate cancer cells it did not depend on inhibition of constitutive active NF-κB *(103)*. There is now strong evidence that the proteasome is involved in nucleotide excision repair *(104)*. Nucleotide excision repair is not considered to have a role in repair of radiation-induced DNA double-strand breaks, but involvement of the proteasome in other, more relevant, repair processes, such as nonhomologous end joining is possible.

At first sight, the use of specific inhibitors to target proteasome function seems to be a new therapeutic approach in cancer therapy. However, a closer look at certain established tumor therapies reveals that some already interfere with proteasome function. In addition to radiation and hyperthermia, chemotherapeutic agents, such as alkaloids *(105)* and anthracyclins (Pajonk et al., submitted) impair proteasome function. Additionally, we (Pajonk et al., submitted) and others *(106)* have recently shown inhibitory effects of proteasome inhibitors on the maturation and pumping function of the multidrug resistance-1 gene product P-glycoprotein, which is responsible for the removal of many chemically unrelated anticancer agents from the cytoplasm and thus the failure of chemotherapy.

Remarkably, drugs like cyclosporine A *(107)*, *N*-acetyl-L-cysteine *(28)*, and HIV-I protease inhibitors *(52,108)* are inhibitors of the proteasome. At least for the latter, it is known that AIDS-related Kaposi's sarcomas can regress when patients are treated with highly active antiretroviral therapy (HAART) regimens *(109)*. In an elegant experimental setting, Sgadari et al. *(110)* were able to demonstrate that this appeared to be caused by inhibition of angiogenesis and not by regained immunologic competence of the host. This explanation is somewhat counterintuitive because inhibition of proteasome function stabilizes HIF-1α, the key transcription factor for hypoxic responses, which enhances VEGF transcription. However, angiogenesis is complex and does not depend only on VEGF but also on endothelial cell proliferation and invasive growth. Thus, Ohkawa et al. *(106)* described complete inhibition of angiogenesis by lactacystein using a chorioallantoic membrane model. On the other hand, Pati and co-workers *(111)* showed that HIV-I protease inhibitors had a direct proapoptotic effect on Kaposi's sarcoma cells, and we have shown recently that they are potent inducers of apoptosis in leukemia, prostate cancer, and glioma cells that is obviously unrelated to HIV. For AIDS-related primary central nervous system lymphoma, the combination of HAART with cranial irradiation increased survival of patients 30-fold compared with cranial irradiation alone *(112)*, suggesting that HIV-I protease inhibitors might be useful as sensitizers in radiation therapy of non-AIDS-related cancers.

Bortezomib is the first specific proteasome inhibitor to enter clinical trials for multiple myeloma *(113)*. Bortezomib has direct antitumor *(13)* as well as radiosensitizing effects *(114,115)* on cancer cells in vitro and in vivo. It seems that other existing drugs, like the HIV-I protease inhibitors, or new proteasome inhibitors modeled on bortezomib, will become valuable adjuncts to existing cancer therapies, especially in combination with conventional chemotherapeutic drugs or radiation therapy. At the same time investigations into the role of the proteasome in cancer is likely to suggest new targets within the ubiquitin–proteasome system, such as regulatory components of the proteasome, the E3 ligases, or the ubiquitination system itself, which may be beneficially manipulated.

5. CONCLUSIONS

There is increasing evidence that proteasome have spatial and structural heterogeneity and that they are functionally responsive to a variety of challenges. Radiation, certain chemotherapeutic agents, hyperthermia, and oxidative stress, as well as cytokines and growth factors can modulate their activity. The impact of changes in proteasome structure, function, and location could critically determine tumor behavior and response to therapy. At the same time the ubiquitin–proteasome system serves as a promising target for intervention, in particular in combination with conventional radiation or chemotherapy.

REFERENCES

1. Druker BJ. STI571 (Gleevec) as a paradigm for cancer therapy. *Trends Mol Med* 2002;8:S14–S18.
2. Marsh D, Zori R. Genetic insights into familial cancers—update and recent discoveries. *Cancer Lett* 2002;181:125–164.

3. Brabletz T, et al. Variable beta-catenin expression in colorectal cancers indicates tumor progression driven by the tumor environment. *Proc Natl Acad Sci USA* 2001;98:10356–10361.

4. Rolfe M, et al. The ubiquitin-mediated proteolytic pathway as a therapeutic area. *J Mol Med* 1997;75:5–17.

5. Pajonk F, McBride WH. The proteasome in cancer biology and treatment. *Radiat Res* 2001;156:447–459.

6. Ichihara AK, et al. Regulation of proteasome expression in developing and transformed cells. *Adv Enzyme Regul* 1993;33:173–180.

7. Shimbara N, et al. Regulation of gene expression of proteasomes (multi-protease complexes) during growth and differentiation of human hematopoietic cells. *J Biol Chem* 1992;267:18100–18109.

8. Kanayama, H K, et al. Changes in expressions of proteasome and ubiquitin genes in human renal cancer cells. *Cancer Res* 1991;51:6677–6685.

9. Kumatori AK, et al. Abnormally high expression of proteasomes in human leukemic cells. *Proc Natl Acad Sci USA* 1990;87:7071–7075.

10. Rock KL, et al. Protein degradation and the generation of MHC class I-presented peptides. *Adv Immunol* 2002;80:1–70.

11. Pallares-Trujillo JN, et al. Does the mechanism responsible for TNF-mediated insulin resistance involve the proteasome? *Med Hypoth* 2000;54:565–569.

12. Ogiso YA, et al. Glucose starvation and hypoxia induce nuclear accumulation of proteasome in cancer cells. *Biochem Biophys Res Commun* 1999;258:448–452.

13. Adams J, et al. Proteasome inhibitors: a novel class of potent and effective antitumor agents. *Cancer Res* 1999;59:2615–2622.

14. Grune T. Oxidative stress, aging and the proteasomal system. *Biogerontology* 2000;1:31–40.

15. Carrard G, et al. Impairment of proteasome structure and function in aging. *Int J Biochem Cell Biol* 2002;34:1461–1474.

16. Meriin AB, et al. Proteasome inhibitors activate stress kinases and induce Hsp72. Diverse effects on apoptosis. *J Biol Chem* 1998;273:6373–6379.

17. Marcu MG, et al. Heat shock protein 90 modulates the unfolded protein response by stabilizing IRE1alpha. *Mol Cell Biol* 2002;22:8506–8513.

18. Bush KT, et al. Proteasome inhibition leads to a heat-shock response, induction of endoplasmic reticulum chaperones, and thermotolerance. *J Biol Chem* 1997;272:9086–9092.

19. Ii K, et al. Immunocytochemical co-localization of the proteasome in ubiquitinated structures in neurodegenerative diseases and the elderly. *J Neuropathol Exp Neurol* 1997;56:125–131.

20. Keller JN, et al. Impaired proteasome function in Alzheimer's disease. *J Neurochem* 2000;75:436–439.

21. Peters PJ, et al. Arfaptin 2 regulates the aggregation of mutant huntingtin protein. *Nat Cell Biol* 2002;4:240–245.

22. Ishii K, et al. Increased A beta 42(43)-plaque deposition in early-onset familial Alzheimer's disease brains with the deletion of exon 9 and the missense point mutation (H163R) in the PS-1 gene. *Neurosci Lett* 1997;228:17–20.

23. Grune T, et al. Proteolysis in cultured liver epithelial cells during oxidative stress. Role of the multicatalytic proteinase complex, proteasome. *J Biol Chem* 1995;270:2344–2351.

24. Reinheckel T, et al. Differential impairment of 20S and 26S proteasome activities in human hematopoietic K562 cells during oxidative stress. *Arch Biochem Biophys* 2000;377:65–68.

25. Reinheckel T, et al. Comparative resistance of the 20S and 26S proteasome to oxidative stress. *Biochem J* 1998;335:637–642.

26. Shringarpure R, et al. Ubiquitin conjugation is not required for the degradation of oxidized proteins by the proteasome. *J Biol Chem* 2003;278:311–318.

27. Shringarpure R, Davies KJ. Protein turnover by the proteasome in aging and disease. *Free Radic Biol Med* 2002;32:1084–1089.

28. Pajonk F, et al. N-acetyl-L-cysteine inhibits 26S proteasome function: implications for effects on NF-kappaB activation. *Free Radic Biol Med* 2002;32:536–543.

29. Luo GJ, et al. Hyperthermia stimulates energy-proteasome-dependent protein degradation in cultured myotubes. *Am J Physiol Regul Integr Comp Physiol* 2000;278:R749–R756.

30. Mathew A, et al. Heat shock response and protein degradation: regulation of HSF2 by the ubiquitin-proteasome pathway. *Mol Cell Biol* 1998;18:5091–5098.

31. Kuckelkorn U, et al. The effect of heat shock on 20S/26S proteasomes. *Biol Chem* 2000;381:1017–1023.

32. Locke JE, et al. Indomethacin lowers the threshold thermal exposure for hyperthermic radiosensitization and heat-shock inhibition of ionizing radiation-induced activation of NF-kappaB. *Int J Radiat Biol* 2002;78:493–502.

33. Pajonk F, McBride WH. Ionizing radiation affects 26s proteasome function and associated molecular responses, even at low doses. *Radiother Oncol* 2001;59:203–212.

34. McBride WH, et al. NF-kappa B, cytokines, proteasomes, and low-dose radiation exposure. *Mil Med* 2002;167(2 suppl):66–67.

35. Bulteau AL, et al. Impairment of proteasome function upon UVA- and UVB-irradiation of human keratinocytes. *Free Radic Biol Med* 2002;32:1157–1170.

36. Conconi M, Friguet B. Proteasome inactivation upon aging and on oxidation-effect of HSP 90. *Mol Biol Rep* 1997;24:45–50.

37. Zaiss DM, et al. PI31 is a modulator of proteasome formation and antigen processing. *Proc Natl Acad Sci USA* 2002;99:14344–14349.

38. Lu X, et al. Heat shock protein-90 and the catalytic activities of the 20 S proteasome (multicatalytic proteinase complex). *Arch Biochem Biophys* 2001;387:163–171.

39. Ottosen S, et al. Transcription. Proteasome parts at gene promoters. *Science* 2002;296:479–481.

40. Ejkova E, Tansey WP. Old dogs and new tricks: meeting on mechanisms of eukaryotic transcription. *EMBO Rep* 2002;3:219–223.

41. Kang Z, et al. Involvement of proteasome in the dynamic assembly of the androgen receptor transcription complex. *J Biol Chem* 2002;277:48366–48371.

42. Yamaguchi R, Dutta A. Proteasome inhibitors alter the orderly progression of DNA synthesis during S-phase in HeLa cells and lead to rereplication of DNA. *Exp Cell Res* 2000;261:271–283.

43. Delic J, et al. The proteasome inhibitor lactacystin induces apoptosis and sensitizes chemo- and radioresistant human chronic lymphocytic leukaemia lymphocytes to TNF-alpha-initiated apoptosis. *Br J Cancer* 1998;77:1103–1107.

44. Pajonk F, et al. Apoptosis and radiosensitization of Hodgkin cells by proteasome inhibition (see comments). *Int J Rad Oncol Biol Phys* 2000;47:1025–1032.

45. Arnold J, Grune T. PARP-mediated proteasome activation: a co-ordination of DNA repair and protein degradation? *Bioessays* 2002;24:1060–1065.

46. Strous GJ, van Kerkhof P. The ubiquitin-proteasome pathway and the regulation of growth hormone receptor availability. *Mol Cell Endocrinol* 2002;197:143–151.

47. Pajonk F, et al. Apoptosis and radisensitization of Hodgkin's cells by proteasome inhibition. *Int J Radiat Oncol Biol* 2000;47:1025–1032.

48. Schenkein D. Proteasome inhibitors in the treatment of B-cell malignancies. *Clin Lymphoma* 2002;3:49–55.

49. Martinelli G, et al. Molecular therapy for multiple myeloma. *Haematologica* 2001;86:908–917.

50. Hideshima T, et al. Novel therapies targeting the myeloma cell and its bone marrow microenvironment. *Semin Oncol* 2001;28:607–612.

51. Almond JB, et al. Proteasome inhibitor-induced apoptosis of B-chronic lymphocytic leukaemia cells involves cytochrome c release and caspase activation, accompanied by formation of an approximately 700 kDa Apaf-1 containing apoptosome complex. *Leukemia* 2001;15:1388–1397.

52. Pajonk F, et al. The human immunodeficiency virus (HIV)-1 protease inhibitor saquinavir inhibits proteasome function and causes apoptosis and radiosensitization in non-HIV-associated human cancer cells. *Cancer Res* 2002;62:5230–5235.

53. Herrmann JL, et al. Prostate carcinoma cell death resulting from inhibition of proteasome activity is independent of functional Bcl-2 and p53. *Oncogene* 1998;17:2889–2899.

54. Tani E, et al. Proteasome inhibitors induce Fas-mediated apoptosis by c-Myc accumulation and subsequent induction of FasL message in human glioma cells. *FEBS Lett* 2001;504:53–58.

55. Bold RJ, et al. Chemosensitization of pancreatic cancer by inhibition of the 26S proteasome. *J Surg Res* 2001;100:11–17.

56. Shah SA, et al. 26S proteasome inhibition induces apoptosis and limits growth of human pancreatic cancer. *J Cell Biochem* 2001;82:110–122.

57. Fan XM, et al. Inhibition of proteasome function induced apoptosis in gastric cancer. *Int J Cancer* 2001;93:481–488.

58. Cusack JC, et al. Enhanced chemosensitivity to CPT-11 with proteasome inhibitor PS-341: implications for systemic nuclear factor-kappaB inhibition. *Cancer Res* 2001;61:3535–3540.

59. Lind DS, et al. Nuclear factor-kappa B is upregulated in colorectal cancer. *Surgery* 2001;130:363–369.

60. Mimnaugh EG, et al. Prevention of cisplatin-DNA adduct repair and potentiation of cisplatin-induced apoptosis in ovarian carcinoma cells by proteasome inhibitors. *Biochem Pharmacol* 2000;60:1343–1354.

61. Oyaizu H, et al. Proteasome inhibitor 1 enhances paclitaxel-induced apoptosis in human lung adenocarcinoma cell line. *Oncol Rep* 2001;8:825–829.

62. Wu LW, et al. The proteasome regulates caspase-dependent and caspase-independent protease cascades during apoptosis of MO7e hematopoietic progenitor cells. *Blood Cells Mol Dis* 1999;25:20–29.

63. Emanuele S, et al. Apoptosis induced in hepatoblastoma HepG2 cells by the proteasome inhibitor MG132 is associated with hydrogen peroxide production, expression of Bcl-XS and activation of caspase-3. *Int J Oncol* 2002;21:857–865.

64. Wolf BB, et al. Calpain functions in a caspase-independent manner to promote apoptosis-like events during platelet activation. *Blood* 1999;94:1683–1692.

65. Borner C, Monney L. Apoptosis without caspases: an inefficient molecular guillotine? *Cell Death Differ* 1999;6:497–507.

66. Kroemer G. (Mitochondrial control of apoptosis). *Bull Acad Natl Med* 2001;185:1135–1142; discussion 1143.

67. Maki CG, Howley M. Ubiquitination of p53 and p21 is differentially affected by ionizing and UV radiation. *Mol Cell Biol* 1997;17:355–363.

68. Fukuchi K, et al. Identification of the regulatory region required for ubiquitination of the cyclin kinase inhibitor, p21. *Biochem Biophys Res Commun* 2002;293:120–125.

69. Delic J, et al. Ubiquitin pathway involvement in human lymphocyte gamma-irradiation-induced apoptosis. *Mol Cell Biol* 1993;13:4875–4883.

70. Soldatenkov VA, Dritschilo A. Apoptosis of Ewing's sarcoma cells is accompanied by accumulation of ubiquitinated proteins. *Cancer Res* 1997;57:3881–3885.

71. Karin M, Lin A. NF-kappaB at the crossroads of life and death. *Nat Immunol* 2002;3:221–227.

72. Karin M, et al. NF-kappaB in cancer: from innocent bystander to major culprit. *Nat Rev Cancer* 2002;2:301–310.

73. Sakai T, et al. Tumor necrosis factor alpha induces expression of genes for matrix degradation in human chondrocyte-like HCS-2/8 cells through activation of NF-kappaB: abrogation of the tumor necrosis factor alpha effect by proteasome inhibitors. *J Bone Miner Res* 2001;16:1272–1280.

74. Ikebe T, et al. Involvement of proteasomes in migration and matrix metalloproteinase-9 production of oral squamous cell carcinoma. *Int J Cancer* 1998;77:578–585.

75. Vaithilingam IS, et al. An extracellular proteasome-like structure from C6 astrocytoma cells with serine collagenase IV activity and metallo-dependent activity on alpha-casein and beta-insulin. *J Biol Chem* 1995;270:4588–4593.

76. Sunwoo JB, et al. Novel proteasome inhibitor PS-341 inhibits activation of nuclear factor-kappa B, cell survival, tumor growth, and angiogenesis in squamous cell carcinoma. *Clin Cancer Res* 2001;7:1419–1428.

77. Tsukamoto T, Nigam SK. Cell-cell dissociation upon epithelial cell scattering requires a step mediated by the proteasome. *J Biol Chem* 1999;274:24579–24584.

78. Park BK, et al. Akt1 induces extracellular matrix invasion and matrix metalloproteinase-2 activity in mouse mammary epithelial cells. *Cancer Res* 2001;61:7647–7653.

79. Li N, Karin M. Ionizing radiation and short wavelength UV activate NF-kappaB through two distinct mechanisms. *Proc Natl Acad Sci USA* 1998;95:13012–13017.

80. Raju U, et al. IkappaBalpha degradation is not a requirement for the X-ray-induced activation of nuclear factor kappaB in normal rat astrocytes and human brain tumour cells. *Int J Radiat Biol* 1998;74:617–624.

81. Johnston CJ, et al. Radiation-induced pulmonary fibrosis: examination of chemokine and chemokine receptor families. *Radiat Res* 2002;157:256–265.

82. Hallahan DE, et al. Increased tumor necrosis factor alpha mRNA after cellular exposure to ionizing radiation. *Proc Natl Acad Sci USA* 1989;86:10104–10107.

83. Chiang CS, et al. Radiation-induced astrocytic and microglial responses in mouse brain. *Radiother Oncol* 1993;29:60–68.

84. Hosoi Y, et al. Induction of interleukin-1beta and interleukin-6 mRNA by low doses of ionizing radiation in macrophages. *Int J Cancer* 2001;96:270–276.

85. Hong JH, et al. Induction of early response genes and tumor necrosis factor (TNF) by irradiation does not appear to occur through map kinase pathway in HL-60 cells. *Int J Radiat Oncol Biol Phys* 1994;30(suppl 1):315.

86. Lu-Hesselmann J, et al. Transcriptional regulation of the human IL5 gene by ionizing radiation in Jurkat T cells: evidence for repression by an NF-AT-like element. *Radiat Res* 1997;148:531–542.

87. Abeyama K, et al. Maruyama, Interleukin 6 mediated differentiation and rescue of cell redox in PC12 cells exposed to ionizing radiation. *FEBS Lett* 1995;364:298–300.

88. Beetz A, et al. Induction of interleukin 6 by ionizing radiation in a human epithelial cell line: control by corticosteroids. *Int J Radiat Biol* 1997;72:33–43.

89. Zhang JS, et al. Ionizing radiation-induced IL-1 alpha, IL-6 and GM-CSF production by human lung cancer cells. *Chin Med J (Engl)* 1994;107:653–657.

90. Woloschak GE, et al. Modulation of gene expression in Syrian hamster embryo cells following ionizing radiation. *Cancer Res* 1990;50:339–344.

91. Haimovitz-Friedman A, et al. Autocrine effects of fibroblast growth factor in repair of radiation damage in endothelial cells. *Cancer Res* 1991;51:2552–2558.

92. Park JS, et al. Ionizing radiation modulates vascular endothelial growth factor (VEGF) expression through multiple mitogen activated protein kinase dependent pathways. *Oncogene* 2001;20:3266–3280.

93. Gorski DH, et al. Blockage of the vascular endothelial growth factor stress response increases the antitumor effects of ionizing radiation. *Cancer Res* 1999;59:3374–3378.

94. Gaugler MH, et al. Late and persistent up-regulation of intercellular adhesion molecule-1 (ICAM-1) expression by ionizing radiation in human endothelial cells in vitro. *Int J Radiat Biol* 1997;72:201–209.

95. Behrends U, et al. Ionization radiation induces ICAM-1 in human cells and organ cultures in vitro as well as in murine organs in vivo. In: *Proceedings of the 42nd Annual Meeting of the Radiation Research Society*, Nashville, TN, 1994.

96. Hallahan D, et al. E-selectin gene induction by ionizing radiation is independent of cytokine induction. *Biochem Biophys Res Commun* 1995;217:784–795.

97. Heckmann M, et al. Vascular activation of adhesion molecule mRNA and cell surface expression by ionizing radiation. *Exp Cell Res* 1998;238:148–154.

98. Iwamoto KS, McBride WH. Radiation induction of lipoxygenase activity in murine macrophages. *Radiat Res* 1992:118.

99. Eisen V, et al. Prostaglandins and complement changes in some conditions related to inflammation. *Agents Actions Suppl* 1977;2:99–108.

100. Fittkau M, et al. A low dose of ionizing radiation increases luminal release of intestinal peptidases in rats. *J Cancer Res Clin Oncol* 2001;127:96–100.

101. Patel S, et al. Ionizing radiation and TNF-alpha and stimulated expression of alpha1-antichymotrypsin gene in human squamous carcinoma cells. *Acta Oncol* 1998;37:475–478.

102. Trott KR, Kamprad F. Radiobiological mechanisms of anti-inflammatory radiotherapy. *Radiother Oncol* 1999;51:197–203.

103. Pajonk F, et al. Inhibition of NF-kappaB, clonogenicity, and radiosensitivity of human cancer cells. *J Natl Cancer Inst* 1999;91:1956–1960.

104. Gillette TG, et al. The 19S complex of the proteasome regulates nucleotide excision repair in yeast. *Genes Dev* 2001;15:1528–1539.

105. Piccinini M, et al. Proteasomes are a target of the anti-tumour drug vinblastine. *Biochem J* 2001;356:835–841.

106. Ohkawa K, et al. Calpain inhibitor causes accumulation of ubiquitinated P-glycoprotein at the cell surface: possible role of calpain in P-glycoprotein turnover. *Int J Oncol* 1999;15:677–686.

107. Meyer S, et al. Cyclosporine A is an uncompetitive inhibitor of proteasome activity and prevents NF-kappaB activation. *FEBS Lett* 1997;413:354–358.

108. Schmidtke G, et al. How an inhibitor of the HIV-I protease modulates proteasome activity. *J Biol Chem* 1999;274:35734–35740.

109. Diz Dios P, et al. Regression of AIDS-related Kaposi's sarcoma following ritonavir therapy. *Oral Oncol* 1998;34:236–238.

110. Sgadari C, et al. HIV protease inhibitors are potent anti-angiogenic molecules and promote regression of Kaposi sarcoma. *Nat Med* 2002;8:225–232.

111. Pati S, et al. Antitumorigenic effects of HIV protease inhibitor ritonavir: inhibition of Kaposi sarcoma. *Blood* 2002;99:3771–3779.

112. Hoffmann C, et al. Survival of AIDS patients with primary central nervous system lymphoma is dramatically improved by HAART-induced immune recovery. *Aids* 2001;15:2119–2127.

113. Adams, J. Development of the proteasome inhibitor PS-341. *Oncologia* 2002;7:9–16.

114. Pervan M, et al. Molecular pathways that modify tumor radiation response. *Am J Clin Oncol* 2001;24:481–485.

115. Russo SM, et al. Enhancement of radiosensitivity by proteasome inhibition: implications for a role of NF-kappaB. *Int J Radiat Oncol Biol Phys* 2001;50:183–193.

10 Radiosensitization and Proteasome Inhibition

Carter Van Waes, John B. Sunwoo,
William DeGraff, and James B. Mitchell

CONTENTS

ABSTRACT

Radiation is an important modality of therapy for a variety of cancers, including squamous cell carcinomas (SCC) of the head and neck and skin. Cell survival and resistance following radiation are mediated by cytoprotective molecules that regulate cell-cycle progression and cell death. Constitutive and radiation-induced activation of the transcription factor nuclear factor-κB (NF-κB) and cell-cycle regulatory proteins have been shown to contribute to differences in resistance of SCC to radiation (Kato et al., *Head Neck* 2000;22:748–759). NF-κB and one of its target genes, cyclin D1, are regulated by signal activation and degradation of inhibitor-κBs by the proteasome. In addition, the proteasome degrades cyclin inhibitors. We investigated the effects of the proteasome inhibitor bortezomib (PS-341, Velcade) on NF-κB activation and cell-cycle regulatory protein expression, as well as cell-cycle and radiosensitizing effects in SCC. Bortezomib produced accumulation of cyclin inhibitor p21 and inhibited activation of NF-κB and cyclin D1. Bortezomib had direct cytotoxic activity, and an accumulation of SCC cells in the radiosensitive G_2/M phase of the cell cycle was accompanied by further radiosensitization. Clinical studies of concomitant therapy with bortezomib and radiation are under way in patients with SCC of the head and neck.

From: *Cancer Drug Discovery and Development: Proteasome Inhibitors in Cancer Therapy*
Edited by: J. Adams © Humana Press Inc., Totowa, NJ

KEY WORDS

Squamous cell carcinoma; radiation; NF-κB; proteasome; cyclin D1; p21; apoptosis.

1. INTRODUCTION

Radiation is an important therapeutic modality in many cancers. Certain cancers, such as squamous cell carcinomas (SCCs) that arise in the upper aerodigestive tract and skin, are sufficiently sensitive to radiation at an early stage that relatively high cure rates comparable to those seen with surgery may be achieved. However, a subset of SCCs and other cancers are found to be relatively resistant to radiation therapy even at relatively early stages. Advanced SCC and other cancers are often resistant to radiation, and the prognosis remains poor even with combined surgical and radiation therapy. As a result, there has been considerable interest in identifying the cellular and molecular factors that contribute to the resistance of cancers to radiation, in the hope of identifying agents that may sensitize cells to radiation. A variety of cellular and molecular factors that contribute to resistance of cancers to radiation have been identified.

Differences in the relative sensitivity to radiation of cells at different phases of the cell cycle has been found to be an important factor contributing to survival of a fraction of cancer cells within the population. Cells in the late growth and mitosis (G_2/M) phase of the cell cycle have been found to be more sensitive to radiation (1). These observations have resulted in the finding that synchronization of cancer cells at more sensitive phases of the cell cycle such as G_2/M using chemotherapy can result in a further decrease in survival of cancer cells treated with the same dose of radiation. For example, taxanes, which dysregulate the microtubular assembly important in mitosis, have been found to promote accumulation of cells in G_2/M and to enhance radiosensitization (2). Consistent with this, recent clinical trials in which taxanes have been given concurrently with radiation have resulted in a high complete response rate in patients with advanced SCC of the head and neck (3).

Recently, there is evidence that common signaling mechanisms contributing to resistance to cell death and enhanced cell survival are also important in determining sensitivity to radiation as well as chemotherapy (4). Several pathways are constitutively activated in SCC and other cancers and may be further induced by hypoxia, nutrient depletion, expression of various cytokines and growth factors, radiation, and cytotoxic chemotherapy agents. One critical pathway, the nuclear factor-κB (NF-κB) signal pathway, may be activated by several important oncogenes, environmental factors, and therapeutic agents (4). NF-κB is constitutively activated in SCC (5,6), and increased activation corresponds to incremental increases in radioresistance (7). Inhibition of constitutive and radiation-induced activation of NF-κB by inhibitor-κB (IκB) results in decreased survival and radiosensitization (7,8). The constitutive and inducible activation of NF-κB has been associated with survival and resistance of other cancers to the cytotoxic effects of radiation and chemotherapy (4).

The proteasome plays an important role in degradation and regulation of proteins that control cell cycling and the activation of the NF-κB signal pathway (9). As outlined in this chapter, proteasome inhibition results in effects on cell cycle, cyclin inhibitors, and cyclins that result in G_2/M block. Proteasome antagonists also inhibit constitutive and radiation-induced activation of NF-κB and decrease the resistance of cancer cells. As a consequence, inhibition of cell-cycle progression and NF-κB activation by proteasome antagonists is associated with direct cytotoxicity and increased radiosensitization.

2. EFFECTS OF PROTEASOME INHIBITION ON PROLIFERATION AND CELL SURVIVAL

We previously reported the effects of the proteasome inhibitor bortezomib (Velcade™; formerly known as PS-341) upon the proliferation and survival of six squamous cell carcinoma lines *(10)*. Bortezomib inhibited proliferation in 6/6 lines in the 10^{-9}–10^{-8} *M* range within 24 h, as measured by a cell densitometric assay. These results are consistent with a study that examined the growth-inhibitory effects of bortezomib using the National Cancer Institute's in vitro cytotoxicity screen, which is comprised of a 60 cell line panel derived from human tumors *(11)*. The concentration at which an average growth inhibition of 50% was observed was 7×10^{-9} *M* in this assay *(11)*. Bortezomib induced massive cell death in cultures of 6/6 SCC lines in the 10^{-7} *M* range, as measured by trypan blue uptake *(10)*. The Caspase-dependent poly-ADP-ribose polymerase (PARP) cleavage characteristic of apoptosis was detected within 12 h, decreased cell viability was detected within 48 h, and over 90% of cells were dead by 72 h. Thus, bortezomib has broad direct antiproliferative and cytotoxic activity in SCC, as well as other cancer cell lines *(10,11)*.

3. EFFECTS OF PROTEASOME INHIBITION ON CELL CYCLE, APOPTOSIS, CYCLIN INHIBITORS P21 AND P27, AND CYCLIN D1

To characterize the effects of proteasome inhibition on the cell cycle and cell death (apoptosis), SCC cells were cultured with bortezomib, and DNA cell cycle analysis was performed by flow cytofluorometry *(2)*. Figure 1 shows increased accumulation of SCC in the G_2/M phase after 24 h of exposure, consistent with the time-course at which decreased proliferation was observed. Loss of the G_2/M peak and the broad sub-G_0/G_1 DNA staining characteristic of the subcellular DNA fragmentation of apoptosis was observed by 72 h, the time at which increased trypan blue uptake was observed *(10)*.

Proliferation of SCC has been associated with decreased expression of various cyclin inhibitors and overexpression of cyclin D1 *(12)*. The proteasome mediates degradation of the cell-cycle inhibitors p21 and p27, as well as IκB, which can inhibit NF-κB-mediated induction of cyclin D1 expression *(9)*. Based on these functions, accumulation of cyclin inhibitors and IκB resulting in inhibition of cyclin activity and cyclin D1 expression would be expected to result from proteasome inhibition. We examined the relationship between the cell-cycle effects of bortezomib and possible changes in proteasome-mediated degradation of the cell-cycle inhibitors p21 and p27, and IκB/NF-κB-dependent expression of cyclin D1. The Western blot in Fig. 2 shows low p21 signal relative to p27 in SCC, and proteasome inhibition by bortezomib resulted in the accumulation of the cell-cycle inhibitor p21, whereas no accumulation of p27 was observed. Conversely, cyclin D1 is expressed in SCC, and cyclin D1 expression was inhibited following a transient rise after exposure of cells to bortezomib. The decrease in cyclin D1 expression was found to follow accumulation of IκB and inhibition of NF-κB by bortezomib. Accumulation of cells in G_2/M in association with p21 has also been reported in prostate PC-3 cells, myeloma cells, and pancreatic cancer cells *(11,13,14)*, indicating that proteasome inhibition had similar effects in several different types of cancer.

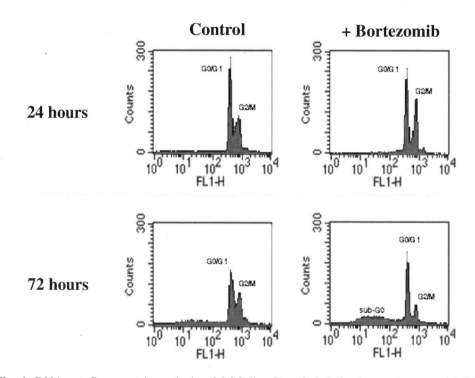

Fig. 1. DNA cytofluorometric analysis of SCC line Pam 212 following proteasome inhibitor bortezomib. Pam 212 cells were exposed to $10^{-7} M$ bortezomib or medium alone, and after 24 and 72 h, the floating and adherent fractions isolated by trypsinization were pooled, fixed, and stained with propidium iodide as previously described. The propidium iodide DNA staining intensity was determined by quantitative flow cytometry (Becton Dickinson, Braintree, MA). The log intensity of DNA staining vs the number of cells for a sample of 10^4 cells is shown. Bortezomib-cultured cells showed an increase in the G_2/M peak at 24 h, and a sub-G_0/G_1 peak by 72 h, compared with the G_0/G_1, S, and G2/M distribution of cells in controls.

4. INHIBITION OF CONSTITUTIVE AND RADIATION-INDUCED ACTIVATION OF NF-κB AND RADIOSENSITIZING EFFECTS OF PROTEASOME INHIBITION

NF-κB is constitutively activated in SCC, but not in normal keratinocytes, and this activation correlates with intrinsic radiation resistance *(7)*. NF-κB may be further induced by radiation as result of DNA double-strand breaks, which activate a cascade involving the phosphotidyl inositol 3-kinase like protein ATM and inhibitor-κB kinase (IKK) *(15,16)*. We previously showed that IκBα mutants deficient in the phosphorylation and ubiquination sites required for proteasome-dependent degradation inhibit constitutive and radiation-induced activation of NF-κB in SCC *(7)*. Based on these observations, we investigated the effects of proteasome inhibition on constitutive and radiation-induced activation of NF-κB. Figure 3 shows that NF-κB DNA binding activity is detected constitutively in SCC and is further induced following 6 Gy of radiation. Proteasome inhibition by bortezomib resulted in a decrease in constitutive and radiation-induced NF-κB DNA binding activity. The effects of bortezomib on constitutive DNA binding shown in Fig. 3 were consistent with the effects on NF-κB DNA binding and functional reporter gene activity in SCC reported previously *(10)*.

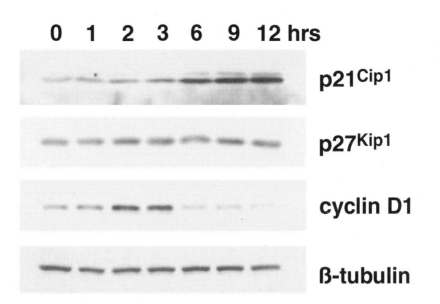

Fig. 2. Western blot analysis of p21, p27, and cyclin D expression in Pam 212 SCC cells treated with the proteaasome inhibitor bortezomib. Cells were incubated with 10^{-7} M bortezomib and lysates were isolated at different time points as shown. Proteins separated by polyacrylamide gel electrophoresis were transferred to nylon membranes and stained using anti-p21, p27, and cyclin D antibodies. β-tubulin was stained as a control.

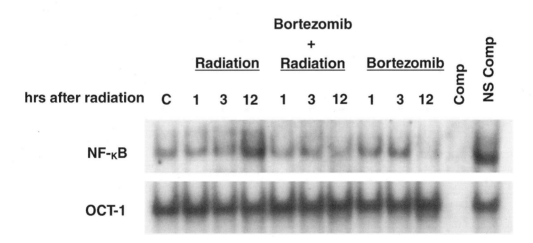

Fig. 3. The proteasome inhibitor bortezomib inhibited radiation-induced and constitutive activation of NF-κB. Nuclear factor-κB (NF-κB) DNA binding was determined by electromobility shift assay as previously described. Constitutive NF-kB DNA binding activity in SCC line Pam 212 (lane C), was enhanced over 12 h following 6-Gy radiation (radiation, lanes 1, 3, and 12). The radiation induced NF-κB DNA binding activity was attenuated in cells pretreated with 10^{-7} M bortezomib (bortezomib + radiation, lanes 1, 3, and 12). Constitutive NF-κB DNA binding activity was also attenuated in cells cultured in medium alone (bortezomib, lanes 1, 3, and 12). NF-κB DNA binding activity was specifically inhibited by unlabeled NF-κB consensus oligonucleotide but not a nonspecific competitor. OCT-1 DNA binding is shown as control.

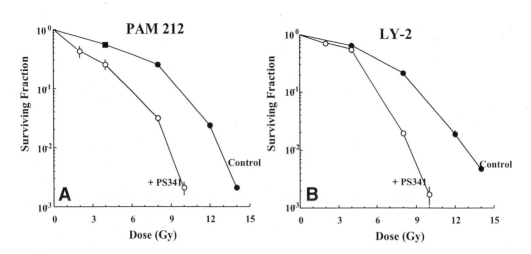

Fig. 4. The proteasome inhibitor bortezomib enhanced radiosensitivity of SCC. Bortezomib and LY-2 cells from stock cultures were plated into a number of 100-mm^2 culture dishes at a concentration of 5×10^5 cells/dish and incubated at 37°C for 24 h. Bortezomib was added to the cells (final concentration, 100 μM), and the cells were incubated an additional 24 h. Following drug treatment, cells were exposed to varying doses of radiation (cobalt-60 irradiator; dose rate = 2.0 Gy/min). After irradiation, the cells were trypsinized, rinsed, counted, and plated (in triplicate) for macroscopic colony formation. Following a 10-d incubation period, colonies were fixed with methanol/acetic acid (3:1) and stained with crystal violet. Colonies with >50 cells were scored and expressed as percentage surviving fraction. The effectiveness of drug alone or in combination with respect to radiation treatment, expressed as a dose effect factor (DEF), was determined for an iso-survival level of 10% by dividing the radiation dose for control cells by the radiation dose for cells treated with drugs. The DEF for PAM 212 cells (**A**) was 1.6, and that for LY-2 cells (**B**) was 1.5 for bortezomib alone.

5. RADIOSENSITIZING EFFECTS OF PROTEASOME INHIBITION

The effects of radiation in the absence and presence of proteasome inhibition on cell survival were examined by colony assays. Figure 4 shows decreased survival of Pam 212 and Pam LY2 SCC cells cultured with bortezomib prior to radiation, resulting in an enhancement in radiosensitization of about 1.5-fold. A requirement for preincubation of SCC with bortezomib for a 24-h interval was consistent with the time interval at which G$_2$/M block and inhibition of radiation-induced activation of NF-κB is observed. Radiosensitizing effects of bortezomib and other proteasome inhibitors have been observed in murine mammary carcinoma, chronic lymphocytic leukemia, Hodgkin's lymphoma, and colon and pancreatic carcinoma cells in vitro *(17–19)*. Combination therapy with bortezomib has also been shown to induce radiosensitization and enhance responses of colon and prostate carcinoma xenografts in vivo *(20,21)*.

6. FUTURE POTENTIAL FOR PROTEASOME INHIBITORS IN RADIOSENSITIZATION

The direct and radiosensitizing cytotoxic effects of proteasome inhibitors on SCC and other cancers indicate that clinical trials are warranted to determine the feasibility and response of concurrent therapy with proteasome inhibitors and radiation. At this writing, a phase I trial of bortezomib and radiation is under way in patients with recurrent SCC of the head and neck, and approval is pending for additional studies.

A number of important questions remain concerning the biologic mechanisms for the direct and radiation cytotoxic effects of proteasome inhibitors. Besides the antiproliferative effects of increasing the concentration of p21 and lowering the concentration of cyclin D, the proteasome contributes to regulation of other cyclins and cyclin-dependent kinase inhibitors *(11)*. For example, it may be interesting to determine whether proteasome inhibitors can restore residual levels of p16, which is frequently decreased by a loss of heterozygosity or hypermethylation in SCC and other epithelial cancers. Degradation of p53 also occurs through the proteasome, and inhibition of the degradation of wild-type p53 could enhance apoptosis in the absence of the antiapoptotic signal mediated by NF-κB. The antiapoptotic effects resulting from inhibition of NF-κB have been associated with a variety of target molecules that inhibit caspase-mediated apoptosis, and the relationship of these candidates to radiation resistance has not been defined. NF-κB activation is likely to be further enhanced in more advanced tumors *(6)*, increasing the antiapoptotic signal, but the penetration, degree of proteasome and NF-κB inhibition, and cytotoxic effects of bortezomib in this setting require further study.

REFERENCES

1. Herscher LL, et al. Principles of chemoradiation: theoretical and practical considerations. *Oncology (Huntingt)* 1998;13(10 suppl 5):11–12.
2. Liebmann J, et al. Changes in radiation survival curve parameters in human tumor and rodent cells exposed to paclitaxel (Taxol). *Int J Radiat Oncol Biol Phys* 1994;29:559–564.
3. Sunwoo JB, et al. Concurrent paclitaxel and radiation in the treatment of locally advanced head and neck cancer. *J Clin Oncol* 2001;19:800–811.
4. Baldwin AS. Control of oncogenesis and cancer therapy resistance by the transcription factor NF-kappaB. *J Clin Invest* 2001;107:241–246
5. Ondrey FG, et al. Constitutive activation of NF-kappaB, AP-1, and NF-IL6 in human head and neck squamous cell carcinoma cell lines that express pro-inflammatory and pro-angiogenic cytokines. *Mol Carcinog* 1999;26:119–129.
6. Dong G, et al. The host environment promotes the constitutive activation of nuclear factor kappaB and proinflammatory cytokine expression during metastatic tumor progression of murine squamous cell carcinoma. *Cancer Res* 1999;59:3495–3504.
7. Kato T, et al. Cisplatin and radiation sensitivity are independently modulated by glutathione and transcription factor NF-kappaB. *Head Neck* 2000;22:748–759.
8. Duffey DC, et al. Expression of a dominant negative inhibitor kappaBalpha of nuclear factor kappaB in human head and neck squamous cell carcinoma inhibits survival, proinflammatory cytokine expression and tumor growth in vivo. *Cancer Res* 1999;59:3468–3478.
9. Adams J, et al. Proteasome inhibition: a new strategy in cancer treatment. *Invest New Drugs* 2000;18:109–121.
10. Sunwoo JB, et al. Novel proteasome inhibitor PS-341 inhibits activation of nuclear factor-kappa B, cell survival, tumor growth, and angiogenesis in squamous cell carcinoma. *Clin Cancer Res* 2001;7:1419–1428.
11. Adams J, et al. Proteasome inhibitors: a novel class of potent and effective anti-tumor agents. *Cancer Res* 1999;59:2615–2622.
12. Dong G, et al. Molecular profiling of transformed and metastatic squamous cell carcinoma cells by differential display and cDNA microarray reveals altered expression of multiple genes related to growth, apoptosis, and angiogenesis and the NF-kappaB signal pathway. *Cancer Res* 2001;61:4797–4808.
13. Hideshima T, et al. The proteasome inhibitor PS-341 inhibits growth, induces apoptosis and overcomes drug resistance in human multiple myeloma cells. *Cancer Res* 2001;3071–3076.
14. Shah S, et al. 26S proteasome inhibition induces apoptosis and limits growth of human pancreatic cancer. *J Cell Biochem* 2001;82:110-122.

15. Li N, Karin M. Ionizing radiation and short wavelength UV activate NF-kappaB through two distinct mechanisms. *Proc Natl Acad Sci USA* 1998;95:13012–13017.
16. Li N, et al. ATM is required for IkappaB kinase (IKKk) activation in response to DNA double strand breaks. *J Biol Chem* 2001;276:8898–8903.
17. Teicher BA, et al. The proteasome inhibitor PS-341 in cancer therapy. *Clin Cancer Res* 1999;5:2638–2645.
18. Masdehors P, et al. Increased sensitivity of CLL-derived lymphocytes to apoptotic death activation by the proteasome-specific inhibitor lactacystin. *Br J Haematol* 1999;105:752–757.
19. Pajonk F, et al. Apoptosis and radiosensitization of hodgkin cells by proteasome inhibition. *Int J Radiat Oncol Biol Phys* 2000;47:1025–1032.
20. Russo SM, et al. Enhancement of radiosensitivity by proteasome inhibition: implications for a role of NF-kappaB. *Int J Radiat Oncol Biol Phys* 2001;50:183–193.
21. Pervan M, et al. Molecular pathways that modify tumor radiation response. *Am J Clin Oncol* 2001;24:481–485.
22. Mitchell JB, et al. Inhibition of oxygen-dependent radiation-induced damage by the nitroxide superoxide dismutase mimic, Tempol. *Arch Biochem Biophys* 1991;289:62–70.

11 Proteasome-Dependent Regulation of NF-κB Activation

Molecular Targeting of Chemotherapy Resistance

James C. Cusack, Jr.

CONTENTS

ABSTRACT

The transcription factor nuclear factor kappa B (NF-κB) is a member of the Rel family of proteins that plays an important role in a variety of cellular response mechanisms including immunity, inflammation, cell growth, and apoptosis. Recent evidence suggests that this transcription factor is induced following exposure of cancer cells to apoptotic stimuli such as tumor necrosis factor (TNF), chemotherapy, and irradiation. The activation of NF-κB involves the proteasome-dependent degradation of an inhibitor of NF-κB and results in a cascade of events leading to the suppression of apoptosis. This mechanism of inducible cancer therapy resistance may be overcome by inhibitors of NF-κB activation. The preliminary studies that led to the development of novel cancer therapies that combine chemotherapy and proteasome inhibition are discussed.

KEY WORDS

Chemotherapy resistance; NF-κB; proteasome inhibition; apoptosis.

1. INTRODUCTION

Recent advances in cancer cell biology have led to the identification of mechanisms responsible for treatment resistance and the development of strategies to overcome treat-

From: *Cancer Drug Discovery and Development: Proteasome Inhibitors in Cancer Therapy*
Edited by: J. Adams © Humana Press Inc., Totowa, NJ

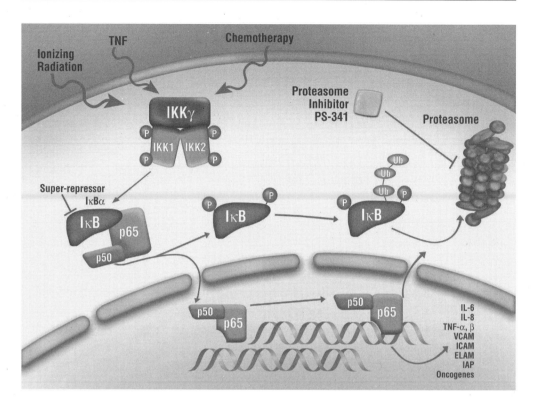

Fig. 1. Mechanism of NF-κB activation. Exposure of cancer cells to apoptotic stimuli such as γ-irradiation, tumor necrosis factor (TNF), or genotoxic chemotherapy results in nuclear localization of the transcription factor NF-κB. DNA binding of NF-κB results in the transcription of a variety of genes involved in inflammation, angiogenesis, and resistance to apoptosis. Inhibition of inducible NF-κB activation by either binding of NF-κB to the super-repressor inhibitor κBα (IκBα) or through the inhibition of proteasomal degradation of the inhibitor IκBα enhances the apoptotic response to these stimuli. ELAM, endothelial leukocyte adhesion molecule; IAP, inhibitor of apoptosis protein; ICAM, intercellular adhesion molecule; IKKγ, IκB kinase γ; IL, interleukin; Ub, ubiquitin; VCAM, vascular cell adhesion molecule.

ment resistance. Among these advances, the transcription factor nuclear factor-κB (NF-κB) has emerged as a principal target partly because of its roles in tumorigenesis and in inducible anticancer therapy resistance. Constitutive activation of NF-κB has been described in a variety of malignancies including cancers of the colon and pancreas (1,2), suggesting that NF-κB may have an important survival function in tumorigenesis. Recent studies have also shown that the inducible activation of NF-κB inhibits the apoptotic response to chemotherapy and irradiation (3). Furthermore, the use of inhibitors of inducible NF-κB has been shown to sensitize cancer cells dramatically to anticancer therapies including certain genotoxic chemotherapy agents (3–13) and γ-irradiation (14,15). The extensive variety of cellular processes that are regulated by NF-κB suggests that the ability to modulate this transcription factor may yield significant improvements in treatments for immune-mediated and inflammatory diseases as well as malignancy (Fig. 1). This chapter, however, focuses on the role of NF-κB in malignancy and the preclinical evidence that has provided the basis for combining NF-κB inhibition with conventional anticancer therapies to treat malignancies derived from solid organs.

2. OVERVIEW OF NF-κB

NF-κB is a member of the Rel family of proteins and is a key transcription factor involved in immune and inflammatory responses as well as cell growth and apoptosis *(8,16,17)*. The five members of the NF-κB family, p65, c-Rel, Rel B, p52, and p50, are able to form various homo- and heterodimeric complexes with a range of transactivation potentials in regulating transcription. The classic form of NF-κB is the heterodimer p50-p65, which binds DNA with high affinity and is a potent activator of gene expression from κB sites due to the strong transactivation domain of p65. NF-κB p50-p65 is the most intensively studied form of NF-κB because of its inducibility by cytokines, lipopolysaccharide (LPS), and T-cell activation signals. Classical NF-κB is regulated primarily through interactions with an inhibitor protein, inhibitor κB (IκB) *(3)*. Activators of NF-κB induce the IκB kinase (IKK) complex to phosphorylate IκB on NH2-terminal serines, leading to ubiquitination and subsequent degradation of the inhibitor by the proteasome. Following IκB degradation, NF-κB translocates to the nucleus, where it regulates a variety of genes involved in cellular processes including the suppression of apoptosis *(16,18)*.

3. REGULATION OF NF-κB ACTIVITY BY THE IκB PROTEINS

The IκB family members, IκBα, IκBβ, IκBε, and Bcl-3, are structurally similar in that they all contain ankyrin repeats. The interaction of the p65 and c-rel NF-κB subunits with IκBα or IκBβ blocks the nuclear localization signal of NF-κB, sequestering these factors in the cytoplasm and thus inhibiting their DNA binding potential. Upon stimulation by a variety of agents (tumor necrosis factor-α [TNFα], IL-1, LPS, and others), IκB molecules are rapidly phosphorylated, leading to subsequent ubiquitination and degradation by proteasome-mediated mechanisms, allowing NF-κB to translocate into the nucleus, where it activates gene expression. Additionally, NF-κB activity can be regulated by control of inherent transcriptional activity. Phosphorylation of NF-κB subunits has been to shown to control whether NF-κB subunits can stimulate transcriptional activity *(16,17)*. This process does not appear to be associated with nuclear translocation (utilizing pre-existing nuclear NF-κB) and thus provides dual control over NF-κB activity. For example, it has been shown that TNF induces the phosphorylation of the p65 subunit of NF-κB on serine 529 and that this stimulates transcriptional potential of at least certain genes *(19)*.

4. ROLE OF THE IκB KINASE (IKK) COMPLEX IN NF-κB ACTIVATION

Activation pathways for NF-κB typically involve ligand-receptor interactions (e.g., TNF and the TNF receptor). Engagement of the receptor by its ligand initiates a signal transduction pathway that ultimately targets the IKK complex that is responsible for phosphorylation of IκB, molecules leading to their degradation and the nuclear translocation of NF-κB *(16,17)*. Additionally, NF-κB can be activated by poorly characterized signal transduction pathways that target the transcriptional activity of certain NF-κB subunits. Some antineoplastic agents such as paclitaxel, doxorubicin, and vincristine have demonstrated a specificity for inducing activation of NF-κB, but not other transcription factors such as activation protein (AP)-1, AP-2, cyclic AMP-responsive element binding protein (CREB), SP-1, or transcription factor II D (TFIID) *(20)*. In the case of paclitaxel, the activation of NF-κB occurs independently of cytokine production *(20)*. How chemotherapy activates NF-κB is poorly understood, but progress has been made at certain levels in understanding the role of the IKK complex in the activation of NF-κB *(21)*. For example, the topoisomerase-I inhibitor camptothecin (CPT) was found by Huang et al. *(22)* to induce transient NF-κB activation in the absence of *de novo* protein synthesis in a variety of cancer cell lines. In addition, NF-κB activation was undetectable in both IKKα- and IKKβ-deficient cells (using embryonic fibroblast cell lines derived from IKKα and IKKβ knockout mice) and was also undetectable in IKKγ-deficient 1.3E2 cells *(22)*. Thus, the authors concluded that the key components of the IKK complex (IKKα/β/γ) are essential for NF-κB activation by CPT, whereas TNF-α was a much weaker activator of NF-κB in IKKβ than IKKκ knockout cells. In contrast to these reported findings, we have found that selective inhibition of IKKβ alone effectively blocked CPT-11–induced activation of NF-κB in colon cancer cells and enhanced tumoricidal response to treatment in colon cancer xenografts (unpublished data). More recently, Tang et al. *(23)* have shown that SN-38- and doxorubicin-induced activation of NF-κB requires nuclear DNA damage and involves both IκBα activation and the IKK complex. The signal leading from DNA damage to IKK activation is not known but has been suggested to involve the ataxia-telangiectasia–mutated (ATM) protein, a member of the high-molecular-weight phosphatidyl inositol 3' (PI3)-kinase-like family, which is mutated in ataxia-telangiectasia patients and is characterized by immunodeficiency and extreme radiosensitivity *(23,24)*.

4.1. Different Classes of Anticancer Therapy May Induce Apoptosis Through Independent Mechanisms

Many cancer therapeutics function by killing cancer cells through induction of the apoptotic pathway. It is therefore not surprising that one effective method cancer cells have developed to protect against these treatments is to resist induction of the death pathway *(25–28)*. Activation of the transcription factor NF-κB by anticancer therapies appears to be a principle mechanism by which cancer cells protect against apoptosis. Wang et al. *(3)* first reported that activation of NF-κB by TNF, ionizing radiation, and the cancer chemotherapeutic compound daunorubicin leads to a functional inhibition of the apoptotic response induced by these stimuli. In addition, it was demonstrated that inhibition of NF-κB leads to a dramatic improvement in the killing response of tumor cells in culture when exposed to these stimuli. Similar results were obtained by other groups relative to TNF and other stimuli *(9,29–31)*. These data indicate that TNF and cytotoxic stimuli activate NF-κB, which provides a cell survival function against a variety of apoptotic stimuli.

The induction of apoptosis controlled by TNF, Fas, and cancer therapies such as chemotherapy or radiation is controlled by induction of the caspase cascade *(25,32,33)*. Apoptosis induced by TNF and Fas typically utilizes caspase-8 as the initiator caspase. However, there are caspase-8–independent mechanisms whereby TNF and Fas can induce apoptosis *(33)*. Activation of caspase-8 is apparently controlled by oligomerization and autoproteolysis, which leads to the activation of other caspases, such as caspase 3/CPP32 *(33)*. Under these conditions members of the interleukin converting enzyme

(ICE) family (caspases) are cleaved by upstream initiators, leading to an expansion of proteolysis of critical cellular proteins, including other members of the caspase family, and ultimately to cell death. TNF-induced apoptosis can be divided into the initiator phase (involving activation of caspase-8) and the effector or "executioner" phase (involving the activation of downstream caspases, such as caspase-3) *(33)*.

4.2. NF-κB Activation Induced by Cancer Therapies Blocks the Induction of Apoptosis Through a Variety of Mechanisms

Recent findings reported by Wang et al. *(34)* indicate that the parallel activation of NF-κB by TNF suppresses the caspase cascade at the level of caspase-8. In contrast, the induction of apoptosis induced by chemotherapy typically does not go through caspase-8 but involves mitochondrial mechanisms leading to release of cytochrome c and the downstream activation of caspase-3 *(32)*. The activation of NF-κB by etoposide leads to the upregulation of A1/Bfl-1, a member of the Bcl-2 family of proteins. A1/Bfl-1 blocks the release of cytochrome c from mitochondria, blocking the downstream activation of caspase-3 *(19)*.

Recently, Gelinas and colleagues *(64)* have provided evidence that Bcl-xL (an antiapoptotic protein that can block Bax proapoptotic function) can be upregulated by NF-κB in response to cytokine treatment. It was shown earlier that Bcl-xL can be upregulated by anticancer drugs *(35)* and that the Jun kinase/stress-activated kinase proteins can interact with Bcl-xL at the level of mitochondria in response to DNA damage *(36)*.

Mammalian inhibitors of apoptosis have been identified and include members of the inhibitor of apoptosis protein (IAP) family of proteins. IAP was originally identified as a baculovirus gene encoding a protein capable of suppressing apoptosis. Now, at least four members of this gene family have been identified: c-IAP1, c-IAP2, XIAP, and NIAP *(37)*. It has been found that c-IAP1 is inducible by TNF and associates with the TNF receptor 1 *(34)*. Recently, Reed and colleagues showed that c-IAP1 and c-IAP2 interact with caspases-3 and -7 to suppress etoposide-induced cell death *(37)*. Wang et al. *(34)* reported that expression of c-IAP1 and c-IAP2 is not sufficient to suppress TNF-induced apoptosis but that activation of TNF-receptor–activated factor (TRAF)1 and TRAF2 are also required; however, c-IAP1 and -2 can block apoptosis induced by etoposide. These results are consistent with the observation that NF-κB suppresses caspase-8 cleavage (the initiating caspase) to block TNF-induced apoptosis and that NF-κB can block apoptosis downstream of caspase-8 as well. Interestingly, IAP proteins have been found in certain tumors *(38)*. More recently, it was shown that the caspase-8 inhibitor Fas-associated death domain (FADD)-like IL-1β converting enzyme (FLICE) inhibitory protein (FLIP) is also an NF-κB–dependent antiapoptotic gene that may be more even efficient than TRAF1, TRAF2, cIAP-1, or c-IAP-2 in protecting against TNF-induced cell death *(39)*.

More recently, in separate reports, Tang et al. *(23)* and De Smaele et al. *(40)* found that one of the ways in which NF-κB protects cells from apoptosis is by substantially blunting the c-Jun-N-terminal kinase (JNK) pathway, part of the mitogen-activated protein kinase (MAPK) family that has been implicated in cell death pathways stimulated by environmental stresses and TNF. Tang et al. *(23)* found that NF-κB negatively modulates TNF-α-mediated JNK activation, partly through NF-κB-induced X-chromosome-linked inhibitor of apoptosis (*XIAP*) gene expression. Importantly, this negative crosstalk, which inhibits apoptosis, was specific to TNF-α signaling and did not affect JNK activation by interleukin-1 (IL-1), demonstrating the specificity of this response for a particular NF-κB activator. De Smaele et al. *(40)* found that Gadd45β, one of the family of genes that encode proteins associated with cell cycle control and DNA repair, was expressed in response to TNF in an NF-κB dependent manner and reduced the activation of JNK.

Just how Gadd45β and XIAP proteins blunt the activation of JNK and suppress apoptosis remains unclear. Kreuz *et al. (41)* found that expression of the caspase-8 homolog FLICE inhibitory protein (cFLIP), a potent negative regulator of death receptor-induced apoptosis, was able to reverse the proapoptotic effect of NF-κB inhibition. Similarly, Micheau et al. *(39)* found that restoration of either the full-length 55-kDa long form of FLIP or an alternatively spliced short form of FLIP in NF-κB null cells inhibits TNF- and FasL-induced cell death efficiently, whereas the expression of IAP or TRAF family members only partially rescues cells from death. It should be noted that under some conditions NF-κB can function proapoptotically. Despite this conclusion, a lack of specificity of the inhibitors used in the experimentation continues. It is clear that NF-κB plays a positive role in T-cell activation-induced cell death through the upregulation of FasL *(42)*. Additionally, it has been proposed that NF-κB functions downstream of p53 in inducing cell death. Nevertheless, our studies indicate that NF-κB functions antiapoptotically when activated by certain chemotherapies.

5. ROLE OF NF-κB IN ONCOGENESIS

Several lines of evidence link NF-κB and IκB family members to cell growth and oncogenesis. First, various viral transforming proteins, including human T-lymphocytic

---

Fig. 2. *(continued on next page)* (**A**) The electrophoresis mobility shift assay (EMSA) was used to evaluate nuclear factor-κB (NF-κB) activation induced by 1 μg/mL SN38 in human colorectal and breast (MCF-7) cancer cell lines. Chemotherapy-induced activation of NF-κB was observed in 11 of 12 cancer cell lines tested, suggesting that NF-κB activation is induced by SN38 in most colorectal cancer cell lines. Positive control (+) was KM12L4 cells treated for 2 h with 10 ng/mL TNF-α (a potent activator of NF-κB). [Reprinted with permission from Cusack JC, Liu R, Baldwin ASJ. Inducible chemoresistance to 7-ethyl-10-(4-(1-piperidino)-1-piperidino)-carbonyloxy-camptothe cin (CPT-11) in colorectal cancer cells and a xenograft model is overcome by inhibition of nuclear factor-κB activation. *Cancer Res* 2000;60:2323–2330.] (**B**) EMSA of nuclear protein extracts obtained from LOVO tumors treated with the super-repressor inhibitor IκBα (IκBα) and camptothecin-11 (CPT-11) demonstrated that NF-κB activation is induced in vivo by treatment with chemotherapy. Inhibition of NF-κB resulted in dramatic enhancement of the apoptotic response to CPT-11 treatment. PBS, phosphate-buffered saline. (A and B reprinted with permission from Cusack JC, Liu R, Baldwin ASJ. Inducible chemoresistance to 7-ethyl-10-(4-(1-piperidino)-1-piperidino)-carbonyloxycamptothecin (CPT-11) in colorectal cancer cells and a xenograft model is overcome by inhibition of nuclear factor-κB activation. *Cancer Res* 2000;60:2323–2330.) (**C**) EMSA was used to evaluate the effect of treatment with the proteasome inhibitor bortezomib (PS-341; 1 μ*M*) on the activation of NF-κB induced by treatment with SN-38 (1 μg/mL) in human colorectal cancer cells. Cell cultures were treated with bortezomib or mock control for 1 h, followed 3 h later by treatment with SN-38. Cells were harvested and assayed for nuclear translocation of NF-κB at 1, 2, and 6 h after chemotherapy treatment. Positive control (+) was KM12L4 cells treated for 2 h with 10 ng/mL TNF-α (a potent activator of NF-κB). (Reprinted with permission from Cusack JC, Liu R, Houston MA, et al. Enhanced chemosensitivity to CPT-11 with proteasome inhibitor bortezomib: implications for systemic NF-κB inhibition. *Cancer Res* 2001;61:3535–3540.

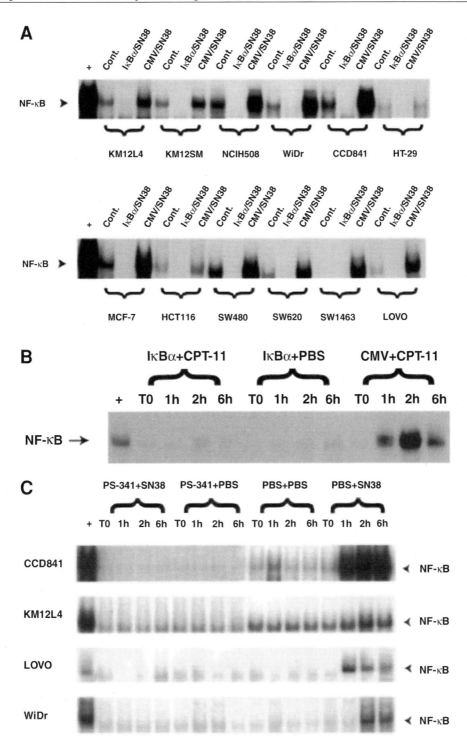

Fig. 2

virus (HTLV)-I Tax and Epstein-Barr virus (EBV) large multifunctional protease (LMP)-1, activate NF-κB *(16,17)*. Second, activated H-Ras *(43)* and the oncoprotein BCR-ABL *(44)* both activate NF-κB. Furthermore, NF-κB activity is required not only for Ras to initiate cellular transformation, but also for BCR-ABL to initiate tumorigenesis *(44)*. Van Waes and colleagues have shown that NF-κB is required for head and neck squamous cell carcinoma *(45)*. NF-κB–mediated transformation may function through the upregulation of gene expression, as several genes that mediate cell growth have been found to be transcriptionally regulated by NF-κB. These genes include *c-myc (16)* and *cyclin D1 (46,47)*. Another important role for NF-κB in oncogenesis is blocking transformation-associated apoptosis. For example, NF-κB blocks the ability of oncogenic Ras to induce apoptosis, allowing successful survival of transformed cells *(48)*. There is also evidence that NF-κB can promote metastasis through the upregulation of certain genes and also can stimulate angiogenesis. One of the NF-κB subunits (p52) was cloned originally as a gene translocated and upregulated in certain lymphomas *(16,17)*, and the founding member of the NF-κB family, c-Rel, is the cellular homolog of the transforming gene of avian reticuloendotheliosis virus *(16,17)*. These data suggest that NF-κB dysregulation may serve as a key component in the early stages of oncogenesis.

5.1. Inhibition of Chemotherapy-Induced NF-κB Activation Enhances the Apoptotic Response to Treatment: Rationale for Combination Anticancer Therapies

It is well known that cancer chemotherapies induce tumor cytotoxicity at least partly through the induction of cell death (apoptosis) *(25–28)*. More recently, some chemotherapy agents have been shown to activate NF-κB. For example, doxorubicin (Adriamycin), cisplatin, gemcitabine, paclitaxel, and 5-fluorouracil (5-FU) have been shown to induce NF-κB nuclear translocation *(5,10,13,49–53)*. We have previously reported that this response is also observed in colorectal cancer xenografts treated with the topoisomerase inhibitor CPT-11 *(7)* (Fig. 2). Activation of NF-κB by some chemotherapy agents may limit the potential apoptotic response to treatment. Findings reported from our laboratory demonstrated that inhibition of chemotherapy-induced NF-κB activation, using a highly selective inhibitor of NF-κB (super-repressor IκBα), in fact enhances apoptosis in vitro and in vivo *(7,54)* (Fig. 3A). Subsequent studies performed in colon cancer cells and a xenograft model similarly demonstrated that nonselective inhibition of NF-κB, using the proteasome inhibitor bortezomib (Velcade®; formerly known as PS-341), enhanced the apoptotic response to CPT-11 and led to a significant tumoricidal response *(8)* (Fig. 3B). Other laboratories have reported similar findings. For example, Lind et al. *(1)* found that gemcitabine hydrochloride's antitumor activity in colon cancer cells was enhanced by inhibition of NF-κB. Similarly Shah et al. *(55)* reported that inhibition of NF-κB in pancreatic cancer xenografts treated with a proteasome inhibitor and CPT-11 significantly inhibited tumor cell proliferation, increased apoptosis, and inhibited tumor cell growth compared with either treatment alone. Taken together, these studies suggest that the antitumor response to chemotherapy agents that induce activation of NF-κB may be significantly enhanced by combining these chemotherapy agents with inhibitors of NF-κB.

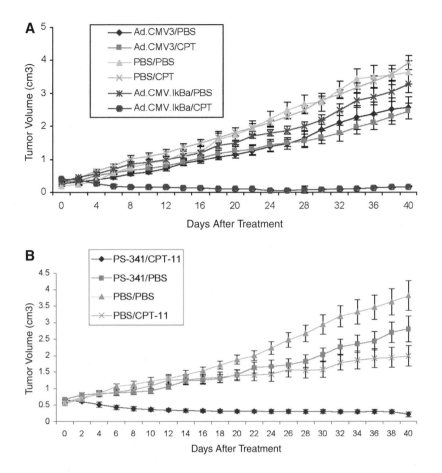

Fig. 3. (A) Tumoricidal response of LOVO tumors to camptothecin-11 (CPT-11) administered in combination with the adenovirus vector expressing the super-repressor IκBα (Ad.CMV.IκBα) compared with control adenovirus (Ad.CMV3), or vehicle alone. Adenovirus was administered as a weekly intratumoral injection of 1×10^{10} PFU/200 μL × 3 wk. CPT-11 (33 mg/kg) was administered iv every 4 d during the 20-d treatment period. Phosphate-buffered saline (PBS) was administered iv as a control. Tumor diameter along two orthogonal axes was recorded every other day. Tumor volume was recorded as the mean ± SE (bars) for each treatment group ($n = 15$–19). (Reprinted with permission from Wang C-Y, Cusack JC, Liu R, Baldwin ASJ. Control of inducible chemoresistance: enhanced antitumor efficacy via increased apoptosis by inhibition of NF-κB. *Nat Med* 1999;5:412–417.) **(B)** The effects of combination therapy using the proteasome inhibitor bortezomib (PS-341) and CPT-11 were assessed in a xenograft model (n = 8–10/group). One-centimeter-diameter LOVO tumors were grown in the flanks of nude mice. The tumoricidal effects of systemic treatment were assessed following pretreatment with bortezomib (1 mg/kg iv bolus injection) or vehicle alone, followed by iv bolus administration of CPT-11 (33 mg/kg) or vehicle. Treatment was administered 2×/wk, and tumor diameter along two orthogonal axes was recorded every other day. (Reprinted with permission from Cusack JC, Liu R, Houston MA, et al. Enhanced chemosensitivity to CPT-11 with proteasome inhibitor bortezomib: implications for systemic NF-κB inhibition. *Cancer Res* 2001;61:3535–3540.)

6. IS THERE A ROLE FOR MONOTHERAPY?
TARGETING CONSTITUTIVE ACTIVATION OF NF-κB

Constitutive activation of NF-κB has been described in a variety of cancer cell lines as well as patient samples of colon cancer (1), pancreatic cancer (2), hepatoma (56), and gastric cancer (57). The high incidence of constitutive NF-κB activation in cancer cells may be explained by the survival role it plays in tumorigenesis. For example, the expression of many early response genes involved in critical aspects of tumor progression such as growth (p21, p27, and cyclin D1), resistance and apoptosis (glutathione-S-transferase, cIAP-1, PEA-15, and Fas ligand), inflammation and angiogenesis (chemokine growth-regulated oncogene 1 [also called KC]), and signal transduction (c-Met, yes-associated protein, and syk) has been associated with NF-κB (58). Modulation of the genes involved in tumorigenesis through the upstream inhibition of NF-κB may offer therapeutic advantages. In hematologic malignancies such as multiple myeloma, recent findings by Anderson and colleagues (59) suggest that the constitutive expression of NF-κB may play a critical survival function that predisposes these cells to be highly sensitive to inhibitors of NF-κB (see Chap. 24). In solid tumor systems, however, the data demonstrating sensitivity to treatment with NF-κB inhibitors alone have been less consistent. In our experience, treatment with either selective or nonselective NF-κB inhibitors alone has resulted in only modest tumor growth inhibition and no significant enhancement of apoptosis (7,8,54). Nonetheless, work reported by Huang et al. (60) suggests that in some solid tumors such as melanoma, inhibition of NF-κB using a dominant-negative mutant inhibitor (IκBα) decreased the level of constitutive NF-κB activity, inhibited tumor growth, and prevented lung metastasis in nude mice. In the case of solid organ malignancies, the role of NF-κB inhibition as an adjuvant to genotoxic chemotherapy has been more compelling.

7. PROTEASOME INHIBITORS ARE POTENT
INHIBITORS OF NF-κB ACTIVATION

Ubiqutin–proteasome–dependent proteolysis plays an essential role in degrading regulatory proteins and thereby controlling processes of cell proliferation and cell death. Recent experiments using cell culture and mouse models have demonstrated that proteasome inhibitors induce cancer cell apoptosis and therefore inhibit tumor growth (61). The proteasome inhibitors have the following features: (1) greater apoptosis-inducing potency than certain anticancer drugs, (2) selectivity toward transformed cells, and (3) the ability to overcome tumor cell resistance to cytotoxic agents. Because proteasome inhibitors block NF-κB activation via inhibition of IκB degradation (61,62), several of the anticancer effects of proteasome inhibition may be attributable to their ability to block NF-κB activation. We have shown that a proteasome inhibitor (bortezomib) strongly synergizes with CPT-11 in inducing an apoptotic response in colorectal tumors grown in nude mice (8) (see Fig. 3B). In these initial studies, the combined use of bortezomib and CPT-11 led to dramatic antitumor responses using the LOVO colorectal tumor model. The use of a nonselective inhibitor of NF-κB, such as the proteasome inhibitor bortezomib, in combination with chemotherapy is currently under investigation in phase I and phase II clinical trials at our institution and others.

It is possible that the anticancer effects of combination chemotherapy and proteasome inhibition are multifactorial. For example, it was recently shown that CPT-induced downregulation of topoisomerase I (TOPI) in tumor cells may contribute to resistance to CPT *(63)*. In these experiments, inhibition of the 26S proteasome, using MG132, effectively blocked CPT-induced downregulation of TOPI. It remains unclear however, whether the downregulation of TOPI is NF-κB–dependent. Other factors such as the stabilization of p53 and the cell cycle regulators p21 and p27 following proteasome inhibition may also contribute to the observed response of enhanced chemosensitivity. Although the mechanisms of response remain to be determined, the observed enhancement of apoptotic response is compelling evidence leading us to explore further the role of proteasome inhibition and other inhibitors of NF-κB as potentially useful adjuvants to conventional chemotherapies.

REFERENCES

1. Lind DS, et al. Nuclear factor-kappa B is upregulated in colorectal cancer. *Surgery* 2001;130:363–369.
2. Wang W, et al. The nuclear factor-κB RelA transcription factor is constitutively activated in human pancreatic adenocarcinoma cells. *Clin Cancer Res* 1999;5:119–127.
3. Wang C-Y, et al. TNF- and cancer therapy-induced apoptosis: potentiation by inhibition of NF-κB. *Science* 1996;274:784–787.
4. Cusack JC, et al. Chemosensitization of human fibrosarcoma xenografts following adenoviral-mediated transfer of the NF-κB super-repressor IκBα gene. *Cancer Gene Ther* 1997;4:S44.
5. Cusack JC, et al. Chemosensitization of colorectal cancer cells by expression of the NF-kB super-repressor IκBα. *Surg Forum* 1997;48:815–817.
6. Cusack JC, et al. NF-κB and chemoresistance: potentiation of cancer chemotherapy via inhibition of NF-κB. *Drug Resistance Updates* 1999;2:271.
7. Cusack JC, et al. Inducible chemoresistance to 7-ethyl-10-(4-(1-piperidino)-1-piperidino)-carbonyloxy-camptothecin (CPT-11) in colorectal cancer cells and a xenograft model is overcome by inhibition of nuclear factor-κB activation. *Cancer Res* 2000;60:2323–2330.
8. Cusack JC, et al. Enhanced chemosensitivity to CPT-11 with proteasome inhibitor PS-341: implications for systemic NF-κB Inhibition. *Cancer Res* 2001;61:3535–3540.
9. Van Antwerp DJ, et al. Suppression of TNF-alpha-induced apoptosis by NF-κB. *Science* 1996;274:787.
10. Bold RJ, et al. Chemosensitization of pancreatic cancer by inhibition of the 26S proteasome. *J Surg Res* 2001;100:11–17.
11. Arlt A, et al. Inhibition of NF-kappaB sensitizes human pancreatic carcinoma cells to apoptosis induced by etoposide (VP16) or doxorubicin. *Oncogene* 2001;20:859–868.
12. Jones DR, et al. Inhibition of NF-kappaB sensitizes non-small cell lung cancer cells to chemotherapy-induced apoptosis. *Ann Thorac Surg* 2000;70:930–936; discussion 936–937.
13. Shah SA, et al. 26S proteasome inhibition induces apoptosis and limits growth of human pancreatic cancer. *J Cell Biochem* 2001;82:110–122.
14. Russo SM, et al. Enhancement of radiosensitivity by proteasome inhibition: implications for a role of NF-kappaB. *Int J Radiat Oncol Biol Phys* 2001;50:183–193.
15. Kato T, et al. Cisplatin and radiation sensitivity in human head and neck squamous carcinomas are independently modulated by glutathione and transcription factor NF-kappaB. *Head Neck* 2000;22:748–759.
16. Baldwin AS, Jr. The NF-kappa B and I kappa B proteins: new discoveries and insights. *Annu Rev Immunol* 1996;14:649–683.
17. Ghosh S, et al. NF-kappa B and Rel proteins: evolutionarily conserved mediators of immune responses. *Annu Rev Immunol* 1998;16:225–260.
18. Ghosh S, et al. Activation in vitro of NF-κB by phosphorylation of its inhibitor IκB. *Nature* 1990;344:678–682.
19. Wang D, et al. Activation of NF-κB-dependent transcription by TNFα is mediated through phosphorylation of RelA/p65 on serine 529. *J Biol Chem* 1998;273:29411–29416.
20. Das KC, et al. Activation of NF-kappaB by antineoplastic agents. Role of protein kinase C. *J Biol Chem* 1997;272:14914–14920.
21. Bottero V, et al. Activation of nuclear factor kappaB through the IKK complex by the topoisomerase poisons SN38 and doxorubicin: a brake to apoptosis in HeLa human carcinoma cells. *Cancer Res* 2001;61:7785–7791.

22. Huang TT, et al. NF-kappaB activation by camptothecin. A linkage between nuclear DNA damage and cytoplasmic signaling events. *J Biol Chem* 2000;275:9501–9509.
23. Tang G, et al. Inhibition of JNK activation through NF-kappaB target genes. *Nature* 2001;414:313–317.
24. Piret B, et al. The ATM protein is required for sustained activation of NF-kappaB following DNA damage. *Oncogene* 1999;18:2261–2271.
25. Thompson CB. Apoptosis in the pathogenesis and treatment of disease. *Science* 1995;267:1456–1462.
26. Schmitt CA, et al. Apoptosis and therapy. *J Pathol* 1999;187:127–137.
27. Kastan MB. Molecular determinants of sensitivity to antitumor agents. *Biochim Biophys Acta* 1999;1424:R37–R42.
28. Fisher DE. Apoptosis in cancer therapy: crossing the threshold. *Cell* 1996;78:539–542.
29. Beg AA, et al. An essential role for NF-κB in preventing TNF-alpha-induced cell death. *Science* 1996;274:782.
30. Arsura M, et al. TGF beta 1 inhibits NF-kappa B/Rel activity inducing apoptosis of B cells: transcriptional activation of I kappa B alpha. *Immunity* 1996;5:31–40.
31. Liu ZG, et al. Dissection of TNF receptor 1 effector functions: JNK activation is not linked to apoptosis while NF-κB activation prevents cell death. *Cell* 1996;87:565.
32. Datta R, et al. Activation of the CPP32 protease in apoptosis induced by 1-beta-D-arabinofuranosylcytosine and other DNA-damaging agents. *Blood* 1996;88:1936–1943.
33. Nicholson DW, et al. Caspases: killer proteases. *Trends Biochem Sci* 1997;22:299–306.
34. Wang C-Y, et al. NF-κB antiapoptosis: induction of TRAF1 and TRAF2 and c-IAP1 and c-IAP2 to suppress caspase-8 activation. *Science* 1998;281:1680–1683.
35. Kojima H, et al. Abrogation of mitochondrial cytochrome c release and caspase-3 activation in acquired multidrug resistance. *J Biol Chem* 1998;273:16647–16650.
36. Kharbanda S, et al. Translocation of SAPK/JNK to mitochondria and interaction with Bcl-x (L) in response to DNA damage. *J Biol Chem* 2000;275:322–327.
37. Ferreira CG, et al. p53 and chemosensitivity. *Ann Oncol* 1999;10:1011–1021.
38. LaCasse EC, et al. The inhibitors of apoptosis (IAPs) and their emerging role in cancer. *Oncogene* 1998;17:3247–3259.
39. Micheau O, et al. NF-kappaB signals induce the expression of c-FLIP. *Mol Cell Biol* 2001;21:5299–305.
40. De Smaele E, et al. Induction of gadd45beta by NF-kappaB downregulates pro-apoptotic JNK signalling. *Nature* 2001;414:308–313.
41. Kreuz S, et al. NF-kappaB inducers upregulate cFLIP, a cycloheximide-sensitive inhibitor of death receptor signaling. *Mol Cell Biol* 2001;21:3964–3973.
42. Kasibhatla S, et al. Regulation of fas-ligand expression during activation-induced cell death in T lymphocytes via nuclear factor kB. *J Biol Chem* 1999;274:987.
43. Finco TS, et al. Oncogenic Ha-Ras-induced signaling activates NF-kappaB transcriptional activity, which is required for cellular transformation. *J Biol Chem* 1997;272:24113–24116.
44. Reuther JY, et al. A requirement for NF-kappaB activation in Bcr-Abl-mediated transformation. *Genes Dev* 1998;12:968–981.
45. Duffey DC, et al. Expression of a dominant-negative mutant inhibitor-kappaBalpha of nuclear factor-kappaB in human head and neck squamous cell carcinoma inhibits survival, proinflammatory cytokine expression, and tumor growth in vivo. *Cancer Res* 1999;59:3468–3474.
46. Hinz M, et al. NF-kappaB function in growth control: regulation of cyclin D1 expression and G0/G1-to-S-phase transition. *Mol Cell Biol* 1999;19:2690–2698.
47. Guttridge DC, et al. NF-kappaB controls cell growth and differentiation through transcriptional regulation of cyclin D1. *Mol Cell Biol* 1999;19:5785–5799.
48. Mayo MW, et al. Requirement of NF-kappaB activation to suppress p53-independent apoptosis induced by oncogenic Ras. *Science* 1997;278:1812–1815.
49. Takizawa K, et al. Synergistic induction of ICAM-1 expression by cisplatin and 5- fluorouracil in a cancer cell line via a NF-kappaB independent pathway. *Br J Cancer* 1999;80:954–963.
50. Rangan GK, et al. Inhibition of nuclear factor-kappaB activation reduces cortical tubulointerstitial injury in proteinuric rats. *Kidney Int* 1999;56:118–134.
51. Byrd CA, et al. Heat shock protein 90 mediates macrophage activation by Taxol and bacterial lipopolysaccharide. *Proc Natl Acad Sci USA* 1999;96:5645–5650.
52. Lee LF, et al. Identification of tumor-specific paclitaxel (Taxol)-responsive regulatory elements in the interleukin-8 promoter. *Mol Cell Biol* 1997;17:5097–5105.

53. Maldonado V, et al. Modulation of NF-kappa B, and Bcl-2 in apoptosis induced by cisplatin in HeLa cells. *Mutat Res* 1997; 381:67–75.
54. Wang C-Y, et al. Control of inducible chemoresistance: enhanced antitumor efficacy via increased apoptosis by inhibition of NF-κB. *Nat Med* 1999;5:412–417.
55. Shah SA, et al. Ubiquitin proteasome inhibition and cancer therapy. *Surgery* 2002;131:595–600.
56. Tai DI, et al. Constitutive activation of nuclear factor kappaB in hepatocellular carcinoma. *Cancer* 2000;89:2274–2281.
57. Sasaki N, et al. Nuclear factor-kappaB p65 (RelA) transcription factor is constitutively activated in human gastric carcinoma tissue. *Clin Cancer Res* 2001;7:4136–4142.
58. Loukinova E, et al. Growth regulated oncogene-alpha expression by murine squamous cell carcinoma promotes tumor growth, metastasis, leukocyte infiltration and angiogenesis by a host CXC receptor-2 dependent mechanism. *Oncogene* 2000;19:3477–3486.
59. Hideshima T, et al. NF-kappa B as a therapeutic target in multiple myeloma. *J Biol Chem* 2002;277:16639–16647.
60. Huang S, et al. Nuclear factor-kappaB activity correlates with growth, angiogenesis, and metastasis of human melanoma cells in nude mice. *Clin Cancer Res* 2000;6:2573–2581.
61. Dou QP, et al. Proteasome inhibition leads to significant reduction of Bcr-Abl expression and subsequent induction of apoptosis in K562 human chronic myelogenous leukemia cells. *J Pharmacol Exp Ther* 1999;289:781.
62. Palombella VJ, et al. Role of the proteasome and NF-kappaB in streptococcal cell wall-induced polyarthritis. *Proc Natl Acad Sci USA* 1998; 95:15671–15676.
63. Desai SD, et al. Ubiquitin/26S proteasome-mediated degradation of topoisomerase I as a resistance mechanism to camptothecin in tumor cells. *Cancer Res* 2001;61:5926–5932.
64. Ravi R., et al. Regulation of death receptor expression and TRAIL/Apo2L-induced apoptosis by NF-kappa B. *Nat Cell Biol* 2001;3:409–416.

12 Bortezomib with Taxanes

Leonard Liebes, Bruce Ng, Yi-He Ling, and Roman Perez-Soler

CONTENTS

INTRODUCTION
MATERIALS AND METHODS
RESULTS
CONCLUSIONS

ABSTRACT

We have examined the use of combinations of bortezomib (PS-341) with docetaxel in in vitro and in vivo studies and have added the use of localized delivery of radiation in in vitro combinations through the use of a ^{90}Y-labeled monoclonal antibody, BrE-3. In in vitro studies, marked cytotoxic effects from the combination of PS-341/docetaxel were seen progressively with the ovarian cell line SKOV3 over the time period of 24–72 h, with additive activity at 48 h and synergistic activity at 72 h. In non-small cell lung cancer (H460 cell) PS-341 induced a 25-kDa Bcl-2 cleavage product different from fragments produced by other anticancer agents. This unique Bcl-2 cleavage product was an early event starting 12 h after PS-341 exposure, followed by DNA fragmentation and cleavage of caspase-mediated PARP and β-catenin at 36 h. Results with ovarian xenograft model showed the beneficial effects of combined treatment with PS-341 and docetaxel: tumor growth was limited for a 30-d period following the cessation of treatment compared with single agents alone. Significant augmentation of cytotoxicity at and below therapeutic levels of PS-341 and docetaxel were observed with radioimmunotherapy studies using ovarian and breast cancer cell lines.

KEY WORDS

PS-341; docetaxel; Bcl-2; cleavage product; H460; SKOV3; MCF-7 cells; ^{90}Y-BrE3; radioimmunotherapy.

1. INTRODUCTION

Bortezomib (Velcade™; formerly known as PS-341), a dipeptide boronic acid derivative, is a potent and reversible inhibitor of the proteasome. It plays a pivotal role in the

From: *Cancer Drug Discovery and Development: Proteasome Inhibitors in Cancer Therapy*
Edited by: J. Adams © Humana Press Inc., Totowa, NJ

degradation of many intracellular regulatory proteins such as inhibitor κB/nuclear factor-κB (IκB/NF-κB), p53, and the cyclin-dependent kinase inhibitors p21 and p27 *(1,2)*. The antineoplastic effect of bortezomib may involve several distinct mechanisms which include inhibition of cell growth signaling pathways, induction of apoptosis, and inhibition of cellular adhesion molecule expression *(2–5)*. Preliminary evidence has also supported the potential radiosensitizing effect of bortezomib *(6)*.

Taxoids have been identified as an important class of cytotoxic agents for the treatment of breast and epithelial ovarian cancer *(7,8)*. Docetaxel is a mitotic spindle poison; it increases tubular polymerization, which promotes microtubule assembly and inhibits tubulin depolymerization and thus stabilizes the microtubules *(9)*. As a result, the cells are blocked in G_2 and M, the phases of the cell cycle most sensitive to ionizing radiation *(10)*. Taxanes have been shown to be useful radiosensitizers alone *(11)* and when combined in-vitro with carboplatin *(12)*.

BrE-3 antibody is a murine IgG1 monoclonal antibody (MAb) that reacts with a polyepitopic 400-kDa moiety of breast epithelial mucin that is a tumor-associated epitope *(13)*. This antibody was developed at the Cancer Research Institute of Contra Costa and has been shown to react with 90% of breast carcinomas as tested by immunopathology as well as with pancreatic carcinoma. We have recently generated immunohistochemical studies (unpublished data) extending work with ovarian cell lines that has shown 95% specificity in ovarian carcinomas compared with paired normal tissue blocks. The utility of this antibody in chemo-radioimmunotherapy (RAIT) combinations for breast and ovarian cancer is currently under investigation *(14,15)*.

We have examined the effects of combinations of docetaxel and bortezomib in in vitro and in-vivo studies with ovarian tumor cell lines. We have also used the non-small cell lung cancer cell line H460 to follow the possible effects on microtubule assembly/disassembly along with the time-course and specificity of the effects of bortezomib on the cleavage of Bcl2. Work is also presented showing the time-course of an observed specific Bcl2 cleavage product with respect to the degree of apoptosis and cleavage of the caspase-3 like target proteins poly-ADP ribose polymerase (PARP) and β-catenin. We also examined the effects of localized radiation using combinations of chemotherapy (bortezomib, docetaxel) with RAIT, employing a ^{90}Y-labeled monoclonal antibody with specificity for breast and ovarian cell lines using the MCF7 and SKOV3 cell lines. Finally, we provide a proposed mechanism that summarizes the pleotrophic apoptotic effects of bortezomib through the action of (1) activated caspases, (2) the cleavage of Bcl2, and (3) cytochrome c release from mitochondria.

2. MATERIALS AND METHODS

2.1. In Vitro Measurement of Cell Proliferation

Bortezomib, docetaxel, and the combination of both together were tested for *in vitro* effects on cell proliferation. The colorimetric [MTT, 3- (4,5-dimethylthiazol-2-yi)-2,5-diphenyl tetrasolium bromide] assay was used to determine cell survival and proliferation; 1×10^4 cells were found to be within the linear range for MTT absorbance readings for both of the ovarian and breast cell lines. Briefly, 1×10^4 cells were plated in 96-well plates overnight in McCoy's 5A modified media with 10% fetal bovine serum (FBS). Previous studies have determined that 0.1 μM of bortezomib is the 20% inhibitory concentration (IC_{20}). Cells were incubated with 0.1 μM bortezomib with or without escalating doses of docetaxel (0.04–5 μM). Cells incubated in media only served as the control. Plates were incubated for 3 d, and MTT was then added and allowed to incubate for an additional 4 h. Cells were lysed with HCl/isopropanol, and absorbance was measured on an enzyme-linked immunosorbent assay (ELISA) plate reader with a test wavelength of 570 nm and a reference wavelength of 630 nm. Percentage cell growth inhibition was calculated by: $[(OD_{control} - OD_{treated})/OD_{control}] \times 100$.

2.2. Determination of Microtubule Assembly–Disassembly

The assessment of microtubule assembly–disassembly was performed as described previously (16). Briefly, the inhibition of microtubule assembly was determined in a reaction solution containing 100 μL of β-tubulin solution (500–600 μg protein/mL), 0.1 M MES, 1 mM EGTA, 0.5 $MgCl_2$, 0.1 mM EDTA, and 2.5 M glycerol. After the addition of either 2 μM bortezomib, 23 μM paclitaxel, or 22 μM vinblastine, 1 mM GTP was added to the reaction system, and the microtubule assembly process was followed by absorbance changes at 350 nm (OD), at room temperature every 5 min, using an Ultrospec III spectrophotometer (Pharmacia LKB, Uppsala, Sweden). The monitoring of the tubulin polymerization required 30 min. For the assay of inhibition of microtubule disassembly, compounds at the indicated concentration were added to a prepolymerized microtubule system as described above and incubated in an ice bath. Changes of OD were monitored at 350 nm for 20 min, until the OD values in the control returned to the starting level, i.e., the completion of assembly–disassembly cycle. Dimethyl sulfoxide (DMSO), added as a control, had no effect in either the assembly or disassembly processes.

2.3. Western Blot Analysis

Cells were scraped from the culture, washed twice with phosphate-buffered saline (PBS), and then suspended in 30 μL of Western blot lysis buffer containing 50 mM Tris-HCl (pH 7.5), 250 mM NaCl, 1 mM EDTA, 1 mM EGTA, 1 mM NaF, 1 mM phenylmethylsulfonyl fluoride (PMSF), 1 mM dithiothreitol (DTT), 20 μg/mL leupeptin, 20 μg/mL aprotinin, 0.1% Triton X-100, and 1% sodium dodecyl sulfate (SDS) at 0–4°C for 15 min. After centrifugation at 1500g for 10 min at 0°C, the supernatants were collected and the proteins were separated on either 12% or 15% SDS-PAGE. Following electrophoresis, protein blots were transferred to a nitrocellulose membrane. The membrane was blocked with 5% nonfat milk in TBST and incubated overnight with the corresponding primary antibodies at 4°C. After washing three times with TBST, the membrane was incubated at room temperature for 1 h, with horseradish peroxidase-conjugated secondary antibody diluted with TBST (1:1000). The detected protein signals were visualized by an ECL reaction system (Amersham, Arlington Heights, IL).

2.4. In Vivo Treatment of Ovarian Tumors in Athymic Nude Mice

Athymic Swiss nude female mice, 8–10 wk old, were obtained from Taconic Animal Laboratory (Germantown, NY). Animals were treated in accordance with the Animal Welfare Act and the NIH Guide for the Care and Use of Laboratory Animals published by the National Institutes of Health. The Institutional Animal Care and Use Committee of New York University School of Medicine approved all experiments. Mice were kept under sterile conditions in a laminar flow room in cages with filter bonnets and were fed a sterilized mouse diet and sterilized tap water *ad libitum*. Housing was temperature controlled, and 12-h light/dark cycles were used.

Athymic female nude mice were inoculated with 10^6 human ovarian tumor cells (SKOV-3) in the left flank. After 21 d, when palpable tumors approximated 100–150 mg, tumor-bearing animals were randomized into prospective treatment groups; untreated control, bortezomib (1 mg/kg iv), docetaxel (8 mg/kg iv), and combined bortezomib and docetaxel. Bortezomib and docetaxel were administered intravenously via the tail vein weekly for 4 wk. Tumor dimensions in three planes were measured with a Vernier caliper, and tumor weights were extrapolated by multiplying the length × width × height and dividing by 1.8.

2.5. In Vitro Combined Treatment With ^{90}Y-BrE3, Docetaxel, and Bortezomib

^{90}Y-BrE3, docetaxel, bortezomib, and the combination were tested for in vitro effects on cell proliferation. The tumor cell line that we utilized for in vitro studies was the SKOV3 human ovarian carcinoma. The SKOV3 cell line expresses the BrE3 epitope. For a comparison with RAIT, from our previous studies with topotecan *(14)*, we also used an MCF-7 breast cancer cell line that also expresses the BrE-3 epitope. An amount of 1×10^4 cells (SKOV3, MCF7) were found to be within the linear range for MTT absorbance readings for both of these cell types. Briefly, 1×10^4 cells were plated in 96-well plates overnight in McCoy's 5A media with 10% FBS. ^{90}Y-BrE3 (1 μCi) was added to half of the wells and incubated for 1 h. Cells were washed three times to remove unbound antibodies. Escalating concentrations of docetaxel or bortezomib (0.001–1 μ*M*) were then added to the appropriate wells. Cells incubated in media only served as the control. Plates were incubated for 3 d, and MTT was then added and allowed to incubate for an additional 4 h. Cells were lysed with HCl/isopropanol, and absorbance was measured on an ELISA plate reader with a test wavelength of 570 nm and a reference wavelength of 630 nm. Percent cell growth inhibition was calculated by: $[(OD_{control} - OD_{treated})/OD_{control}] \times 100$.

3. RESULTS

3.1. In Vitro Cytotoxicity

Figure 1 contains the results from a series of dose-escalating studies of the cytotoxic effects of docetaxel over the concentration range of 0.04–5 μ*M*. The addition of 0.1 μ*M* bortezomib was found to enhance the cytotoxicity significantly for each of the docetaxel doses examined. The effects of combinations of docetaxel/bortezomib were more discernable and additive at the 48-h test point compared with the 24-h exposure for the combination of these two drugs (Fig. 1B). After 72 h of exposure, the effects of the combination bortezomib and docetaxel exposures were more dramatic and appeared to show synergistic activity, particularly at concentrations in the range of 0.04–1 μ*M* docetaxel (Fig. 1C).

Fig. 1. *(Continued on next page)* Comparison of duration of exposure of the combination bortezomib (PS-341) and docetaxel (taxotere) on the cytotoxicity of SKOV3 cells at time points ranging from 24 to 72 h. **(A)** 24 h; **(B)** 48 h; **(C)** 72 h.

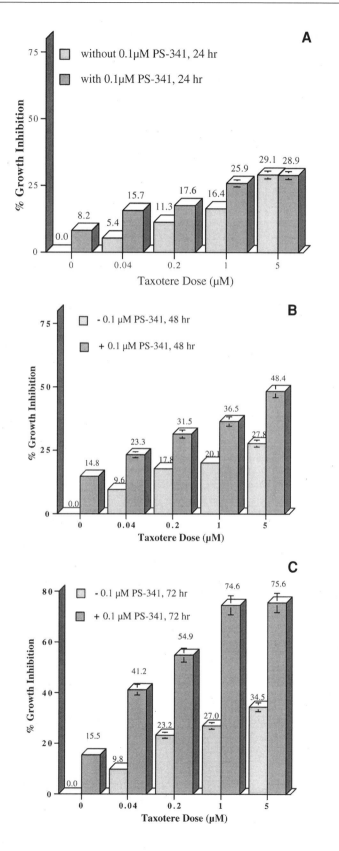

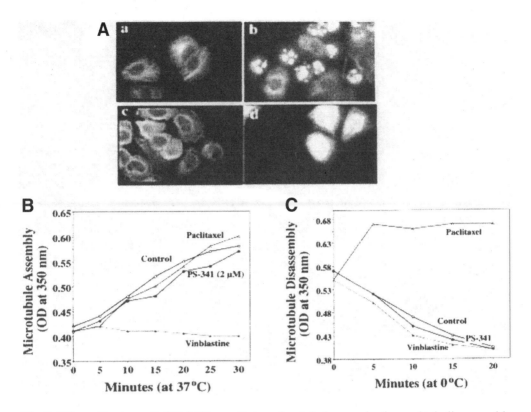

Fig. 2. Effect of bortezomib (PS-341) on cellular microtubule organization and tubulin assembly-disassembly. (**A**) Immunocytochemical study of cellular microtubule organization in H460 cells treated with 0.5 μ*M* paclitaxel (**b**) 0.1 μ*M* vinblastine (**c**) 0.1 μ*M* bortezomib (**d**) or with PBS as a control (**a**). After 24 h of treatment, cells were harvested and fixed with methanol at $-20°C$ for 5 min. Cells were incubated with anti-β-tubulin antibody for 90 min. After being washed three times with PBS solution, cells were reincubated with FITC-conjugated secondary antibody for 30 min. The microtubule arrays were observed with a Nikon 200 fluorescence microscope. Tubulin assembly (**B**) and tubulin disassembly (**C**) were determined in a 100-μL reaction mixture containing purified β-tubulin, 1 m*M* GTP, reaction buffer, and the testing agents, including pacliteaxel, vinblastine, and bortezomib. Tubulin assembly and disassembly were monitored by spectrophotometric measurements at 350 nm as described in Materials and Methods. Each point represents the mean of two independent experiments.

3.2. Effect of Bortezomib on Microtubule Assembly–Disassembly

Given the specific effects of arresting cells at M phase, the morphologic changes in bortezomib IB-treated cells appear similar to those in cells that had been treated with antitubulin agents such as drugs from the taxane family as well as vinblastine. We examined whether the exposure of cells (H460) to bortezomib could directly affect microtubule assembly or disassembly in several test systems. Our first observations on a cellular level (Fig. 2A) revealed that in bortezomib-exposed H460 cells (Fig. 2D), the microtubules were observed to display a normal structure and arrangement comparable to that of control cells (Fig. 2A). In comparison, the results with the positive controls paclitaxel and vinblastine showed, respectively, microtubule polymerization (Fig. 2B) and microtubule

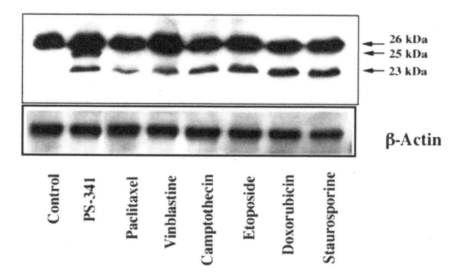

Fig. 3. Bcl2 proteolytic cleavage by bortezomib (PS-341) and other different anticancer agents. H460 cells were treated with 0.1 μM bortezomib, 0.5 μM paclitaxel, 0.1 μM vinblastine, 1 μM camptothecin, 5 μM etoposide, 0.25 μM doxorubicin, 1 μM staurosporine, or with the same volume of PBS solution as control. After 48 h of incubation, cells were lysed with lysis buffer, and protein amount was assessed with a Bio-Rad DC protein assay kit as described in Materials and Methods. Equal amounts (50 μg of protein) of lysate were subjected to a 15% SDS-PAGE. After electrophoresis, protein blots were transferred on a nitrocellulose membrane, and Bcl-2 protein was probed by a monoclonal anti-Bcl2 antibody. β-Actin was used as a sample loading control.

depolymerization (Fig. 2C). The results from a cell-free system using purified tubulin to assess the effects of bortezomib on tubulin assembly and disassembly were parallel to the cellular observations. Exposures to bortezomib did not affect microtubule assembly and disassembly even at concentrations of 2 μM, which were 20 times higher than the IC$_{50}$ in cell culture (Figs. 2B and C).

3.3. Bortezomib Induces a Specific Cleavage Fragment of Bcl-2 Protein

We carried out a series of studies examining the integrity of Bcl-2 that were intended to extend findings described in the literature that Bcl-2 protein can be cleaved into a 23-kDa fragment by several stimuli, such as virus infection, treatment with etoposide, and the proteasome inhibitor MG-132 (17–19). We proceeded to examine the degree of specificity for the induction of an additional cleavage fragment of Bcl-2 (a 25-kDa product) with respect to a smaller cleavage product (23 kDa) that normally results from exposures with other types of anticancer agents at comparable cytotoxic concentrations. As shown in Fig. 3, exposures of H460 cells to bortezomib result in the induction of two cleavage fragment bands. In contrast, only a 23-kDa Bcl-2 cleavage fragment was produced from the exposure of H460 cells to a variety of anticancer agents that ranged from the antitubulin agents paclitaxel and vinblastine; the topoisomerase I inhibitor camptothecin; the topoisomerase II inhibitor etoposide; the anthracycline antibiotic doxorubicin; and the protein kinase C (PKC) inhibitor staurosporine. It is apparent that

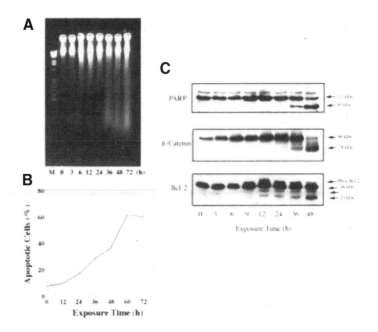

Fig. 4. Time-course studies on bortezomib -induced DNA fragmentation, apoptosis, and cleavage of poly-ADP ribose polymerase (PARP) β-catenin, and Bcl2 protein. H460 cells were treated with 0.1 μ*M* bortezomib for the indicated time. After treatment, cells taken from culture were divided into three parts. (**A**) One was prepared for determination of DNA fragmentation using agarose gel electrophoresis. (**B**) The second part was prepared for determination of apoptosis by flow cytometry after cells were stained with propidium iodide. (**C**) The third was prepared for the determination of cleavage of PARP, β-catenin, and Bcl2 by Western blot analysis. Each point in B represents the mean ± SD of three independent experiments.

only agents acting as proteasome inhibitors are able to produce the observed specific and unique Bcl-2 25-kDa cleavage fragment.

3.4. Bcl-2 Cleavage is an Early Event Mediated by Initiator Caspases in Bortezomib-induced Apoptosis

The time-course of the Bcl-2 cleavage using the H460 non-small cell lung cancer cell line was compared with the time-course of DNA fragmentation and cleavage of caspase-3-like–mediated target proteins PARP and β-catenin, following exposure to 0.1 μ*M* bortezomib. The results from the assessment of DNA fragmentation using agarose gel electrophoresis from a time-course study show that bortezomib-induced DNA fragmentation could be detected after 36 h of exposure and peaked over the period 48–72 h. These results correlate with the plot in Fig. 4B showing the assessment of apoptotic cells by flow cytometry. The Western blot time-course studies summarized in Fig. 4C reveal that Bcl-2 cleavage starts occurring at 12 h, with more discernable effects at 36–48 h after treatment, whereas the cleavage of PARP and β-catenin proteins can be observed at 36 h.

3.5. In Vivo Ovarian Tumor Xenograft Model

We proceeded to build on the data presented in Fig. 1, with an in vivo model that examined the antitumor effect of combined docetaxel and bortezomib treatment in an ovarian tumor xenograft. After the tumors were well established to a 100–150-mg size

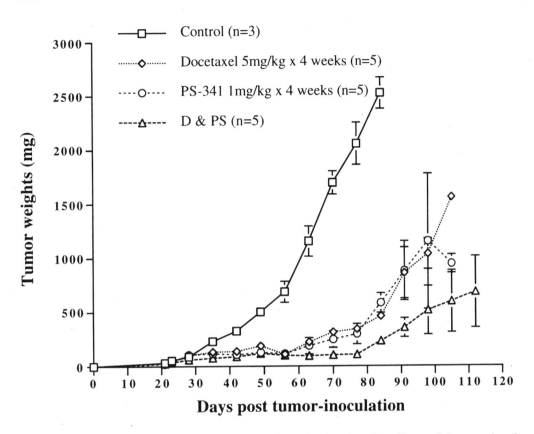

Fig. 5. Results from an ovarian tumor xenograft study showing the effects of docetaxel and bortezomib (PS-341) over 3.7 mo. Combination treatments (D & PS) using four weekly injections kept tumor growth in check for 30 d following the cessation of treatments.

at d 21, a series of four weekly treatment arms (depicted in Fig. 5) was evaluated. During the course of the treatments and following the last treatment on d 42 for the period 42–56 d, a comparable retardation in tumor growth was seen for both of the single-agent treatment arms of bortezomib and docetaxel, as well as for the combination of bortezomib and docetaxel. However starting with d 56, tumor growth was observed to start for each of the single-agent arms but was still held in check with the bortezomib/docetaxel combination until d 78. At this time point, tumor growth could now be detected but at a reduced rate for the docetaxel/bortezomib combination, compared with either the docetaxel or bortezomib treatment arms alone. The use of four weekly administrations of docetaxel (8 mg/kg iv) and bortezomib (1 mg/kg iv) significantly reduced the ovarian tumor xenograft growth compared with untreated tumor-bearing animals (on d 84; 460 ± 67 mg, 584 ± 91 mg vs 2525 ± 146 mg, $p < 0.001$). The combination of docetaxel and bortezomib further reduced tumor growth compared to either of the single-agent administrations alone (232 ± 68 mg, $p < 0.05$). Thus, in summary, the benefits of the combined treatment effects of the SKOV3 tumor reduction were maintained for 30 d after cessation of the four weekly combination treatments compared with the same treatments with the single agents alone when examined over the course of a 112-d observation period until the experiment was terminated.

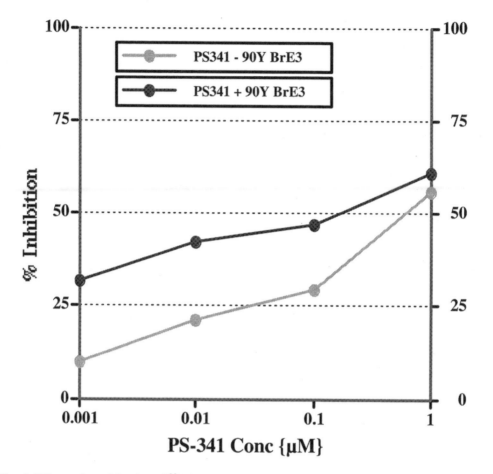

Fig. 6. Effects of combination of ^{90}Y huBrE3 with docetaxel and bortezomib (PS-341) on cytotoxic activity in SKOV3 cells.

3.6. In Vitro Cytotoxic Effects of RAIT Combinations With Docetaxel/Bortezomib

Based on earlier studies, we had seen effects of chemotherapy with topotecan and RAIT with ^{90}Y-HuBrE-3 on the cytotoxicity and induction of apoptosis with the human mammary carcinomas cell lines MDA-MB-435 and MDA-MB-157 *(14)*, in which the effects were most pronounced with the MDA-MB-435 cell line, which expresses the BrE-3 epitope. We decided to extend these observations for MCF-7 and SKOV-3 cells (which also express the BrE-3 epitope) and carried out a series of combinations of RAIT with docetaxel and bortezomib. Figures 6 and 7 contain a summary of preliminary studies with the SKOV-3 ovarian cell lines. Figure 7 shows the positive modulation of bortezomib on the cytotoxicity of ^{90}Y-huBrE-3. The most dramatic effect was observed with a 1 n*M* concentration of bortezomib: a threefold increase in cytotoxicity was detected. With respect to the modulation effects of RAIT with docetaxel combinations, the data in Fig. 7 show a similar positive modulation to that seen with bortezomib: a twofold increase in cytotoxicity evident at a 1 n*M* concentration of docetaxel. Figures 8 and 9 contain summaries with the breast cancer cell line MCF-7. Similar to what we saw in the ovarian SKOV3 cancer cells, ^{90}Y-huBrE-3 potentiates the cytotoxic activity of docetaxel and

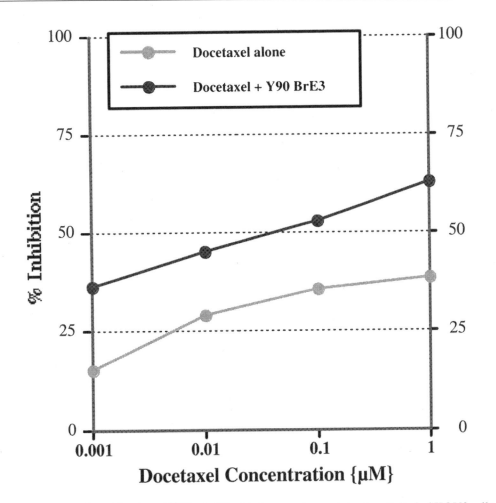

Fig. 7. Effects of combination of ^{90}Y huBrE3 with docetaxel on cytotoxic activity in SKOV3 cells.

bortezomib, particularly at the modest 1-nM levels, at which one could expect little if any cytotoxic activity in the absence of ^{90}Y-huBrE-3. Similar increased cytotoxic activity was observed with bortezomib. Based on our experience from a recently completed CTEP sponsored phase I study with 41 patients, the 20–30% increase in cytotoxic activity observed in the above preliminary studies is at 10–100-fold lower levels than the 0.1-μM levels at which clinical activity was seen *(20)*.

4. CONCLUSIONS

The results of the studies described above have a common theme in that the combination of bortezomib and docetaxel was shown to have additive cytotoxic effects in vitro, and these findings were extended to an in vivo ovarian xenograft model. In addition, in vitro combinations with bortezomib and docetaxel employing receptor-positive cells for RAIT also showed cytotoxic effects at a concentration of each agent that was below any activities seen with single agents alone. In addition, this combination has a good potential for chronic treatment in ovarian cancer, given the lack of multicellular drug resistance

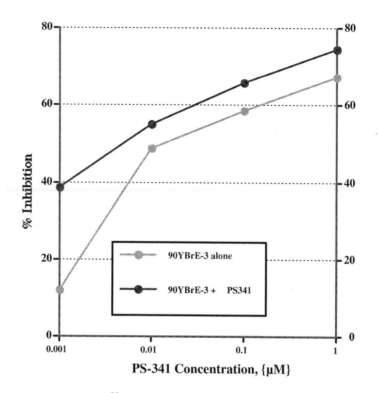

Fig. 8. Effects of combination of ^{90}Y huBrE3 with bortezomib (PS-341) on cytotoxic activity in MCF7 breast cancer cells.

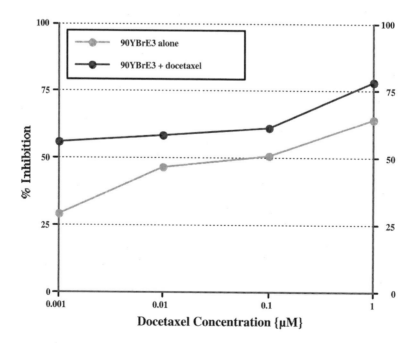

Fig. 9. Effects of combination of ^{90}Y huBrE3 with docetaxel on cytotoxic activity in MCF7 breast cancer cells.

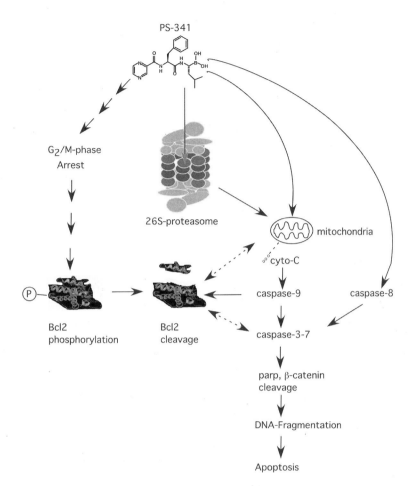

Fig. 10. Pleotropic activity of bortezomib (PS-341) showing parallel effects on G_2/M phase arrest that lead to Bcl2 phosphorylation and cleavage. Perturbations on mitochrondria lead to the release of cytochrome C and subsequent cleavage of procaspase-9. The activated caspase-9 further cleaves procaspase-3 and -7 and subsequently leads to the cleavage of poly-ADP ribose polymerase (PARP) and β-catenin, DNA fragmentation, and cell apoptosis. The Bcl-2 can be cleaved either by caspase-9 at the initiation stage or by caspase-3 or -7 at the execution stage. The Bcl-2 cleavage products can act on the mitochondria to induce cytochrome c release and further increase the activity.

observed with ovarian and prostate cells in a recent study by Frankel and collaborators *(21)*. A common element may be effects on Bcl-2 phosphorylation. Docetaxel has been found to be a highly effective inducer of Bcl-2 phosphorylation and apopotic cell death in a number of cell types *(22)*. Both docetaxel and bortezomib induce Bcl-2 phosphorylation, and bortezomib also induces a unique 25-kDa cleavage fragment *(23)*. In our previous work, the bortezomib-induced G_2/M phase arrest was correlated to Bcl-2 phosphorylation whose extent was coincident with the accumulation of substantial cell numbers at G_2/M phase, an activity similar to that of antitubulin agents such as paclitaxel and vinca alkaloids. The Bcl-2 phosphorylation was not exclusively implicated in the disturbance of microtubule events related to G_2/M phase arrest. However, it is conceivable that the activity of docetaxel may help potentiate the apoptotic activity of bortezomib through the combined phosphorylation effects as well as the dual cleavage products.

The cytotoxic activities of docetaxel and bortezomib were augmented with combination radioimmunotherapy using a specific antibody (HuBrE-3) directed to a specific mucin epitope on ovarian and breast cancer cells. A key mechanism for this induced cytotoxicity could be related to the inhibition of NF-κB activation in a manner similar to that described by Russo and collaborators with irradiated LOVO colorectal cancer cells *(6)*.

Figure 10 shows a graphic summary of observed points of activity of bortezomib based on our recent observations with H460 cells *(23,24)*. One working hypothesis is that the activated caspases (-3, -7, and -9) through bortezomib effects on mitochondria, could cleave Bcl2 and convert its antiapoptotic form to the truncated Bcl2 molecule with a proapoptotic function. The cleaved Bcl-2 could induce cytochrome c release from mitochondria, and the subsequent activation of caspases-3 and -7. The released cytochrome c and activated caspases-3 and -7 would further enhance the cleavage of Bcl-2 and other target proteins. Such a feedback loop could lead to an amplification of bortezomib-induced apoptotic cascades that are further potentiated by the lack of NF-κB activation by the localized ionizing radiation.

REFERENCES

1. Adams J, et al. Potent and selective inhibitors of the proteasome: dipepidyl boronic acids. *Bioorg Med Chem Lett* 1998;8:333–338.
2. Adams J, et al. Proteasome inhibitors: a novel class of potent and effective antitumor agents. *Cancer Res* 1999;59:2615–2622.
3. Shah SA, et al. 26S proteasome inhibition induces apoptosis and limits growth of human pancreatic cancer. *J Cell Biochem* 2001;82:110–122.
4. An W, et al. Protease inhibitor-induced apoptosis: accumulation of wt p53, p21WAF1/CIP1, and induction of apoptosis are independent markers of proteasome inhibition. *Leukemia* 2000;14:1276–1283.
5. Wu Y, et al. The proteasome controls the expression of a proliferation-associated nuclear antigen Ki-67. *J Cell Biochem* 2000;76:596–604.
6. Russo S, et al. Enhancement of radiosensitivity by proteasome inhibition: implication for a role of NF-κB. *Int J Radiat Oncol Biol Phys* 2001;50:183–193.
7. Dieras V. Taxanes in combination with doxorubicin in the treatment of metastatic breast cancer. *Semin Oncol* 1998;5(suppl 12):18–22.
8. Kavanagh JJ, et al. Phase II study of docetaxel in patients with epithelial ovarian carcinoma refractory to platinum. *Clin Cancer Res* 1996;2:837–842.
9. Gueritte-Voegelein F, et al. Relationships between structure of taxol analogues and their antimitotic activity. *J Med Chem* 1991;34:992–998.
10. Creane M, et al. Radiobiological effects of docetaxel (Taxotere): a potential radiation sensitizer. *Int J Radiat Biol* 1999;75:731–737.
11. Hennequin C, Giocanti N, Favaudon V. Interaction of ionizing radiation and paclitexel (Taxol) and docetaxel (Taxotere) in HeLa and SQ20B cells. *Cancer Res* 1996;56:1842–1850.
12. Amorino G, Hamilton V, Choy H. Enhancement of radiation effects by combined docetaxel and carboplatin treatment in vitro. *Radiat Oncol Invest* 1999;7:343–352.
13. Ceriani RL, et al. Levels of expression of breast epithelial mucin detected by monoclonal antibody BrE-3 in breast-cancer prognosis. *Int J Cancer* 1992;51:343–354.
14. Ng B, et al. Radiosensitization of tumor-targeted radioimmunotherapy with prolonged topotecan infusion in human breast cancer xenografts. *Cancer Res* 2001;61:2996–3001.
15. Liebes L, et al. Treatment of an ovarian tumor xenograft with combined chemo-radimmunotherapy (RI) using 90Y-BrE-3 antibody and intraperitoneal (IP) administration of topotecan (TPT). In: *Proceedings of the Society of Gynecologic Oncologists*, New Orleans, 2003.
16. Jiang J, et al. 3-(Iodoacetmido)-bezoylurea: a novel cancericidal tubulin ligand that inhibits microtubule polymerization, phosphorylates bcl-2, and induces apoptosis in tumor cells. *Cancer Res* 1998;58:5398–5395.
17. Grandgirard D, et al. Alphaviruses induce apoptosis in Bcl-2 overexpressing cells: evidence for a caspase-mediated, proteolytic inactivation of Bcl-2. *EMBO J* 1998;17:1268–1278.

18. Zhang XM, et al. Inhibition of ubiquitin-proteasome pathway activates caspase-3-like protease and induces Bcl-2 cleavage in human M-07e leukaemic cells. *Biochem J* 1999;340:127–133.
19. Fadeel B, et al. Cleavage of Bcl-2 is an early event in chemotherapy-induced apoptosis of human myeloid leukemia cells. *Leukemia* 1999;13:719–728.
20. Hamilton A, et al. in *Proc Am Soc Clin Onc* 2001. San Francisco: *ASCO*, 2001.
21. Frankel A, et al. Lack of multicellular drug resistance observed in human ovarian and prostate carcinoma treated with the proteasome inhibitor PS-341. *Clin Cancer Res* 2000;6:3719–3728.
22. Gianni LD, et al. Cardiac function following combination therapy with paclitaxel and doxorubicin: an analysis of 657 women with advanced breast cancer. *Ann Oncol* 2001;12:1067–1073.
23. Ling YH, et al. PS-341, a novel proteasome inhibitor, induces bcl2 phosphorylation and cleavage in association with G2-M phase arrest and apoptosis. *Mol Cancer Ther* 2002;1:841–849.
24. Ling YH, et al. Mechanisms of proteasome inhibitor PS-341-induces G2/M phase arrest and apoptosis in human non-small cell lung cancer cell lines. *Clin Cancer Res* 2003;9:1145–1154.

13 Proteasome Inhibitor Therapy in a Brain Tumor Model

Jeffrey J. Olson, Geoffrey Bowers,
and Zhoabin Zhang

CONTENTS

ABSTRACT

Bortezomib (formerly known as PS-341) inhibits the ubiquitin–proteasome pathway with a hypothesized high degree of specificity for cell-cycle proteins. Preclinical activity has been observed in prostate and mammary cancer. Phase I data have defined tolerable toxicity, and thus analysis for brain tumor therapy is warranted. A rat intracranial 9L gliosarcoma model was given 1.0 mg/kg iv of C-14-labeled bortezomib to assess distribution. Intravenous and intratumoral bortezomib administration 10 d after implant was used to assess efficacy. At 1 h, tumor penetration reached 0.2–0.4 μM concentrations with negligible amounts found in the contralateral normal hemisphere. Survivals of rats given bortezomib 0.1 mg/kg iv twice a week and of controls were 20.8 ± 0.5 and 18.5 ± 0.7 d ($p = 0.014$), respectively. At 0.2 mg/kg, the bortezomib and control survivals were 22 ± 1.5 and 16 ± 0.9 d ($p = 0.0045$), respectively. The single iv median lethal dose was 0.4 mg/kg. Intratumoral injections had less toxicity than systemic injections, and 0.2 mg/kg of bortezomib given intratumorally provided benefit over vehicle injection, with survivals of 28 ± 6.4 d and 16.5 ± 0.6 d ($p = 0.0013$), respectively. In vivo, a single iv dose of 0.2 mg/kg of bortezomib increased 9L tumor p21 protein content 6–24 h after exposure; baseline was reached at 48 h, supporting its impact on the cell cycle. Quantification of intrinsic 20 S proteasome activity in human brain tumors may offer insight into which tumors might respond to inhibitors. Mean 20S proteasome specific activity values (in pmol/s/mg protein) from a small series of frozen fresh human specimens of glioblastoma (GBM), anaplastic astrocytoma, oligodendroglioma, adenocarcinoma, schwannoma, and meningioma were 5.0, 4.6, 5.2, 8.3, 12.0, and 14.3, respectively. A range of values (3.5–

From: *Cancer Drug Discovery and Development: Proteasome Inhibitors in Cancer Therapy*
Edited by: J. Adams © Humana Press Inc., Totowa, NJ

8.2), occurred for GBM ($n = 5$). It is hypothesized that this measurement may be predictive of the responsiveness of GBM to bortezomib. As a first step, a phase I study of the safety and tolerability of bortezomib has been initiated to determine a maximum tolerated dosage (MTD). In the 9L model bortezomib clearly enhances survival, but at high enough doses systemic bortezomib is not without toxicity. The hypothesized function inhibited by the drug, proteasome activity, is measurable. Therefore, with a MTD in hand, a study correlating this quantity as a predictive surrogate marker with efficacy is possible.

KEY WORDS

Brain tumors; proteasome; 9L gliosarcoma.

1. INTRODUCTION

Despite the numerous advances in our understanding of tumor physiology and the treatment of cancer patients in the past two decades, it is discouraging that the prognosis of patients with malignant primary brain tumors has changed very little. In patients with anaplastic astrocytoma or glioblastoma multiforme, the overall 5-yr survival following diagnosis is less than 20% *(1,2)*. This is true whether patients are treated by biopsy followed by radiation therapy alone or by surgical resection combined with radiation therapy, and chemotherapy. Thus, irrespective of treatment, the survival curves after any of these treatments for the most common histologic type, glioblastoma multiforme, converge after 18–24 mo, showing no clear long-term benefit of complex over simple therapies *(3)*.

Because cure by surgery, radiation, chemotherapy, or a combination of these approaches remains elusive, this set of difficult problems warrants assessment of novel agents for treatment of these tumors. Bortezomib (Velcade™; formerly known as PS-341) is a proteasome inhibitor chemically characterized as a dipeptidyl boronic acid analog with minor activity toward serine and thiol proteases *(4,5)*. Bortezomib has potent and reversible inhibitory activity against the hydrolysis of polypeptide substrates by the 20S proteasome and hydrolysis of ubiquinated proteins by the 26S proteasome *(6)*. The proteasome is a final degradative enzyme in the catabolic pathway for many intracellular regulatory proteins including the inhibitor κB/nuclear factor-κB (IκB/NF-κB), p53, and the cyclin-dependent kinase inhibitors p21 and p27 *(7–10)*. By stabilizing cytoplasmic IκBα bortezomib has shown an inhibitory effect on transactivation of NF-κB in vitro and in vivo *(11)*. The antineoplastic effect of bortezomib may involve several distinct mechanisms including inhibition of cell growth signaling pathways, induction of apoptosis, and inhibition of cellular adhesion molecule expression *(12,13)*.

In the following work, it was hypothesized that the bortezomib would have an inhibitory effect on brain tumor proteasome 20S activity and would be useful for treatment of malignant brain tumors in a preclinical setting. To assess this hypothesis, the intracranial distribution of ^{14}C-labeled bortezomib was tested. Then efficacy was tested by intravenous and intratumoral injection of bortezomib. Lastly, the effect of bortezomib on rodent brain tumor 20S proteasome activity was assessed.

2. METHODS

2.1. Tumor Implantation

Fisher 344 rats with intracranial 9L brain tumor isografts were used for the rodent intracranial brain tumor model. 9L tumor cells were cultured at 37°C in a CO_2 incubator in Dulbecco's modified Eagle's medium (DMEM) with 10% fetal calf serum and standard antibiotic and antifungal supplements. After induction of anesthesia with 13 mg/kg xylazine and 87 mg/kg ketamine intramuscularly, the 125–175-g rats were placed in a standard David Kopf stereotactic head holder for rodents. Utilizing an aseptic technique, the scalp was prepared, and a sagittal midline incision was made from 5 mm anterior to the bregma to the occiput. The scalp was bluntly elevated in the subgaleal plane on the right side of midline. A 2-mm drill was used to form a burr hole in the skull 3 mm to the right and 1 mm anterior to the bregma. The dura was pierced with a 23-gauge needle. Through this opening a Hamilton syringe with 4 μL of tumor suspension (10^4 cells/μL in serum-free DMEM) was advanced to a depth of 4 mm. Here the tumor cells were injected over 2 min, and then the needle was withdrawn over 1 min. The burr hole was filled with bone wax, the subgaleal space was irrigated with sterile saline, and the scalp was closed with 3-0 absorbable suture. The animals were then removed from the head holder and allowed to recover in a cage warmed by an indirect heat lamp.

2.2. ^{14}C Distribution Study

The assessment of the distribution of ^{14}C-labeled bortezomib was carried out in animals with tumors established by the above method. Fourteen days after tumor inoculation the animals underwent intravenous administration of bortezomib over a range of doses. Based on toxicities seen, doses of 0.2 or 1.0 mg/kg of bortezomib labeled with ^{14}C were chosen for this portion of the study. The animals were anesthetized with a combination of 13 mg/kg xylazine and 87 mg/kg ketamine im. They underwent injection of the ^{14}C-labeled bortezomib via tail vein injection or by femoral vein cutdown. Animals undergoing femoral vein injection were placed supine, and the cutdown was carried out with an aseptic technique. The femoral vein was immobilized with a 3-0 silk suture, and a 25-gauge needle was used to inject ^{14}C- bortezomib intravenously. The needle was withdrawn, and the minor hemorrhage from the entry site was controlled with gentle tamponade. The wound was repaired with 3-0 vicryl, and the animals were allowed to recover with an indirect heat lamp. They were sacrificed with pentobarbital (75 mg/kg ip) 1 h after the injection time. At that time the brain tumor, contralateral cerebral hemisphere, and blood by cardiac stick were harvested for weighing and counting to assess ^{14}C- bortezomib distribution.

2.3. Assessment of Bortezomib Efficacy via Systemic Administration

Intracranial tumor implantation of 9L tumor in rats was carried out as noted above. Seven days later intravenous administration of bortezomib began, with doses twice a week. Animals were observed daily for eating habits and diarrhea and were weighed twice a week. The animals were observed until spontaneous death or until sacrifice was carried out for inability to eat over 1 d, or for a decrease in weight of more than 25% from baseline. An additional group of five tumor-bearing animals was treated with vehicle (phosphate-buffered normal saline) on the same schedule.

2.4. Assessment of Bortezomib Efficacy via Direct Intracranial Administration

Because of concern about potential limitations of systemic delivery of treatment compounds to the brain, direct administration of bortezomib to a brain tumor was studied. Intracranial tumor implantation of 9L tumor in rats was carried out as noted above. Seven days later bortezomib was administered intratumorally at the same stereotactic coordinates as were utilized for tumor implantation. Control injections consisted of vehicle media (phosphate-buffered normal saline). The animals were observed for daily eating habits, diarrhea, and new neurologic deficits and were weighed twice a week. Animals were observed until spontaneous death or until sacrifice was carried out for inability to eat over 1 d, or for decrease in weight of more than 25% from baseline.

2.5. Tumor and Normal Brain Proteasome Activity Analysis

To show that bortezomib had an effect on proteasome activity in this model, such activity was measured in animals with 9L tumors who were given bortezomib intravenously. Intracranial tumor implantation of 9L tumor in five Fisher 344 rats was carried out as noted above. Fourteen days later four animals were given bortezomib at 0.2 mg/kg. They were sacrificed with pentobarbital 75 mg/kg ip at 1, 6, 24, or 48 h after injection. One animal that did not receive the bortezomib injection was sacrificed 14 d after tumor injection to serve as a time zero control. The brain tumor and contralateral hemisphere were harvested from all animals immediately after sacrifice. The tissues were processed for 20S proteasome activity. This was accomplished by tissue sample homogenization and measurement of proteasome 20S activity using fluorometric analysis (14). The assay was carried out at Millennium Pharmaceuticals (Cambridge, MA).

2.6. Data Analysis

Dosage and administration route, toxicity, relative ^{14}C-labeled bortezomib tumor and brain uptake, proteasome 20S activity results for brain tumor, and brain were tabulated utilizing simple descriptive statistics. Analysis of variance was utilized for simple comparisons. The survival times/times to sacrifice (due to weight loss or other untoward effects) of the bortezomib- or vehicle-treated groups were expressed with the Kaplan–Meier survival curve method and compared with log-rank (Mantel–Cox) statistics. Significance for any analysis of variance or log rank comparisons was accepted at the $p \leq$ 0.05 level.

3. RESULTS

3.1. ^{14}C Distribution Study

Test injections of intravenous bortezomib were utilized in animals with 9L tumors that had been established for 14 d using doses beginning at 0.1-mg/kg and increasing by 0.1 mg/kg increments to 1.0 mg/kg. At the highest dose, animals died within 3 h of injection. This dose was therefore judged to be the extreme limit of tolerability of bortezomib in animals with the intracranial 9L tumor model. This dose was utilized for the ^{14}C-labeled bortezomib distribution study at 1 h to allow the largest amount of ^{14}C to be delivered. At the 0.3-mg/kg iv dose, one animal died within 24 h of injection, and others appeared ill for at least 3 h. This apparent toxicity was manifest as decreased movement about the cage, hunching, and some mattering about the eyes, but without overt diarrhea or perioral crusting. Thus, this dose was interpreted as the level at which dose-limiting toxicity occurred in the 9L intracranial tumor model, and 0.2 mg/kg was chosen as the maximum tolerated dose.

The ratio of tumor/brain ^{14}C-labeled bortezomib was 3.8 for the 0.2-mg/kg dose and 2.6 for the 1.0-mg/kg dose. Thus, in this model system, bortezomib does reach the tumor in

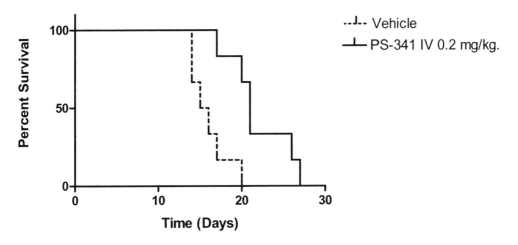

Fig. 1. Survival curves of Fisher 344 rats with intracranial 9L tumors receiving intravenous bortezomib compared with those receiving vehicle, showing the extent of improvement with bortezomib.

greater amounts than the brain. Representative ratios of circulating serum bortezomib in brain and tumor were 13.4 and 3.5, respectively, for the 1.0-mg/kg dose. Representative ratios of circulating serum bortezomib in brain and tumor were somewhat less, at 8.4 and 3.2, respectively, for the 0.2-mg/kg dose. The mean intratumoral concentration of bortezomib in three animals receiving 0.2 mg/kg was 0.074 ± 0.015 (SD) nM. For the contralateral normal cerebral hemisphere, the mean concentration was 0.021 ± 0.02 nM. Although the concentrations are different ($p < 0.05$), the number of subjects is small ($n = 2$) and did not take into account potential gray and white matter differences in normal tissue.

3.2. Assessment of Bortezomib Efficacy via Systemic Administration

In normal animals, iv injections of 0.4 mg/kg bortezomib resulted in lethargy as well as gait unsteadiness for more than 24 h followed by resumption of normal activity, eating habits, and weight gain. At 0.3 mg/kg, the animals were hunched and inactive for approx 3 h and then resumed normal activity, eating habits, and weight gain. As mentioned above, one animal in the above initial distribution studies died within 24 h of this dose. Therefore, 0.3 mg/kg was judged as the dose at which dose-limiting toxicity occurred for the purposes of this preclinical study, and 0.2 mg/kg was chosen as the maximum tolerated intravenous dose.

Mean survival with 0.2 mg/kg of bortezomib injected twice a week beginning 7 d after 9L implantation was 22 ± 1.5 (SE) days compared with 16 ± 0.9 d in the vehicle injection group ($p = 0.0045$; Fig. 1). Mean survival with 0.1 mg/kg of bortezomib injected twice a week beginning 7 d after 9L implantation was less, at 20.8 ± 0.4 d compared with 18.5 ± 0.7 d in the vehicle injection ($p = 0.0136$). No difference was seen in the bortezomib and control groups when a dose of 0.3 mg/kg iv was assessed, which may have been due to drug toxicity.

3.3. Assessment of Bortezomib Efficacy via Direct Intratumoral Administration

In normal animals, intracerebral injections of 0.4 mg/kg bortezomib resulted in lethargy and gait unsteadiness for more than 24 h followed by resumption of normal activity,

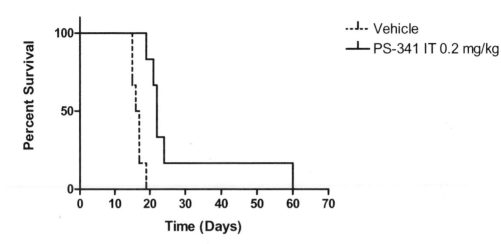

Fig. 2. Survival curves of Fisher 344 rats with intracranial 9L tumors receiving a single intratumoral injection of bortezomib compared with those receiving vehicle injection. Improvement of survival with bortezomib is noted.

eating habits, and weight gain. At the 0.3-mg/kg bortezomib dose, the animals were hunched and inactive for approximately 3 h and then resumed normal activity, eating habits, and weight gain. No deaths occurred. Therefore 0.3 mg/kg was judged as the maximum tolerated dose for the purposes of this preclinical study. It is possible that higher doses may have been tolerated, but it is doubtful that early toxicity would have been any less.

Mean survival with 0.2 mg/kg of bortezomib injected 7 d after 9L implantation was 28 ± 6.4 d compared with 16.5 ± 0.6 d in the vehicle injection curves ($p = 0.0013$; Fig. 2). Mean survival with 0.3 mg/kg of bortezomib injected 7 d after 9L implantation was less impressive, at 19.3 ± 1.1 d compared with 16.5 ± 0.8 d in the vehicle injection, with the difference not reaching significance ($p = 0.08$). This lesser survival for the higher dose was attributed to a combination of tumor progression and drug toxicity that could not be overcome by the animals in this model. There was no difference in the groups when a dose of 0.1 mg/kg was utilized.

3.4. Tumor and Normal Brain Proteasome Activity Analysis

The 20S proteasome activity, expressed as spectral activity, was clearly reduced in the tumors of animals receiving bortezomib 1 h before sacrifice, harvest, and freezing. A gradual return toward baseline then occurred over the subsequent 47 h. At all time periods, 20S proteasome activity of the tumor remained greater than that of the contralateral occipital lobe. There was a small decrement in 20S proteasome activity in the contralateral occipital lobe at 1 h; however, this value had returned to baseline by 48 h (Fig. 3). The data are from five different animals and therefore should be considered preliminary as this reflects only one animal per time point.

4. DISCUSSION

Primary malignant brain tumors do not metastasize widely but rather tend to grow locally within the brain, resulting in progressive brain injury and eventual death (*15–17*).

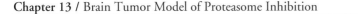

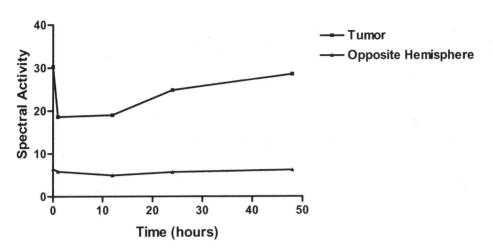

Fig. 3. Proteasome activity in an intracranial 9L tumor and the normal brain of the contralateral hemisphere as measured over time as spectral activity in pmol AMC (7-amino-4-methylcoumarin)/s/mg protein after administration of bortezomib 0.2 mg/kg iv.

Aggressive local therapies have been undertaken in an effort to minimize local recurrence. These have included wide surgical excision, implanted radioactive sources *(18)*, high doses of chemotherapeutic agents *(19,20)*, regional hyperthermia *(21)*, and focused external beam radiation such as stereotactic radiosurgery *(22)*. In selected populations each of these modalities has had efficacy. However, none have been shown to be better for the newly diagnosed individual than careful surgical resection followed by X-radiation, and none are reliably curative. This is inherent in glial tumors because the tumor cells frequently infiltrate and intermingle with normal tissue including neurons, astrocytes, and vascular endothelia *(23–25)*. Surgical resection cannot remove these cells selectively, and thus alternative modes of therapy are necessary.

Because of its method of inhibiting tumor proliferation by mechanisms different from those of standard cytotoxic agents, bortezomib has been assessed on a preclinical basis in a number of tumor types. Activity has been found using bortezomib in a murine model of adult T-cell lymphoma, in which NF-κB is indispensable in the maintenance of the malignant phenotype Bortezomib was used in combination with humanized anti-interleukin-2 receptor α antibody in this model, and survival was enhanced compared with animals that received the antibody alone *(5,26)*. In a model of squamous cell carcinoma, bortezomib has been shown to inhibit activation of NF-κB pathway components related to cell survival, tumor growth, and angiogenesis *(12)*.

The mechanism by which bortezomib functions is probably broad in nature, as so many proteins are involved in its metabolic purview. It has been shown to slow the normal breakdown of p53 and cell cycle proteins such as p21 *(27)*. Notably, bortezomib induces apoptosis in cells that overexpress bcl-2, a genetic trait that confers unregulated growth and resistance to conventional chemotherapeutics. In addition, bortezomib has cytotoxic activity in a variety of xenograft tumor models. Systemic and direct administration of bortezomib in mice bearing the PC-3 prostate xenograft resulted in 60–70% reduction in tumor growth *(14)*. Bortezomib induces tumor growth delay and reduces the number of lung metastases over a given period in mice inoculated with the Lewis lung carcinoma *(28)*. Peak concentration after intravenous administration occurs in less than 10 min, and peak effects in human white cell measurements occur after 1 h *(29)*. The relatively rapid effect is substantiated in our data: proteasome activity in the tumor is substantially decreased in just 1 h. In rodent evaluations it is eliminated from the circulation rapidly and by 120 h after administration, 10% has been excreted in the urine and 40% in the feces, presumably via a biliary route. The remaining drug was still bound in tissues. Toxicity events in rats have been decreased food consumption, diarrhea, and weight loss *(14)*.

The 7-d period that was chosen as the time to start the intravenous regimen was based on this being the earliest time point that visible tumor is usually present in the intracranial 9L model. This was advantageous for purposes of necropsy and, knowing the usual characteristics of this tumor, would also allow at least two doses to be delivered to most animals as average survival is in the range of 20 d. The 14-d interval was chosen for the intratumoral injection study as the tumor has reached a substantial size that maximizes the likelihood of actually delivering bortezomib to the tumor and still not having so large a lesion as to preclude the animal's ability to survive the brief anesthesia necessary for injection in its debilitated state. As is well recognized, the intracranial 9L tumor is a small lesion compared with human brain tumors. Additionally, it is minimally invasive and grows as a relatively solid tumor mass, which is not a characteristic of all human tumors *(30)*. However, its reliability and economy allow it to serve as an excellent point of departure for preclinical analysis of new brain tumor therapies.

Little intratumoral administration of bortezomib has been undertaken in other tumor types, and therefore the preclinical data reported here are of note. The intratumoral route was used to address ever present concerns about blood-brain barrier limitation of delivery of systemically administered compounds *(31)*. In fact, the best responses/survivals to bortezomib were via this route.

Toxicities clearly did occur with the use of bortezomib in this model. At the highest intravenous dose used (1.0 mg/kg), tumor-bearing animals died after 3 h. At substantially lower doses, the drug was better tolerated, with only one of the animals that received 0.3 mg/kg iv dying of apparent drug-related effects at 24 h. Below this dose the tumor-bearing animals seemed to have no toxicities that were not already expected due to tumor growth. Temporary general decline in function occurred with direct intratumoral bortezomib injection at 0.4 mg/kg. Higher doses via this route may have been tolerable and efficacious and warrant future evaluation. Ubiquitin–proteasome proteolysis is the principal pathway for intracellular turnover of numerous key regulatory proteins in all eukaryotic cells, and therefore the inhibition of this widespread pathway may inevitably be accompanied by severe side effects if its activity is inhibited enough *(5,32)*. Prior reports have noted that dose-limiting toxicity was in the range of 0.8 mg/m^2 in rats and primates. This toxicity was manifest as anorexia, diarrhea, nausea, and vomiting *(1)*. To work with lower doses of bortezomib and avoid its toxicities, it may be necessary to combine this agent with other forms of chemotherapy that may also be able to exploit possible useful drug interactions *(12,13,28)*.

In summary, tumor types in which bortezomib has shown the greatest degree of promise with some form of antagonistic effect have been prostate *(14,33,34)*, multiple myeloma *(13)*, and ovarian carcinoma *(33)*. Phase I studies to define the pharmacokinetics better in advanced solid tumor cases have also been completed *(35,36)*. The promise of proteasome inhibition in tumor control is reflected by reports of other compounds with similar mechanisms of action *(37)*. The data in the present report, describing another tumor type that might be responsive to bortezomib, must be recognized as preliminary preclinical data. The proteasome activity data represent only one animal per time point, and this needs to be extended. Interestingly, the rapid dropoff in tumor proteasome activity followed by approx 50% recovery at 24 h supports clinical information developed thus far *(38)*.

Bortezomib demonstrated preference for distribution into and effect on the 9L tumor over normal brain. Interestingly, the greatest effect seems to be by direct intracranial injection. The exact mechanism of bortezomib's effect on brain tumors remains to be determined. Certainly more can be learned about bortezomib from in vitro and in vivo investigations. However, to determine whether this information extrapolates to human primary malignant brain tumors, it will be necessary to carry out phase I and II clinical trials of the agent to evaluate toxicity and efficacy, respectively.

ACKNOWLEDGMENTS

The authors would like to acknowledge the fine technical work on the 20S proteasome activity assays by Christine Pien. Assistance in obtaining bortezomib and review of the initial experimental plan by Peter Elliott are greatly appreciated.

REFERENCES

1. Elliott PJ, et al. Clinical development of the first proteasome inhibitor. *Proc ASCO* 1999;18:209.
2. Berens ME, et al. Role of surgery in brain tumor management. In: *Neurosurgery Clinics of North America*, vol 1 (Rosenblum ML, ed.). WB Saunders, Philadelphia, 1990:1–18.
3. Salcman M. Survival in glioblastomas. *Neurosurgery* 1980;7:435–439.
4. Adams J, et al. Potent and selective inhibitors of the proteasome: dipeptidyl boronic acids. *Bioorg Med Chem Lett* 1998;8:333–338.
5. Tan C, Waldmann A. Proteasome inhibitor PS-341, a potential therapeutic agent for adult T-cell leukemia. *Cancer Res* 2002;62:1083–1086.
6. Gardner RC, et al. Characterization of peptidyl boronic acid inhibitors of mammalian 20S and 26S proteasomes and their inhibition of proteasomes in cultured cells. *Biochemistry* 2000;346:447–454.
7. Goldberg AL, et al. New insights into proteasome function: from Archaebacteria to drug development. *Chem Biol* 1995;2:503–508.
8. Coux O, et al. Structure and function of the 20S and 26S proteasomes. *Annu Rev Biochem* 1996;65:801–847.
9. King RW, et al. How proteolysis drives the cell cycle. *Science* 1996;274:1652–1659.
10. Adams J, et al. Proteasome inhibitors: a novel class of potent and effective antitumor agents. *Cancer Res* 1999;59:2615–2622.
11. Palmobella VJ, et al. Role of the proteasome and NF-κB in streptococcal cell wall-induced polyarthritiis. *Proc Natl Acad Sci USA* 1998;95:15671–15676.
12. Sunwoo JB, et al. Novel proteasome inhibitor PS-341 inhibits activation of nuclear factor-κB, cell survival, tumor growth and angiogenesis in squamous cell carcinoma. *Clin Cancer Res* 2001;7:1419–1428.
13. Hideshima T, et al. The proteasome inhibitor PS-341 inhibits growth, induces apoptosis and overcomes drug resistance in human multiple myeloma cells. *Cancer Res* 2001;61:3071–3076.
14. Adams J, et al. Proteasome inhibitors: a novel class of potent and effective antitumor agents. *Cancer Res* 1999;59:2615–2622.
15. Bashir R, et al. Regrowth pattterns of glioblastoma multiforme related to planning of interestial brachytherapy radiation fields. *Neurosurgery* 1988;23:27–30.
16. Shiffer D, et al. Histological observations on the growth of malignant gliomas after radiotherapy and chemotherapy. *Acta Neuropathol* 1982;58:291–299.
17. Tsuboi K, et al. Regrowth patterns of supratentorial gliomas: estimation from computed tomographic scans. *Neurosurgery* 1986;19:946–951.

18. Larson DA, Gutin PH. Brachytherapy. In: *Rationale, Techniques and Expectations in Malignant Cerebral Glioma* (Apuzzo MJ, ed.). AANS, Park Ridge, IL, 1990:173–180.
19. Greenberg HS, et al. Intra-arterial BCNU chemotherapy for treatment of malignant gliomas of the central nervous system. *J Neurosurg* 1984;61:423–429.
20. Brem H, et al. Interstitial chemotherapy with drug polymer implants for the treatment of recurrent gliomas. *J Neurosurg* 1991;74:441–446.
21. Sneed PK, et al. Interstitial irradiation and hyperthermia for the treatment of recurrent malignant brain tumors. *Neurosurgery* 1991;28:206–215.
22. Leksel DG. In: *Stereotactic Neurosurgery* (Heilbrun MP, ed.).Williams & Wilkins, Baltimore, 1998:195–209.
23. Marks JE, Baglan RJ, Wong J. In: *Biology of Brain Tumors* (Walker MD, Thomas DGT, eds.) Martinus Nijhoff, Netherlands, 1986:325–339.
24. Matsukado Y, MacCarty CS, Kernohan JW. J *Neurosurg* 1981;18:636–644.
25. Schiffer D. In: *Neurobiology of Brain Tumors* (Salcman M, ed). Williams & Wilkins, Baltimore, 1991:85–135.
26. Kitajima I, et al. Ablation of transplanted HTLV-1 Tax transformed tumors in mice by antisense inhibition of NF-κB. *Science* 1992;258:1792–1795.
27. Maki CG, et al. In vivo ubiquitination and proteasome-mediated degradation of p53. *Cancer Res* 1996;56:2649–2654.
28. Teicher BA, et al. The proteasome inhibitor PS-341 in cancer therapy. Clin *Cancer Res* 1999;5:2638–2645.
29. Nix D, et al. Clinical development of a proteasome inhibitor, PS-341, for the treatment of cancer. *ASCO Proc* 2001;20:86a.
30. Barth RF. Rat brain tumor models in experimental neuro-oncology: the 9L, C6, T9, F98, RG2 (D74), RT-2 and CNS-1 gliomas. *J Neurooncol* 1998;36:91–102.
31. Englehard HH, Groothius DG. The blood-brain barrier: structure, function, and response to neoplasia. In: *The Gliomas* (Berger MS, Wilson CB, eds). WB Saunders, Philadelphia, 1999:115–121.
32. Ciechanover A. The ubiquitin-proteasome pathway: on protein death and cell life. *EMBO J* 1998;17:7151–7160.
33. Frankel A, et al. Lack of multicellular drug resistance observed in human ovarian and prostate carcinoma treated with the proteasome inhibitor PS-341. *Clin Cancer Res* 2000;6:3719–3728.
34. Logothetis CJ, et al. Dose dependent inhibition of 20S proteasome results in serum IL-6 and PSA decline in patients with androgen-independent prostate cancer treated with the proteasome inhibitor PS-341. *Proc ASCO* 2001;20:186a.
35. Erlichman C, et al. A Phase I trial of the proteasome inhibitor PS-341 in patients with advanced cancer. *Proc ASCO* 2001;20:85a.
36. Aghajanian C, et al. A phase I trial of the novel protesome inhibitor PS-341 in advanced solid tumor malignancies. *Proc ASCO* 2001;20:85a.
37. Sun J, et al. CEP1612, a depeptidyl proteasome inhibitor, induces p21WAF1 and p27KIP1 expression and apoptosis and inhibits the growth of the human lung adenocarcinoma A-549 in nude mice. *Cancer Res* 2001;61:1280–1284.
38. Hamilton AL, et al. Phase I study of a novel proteasome inhibitor with pharmacodynamic endpoints. *Proc ASCO* 2001;20:85a.

14 Anthracyclines and Bortezomib

Robert Z. Orlowski

CONTENTS

ABSTRACT

Anthracycline chemotherapeutics display activity against a broad range of cancers and are therefore in clinical use for therapy of patients with both hematologic malignancies and solid tumors. However, these drugs have the ability to activate pathways such as nuclear factor-κB and p44/42 mitogen-activated protein kinase which play roles in inducible chemoresistance and promote tumor cell survival. Because proteasome inhibitors block activation of these pathways, it is possible that combinations of an anthracycline and a proteasome inhibitor could induce higher levels of tumor cell apoptosis. Furthermore, other mechanisms of resistance to anthracyclines, such as P-glycoprotein expression and downregulation of topoisomerase II, may also be abrogated by proteasome inhibitors, further supporting the development of such regimens. This chapter describes some of the molecular mechanisms by which addition of a proteasome inhibitor to an anthracycline could result in enhanced antitumor efficacy. In addition, the available preclinical and early clinical data are critically reviewed, to afford the reader some insight into the promise of this area of investigation.

KEY WORDS

Proteasome, multicatalytic proteinase complex, proteasome inhibitor, bortezomib, PS-341, Velcade, anthracycline, doxorubicin, apoptosis, NF-κB, IκB, p44/42 MAPK, MKP-1, P-glycoprotein, topoisomerase II, chemotherapy, clinical trial, phase I

1. INTRODUCTION

Anthracyclines comprise a group of compounds that are some of the more commonly used drugs in cancer chemotherapy. The original agents in clinical use, doxorubicin and

From: *Cancer Drug Discovery and Development: Proteasome Inhibitors in Cancer Therapy*
Edited by: J. Adams © Humana Press Inc., Totowa, NJ

daunomycin, were first isolated from species of *Streptomyces*, but newer compounds that have been introduced into clinical practice, including epirubicin and idarubicin, are synthetic. As a result of their significant antitumor activity, they have become important components of many chemotherapeutic regimens. Salient examples include the use of doxorubicin (Adriamycin) and cyclophosphamide, with or without a taxane, as adjuvant therapy for breast cancer; the application of cytarabine with either doxorubicin or idarubicin in both induction and consolidation therapy of acute myelogenous leukemia; and the combination of doxorubicin with cyclophosphamide, vincristine, and prednisone for therapy of non-Hodgkin's lymphoma. In addition, these agents have significant activity as part of regimens in small cell lung carcinoma, germ cell tumors, sarcomas, and several other malignancies. This broad spectrum of action alone makes anthracyclines interesting candidates for the development of combinations with novel investigational agents, such as the proteasome inhibitor bortezomib (Velcade™; formerly known as PS-341).

Although structural variations between the anthracyclines can result in some different properties, most of their cytotoxicity has been thought to occur because of their effect on nuclear structures in general, and on DNA in particular. These agents can intercalate between DNA base pairs and generate toxic oxygen free radicals that cause single- or double-stranded DNA breaks. Such strand breaks also occur as a result of the ability of anthracyclines to induce formation of covalent topoisomerase II–DNA complexes, which prevent DNA religation after the initial strand scission. This DNA damage inhibits DNA transcription and protein translation, and free-radical damage to other cellular structures such as proteins and membrane lipids also contributes to cytotoxicity *(1)*. Based on what is known about these mechanisms of action and about those by which proteasome inhibitors act, there is particular reason to be excited about the potential activity of such combination regimens. Some of the potential areas of synergy between proteasome inhibitors and anthracyclines are discussed below, followed by an overview of the laboratory and preclinical studies that have been performed to date. Finally, because such combinations are already being evaluated in phase I clinical trials, the available preliminary data from this arena are presented, to highlight the rapid steps being taken to translate this promising field of research into improved care of patients with cancer.

2. SCIENTIFIC RATIONALE

Evidence already exists suggesting that the proteasome plays an important role in anthracycline-mediated cytotoxicity. Doxorubicin appears to be able to bind to several of the subunits of the 20S proteasome *(2)*, after which this complex translocates to the nucleus in L1210 murine leukemia cells *(2,3)*. Both the expression of proteasome subunits and the activity of the proteasome have been noted to be increased in some transformed and proliferating cells, compared with controls *(4–6)*. This has been hypothesized to contribute to the differential effects of doxorubicin on transformed cells *(3)*, because a greater content of proteasome subunits would theoretically result in enhanced delivery of doxorubicin to the nucleus. After translocation, there appears to be an increase in nuclear proteasome function *(7)*, and in cardiac myocytes this appears to result in specific degradation of the p300 coactivator protein *(8)*. It is also interesting to note that the anthracycline aclarubicin has itself been noted to inhibit the proteasome *(9,10)*, although this occurs at concentrations that are probably not clinically relevant *(11)*. One subunit of the 26S proteasome, Poh1, when overexpressed appears to confer resistance to ultraviolet light and several chemotherapeutic drugs, including doxorubicin *(12)*. In addition to these areas of overlap, however, there are several mechanisms by which the combination of a proteasome inhibitor and an anthracycline could have at least additive, and possibly even synergistic antitumor efficacy. These have been divided into two categories: proteasome inhibitor-mediated blockade of anthracycline-activated antiapoptotic pathways and reversal of inherent drug resistance pathways.

2.1. Blockade of Antiapoptotic Pathways

2.1.1. NF-κB

While it is likely that proteasome inhibitors such as bortezomib induce apoptosis of transformed cells by impacting on several cell-death associated pathways, clearly one of the more important of these is the transcription factor nuclear factor-κB (NF-κB). Many studies have shown that activation of NF-κB leads to the induction of an antiapoptotic gene program, including tumor necrosis factor receptor-activated factor (TRAF)-1 and -2, inhibitor of apoptosis (IAP)-1 and -2, and several Bcl-2 homologs, such as A1/Bfl-1 and Bcl-X_L *(13)*. This finding has particular relevance to oncology in that several of the more commonly used classes of cytotoxic drugs induce NF-κB and would therefore seem in part to subvert their own ability to induce tumor cell death. Consistent with this possibility, blockade of NF-κB activation, with interventions such as the use of dominant negative constructs of the inhibitory protein IκBα, which prevents nuclear translocation of NF-κB, enhances apoptosis *(14)*. Proteasome inhibitors have been used to block NF-κB nuclear localization as well, since they inhibit IκBα degradation, and they may also interfere with NF-κB activity because the proteasome is involved in processing of the NF-κB p105 precursor *(15)*. This rationale has been used by several investigators to test combinations of bortezomib with chemotherapeutic agents that activate NF-κB, such as campothecin (CPT)-11 *(16)*, and an enhanced antitumor efficacy was demonstrated. Similar findings have been reported using combinations of bortezomib with ionizing radiation in preclinical studies *(17)*, since the latter can also activate NF-κB. Anthra-cyclines are themselves potent activators of NF-κB *(18)*, and the addition of bortezomib has the potential, therefore, to enhance similarly the antitumor activity of this class of drugs.

2.1.2. p44/42 MAPK

Another mechanism by which proteasome inhibitors induce apoptosis is through the induction of the mitogen-activated protein kinase (MAPK) phosphatase-1 (MKP-1), which dephosphorylates p44/42 MAPK *(19)*. The p44/42 signal transduction pathway carries important growth and survival signals and is also involved in resistance to certain chemotherapeutic agents and radiation *(20–22)*. These tumor cell survival and chemotherapy resistance signals may be transduced from p44/42 MAPK to p90-RSK, and then to the protein Bad. When Bad is phosphorylated, it is sequestered in the cytoplasm by the 14-3-3 protein and cannot reach mitochondria, where it would otherwise form proapoptotic heterodimers with Bcl-2 and Bcl-X_L proteins *(23,24)*. Thus, MAPK inhibition should lead to Bad hypophosphorylation and induction of Bad-mediated apoptosis, which has been demonstrated by some investigators *(25,26)*. Anthracyclines such as doxorubicin have been noted to activate p44/42 MAPK *(27)*, and preliminary evidence from studies in our laboratory indicates that this activation is also antiapoptotic. If a proteasome inhibitor could inhibit doxorubicin-mediated activation of p44/42 MAPK,

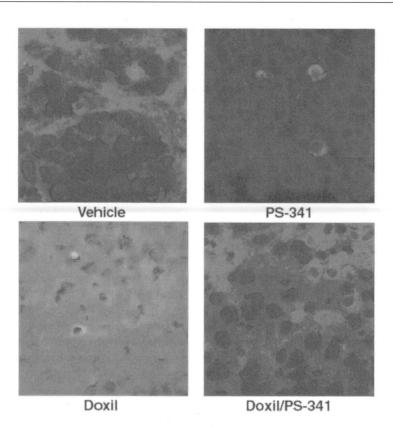

Fig. 1. The effect of bortezomib (PS-341) and Doxil® on MAPK activation in vivo. Using a murine xenograft model of human breast cancer, the impact of vehicle, bortezomib alone, Doxil® alone, and the combination was studied by immunofluorescence. MAPK activation status was evaluated in tumor sections by staining for activated, dually phosphorylated p44/42 MAPK using a phospho-specific antibody (in gray). A counterstain (black) shows nuclear DNA.

therefore, apoptosis could be enhanced. Consistent with this possibility, bortezomib indeed not only decreased the basal level of activated, dually phosphorylated p44/42 MAPK in tumor tissue, but also decreased the induction of this activation by doxorubicin in laboratory studies (Fig. 1). This may be another anthracycline-activated cell survival pathway, therefore, that can be inhibited in combination with a proteasome inhibitor, potentially resulting in enhanced antitumor activity.

2.2. Reversal of Drug Resistance

2.2.1. P-GLYCOPROTEIN

Despite the broad spectrum of antineoplastic activity of anthracyclines, some tumors are resistant to therapy, and resistance can develop during or after therapy in others. One of the most common mechanisms of anthracycline resistance is by the expression of the multidrug resistance (MDR) phenotype. This is generally due to the presence on the cellular surface of the P-glycoprotein (P-gp), or one of several related membrane proteins, which function as pumps that can extrude many xenobiotics such as anthracyclines *(28,29)*. Blockade of this activity would have the potential benefit of increasing intracellular doxorubicin levels and thereby increasing its antitumor efficacy. Many laboratory studies have supported the validity of this hypothesis, and clinical trials have shown that MDR modulators such as cyclosporin can impact on doxorubicin metabolism *(30)*. In addition, combinations such as dexverapamil with doxorubicin may induce responses in previously anthracycline-resistant patients *(31)*, but the toxicity of some of these currently available MDR modulators has limited their clinical applicability. Bortezomib, by contrast, was well tolerated by patients in phase I and II trials, and this is relevant since the proteasome is important in the biology of P-gp. Because proteasome inhibition prevents mature P-gp from reaching surface membranes *(32,33)*, bortezomib may have the ability to enhance the antitumor activity of MDR substrates such as anthracyclines, while itself contributing minimally to toxicity. This possibility merits further clinical investigation.

2.2.2. TOPOISOMERASE II

Another mechanism used by cancer cells to avoid toxicity induced by topoisomerase II (Top II)-directed drugs is either to mutate this target protein or to downregulate its expression *(34)*. The latter mechanism is particularly interesting in that chronic hypoxia and low glucose levels, conditions that are present in some regions of solid tumors, decrease Top II expression and induce resistance to drugs such as etoposide and doxorubicin *(35)*. Because the proteasome is involved in degradation of Top II *(36,37)*, one might expect that inhibition of the proteasome would increase Top II levels and thereby increase sensitivity to drugs that target this protein. Recent laboratory studies have indeed shown that the proteasome inhibitor lactacystin can attenuate Top II depletion induced by hypoxia and glucose starvation and that sensitivity to etoposide is then increased *(38)*. Furthermore, drugs such as doxorubicin trap Top II in a so-called cleavable complex in which each Top II subunit is covalently linked to DNA, and these complexes trigger DNA damage responses, including p53 stabilization, which contribute to apoptosis *(39)*. The 26S proteasome is involved in degradation of these complexes in preparation for their repair *(40)*, and it is therefore possible that proteasome inhibition would delay the time to repair, prolong cell cycle arrest, and perhaps thereby increase apoptosis.

Because the mechanisms by which proteasome inhibitors induce apoptosis and modify drug resistance are under active investigation, and anthracyclines impact on several signaling pathways *(41)*, it is likely that such combinations will be shown to interact in many ways. The possibility that some of these may actually decrease antitumor efficacy will need to be considered as well, however. For example, proteasome inhibitors activate the c-Jun-N-terminal kinase *(42)*, as does doxorubicin *(41)*. Since this is felt to be an important step in the induction of apoptosis by many drugs *(22)*, if maximal activation is achieved with one agent then the addition of another drug working through a similar mechanism may result in less than additive cell death. Also, bortezomib *(43)*, as well as other apoptosis-inducing proteasome inhibitors like lactacystin *(44)*, are targeted in part against the chymotrypsin-like activity of the proteasome. Since the proteasome may ferry anthracyclines to the nucleus, if such inhibitors would block binding of doxorubicin they could inhibit the induction of apoptosis. In this regard there are data showing that lactacystin does not impact on the accumulation of doxorubicin inside HT-29 colon carcinoma cells *(38)*. Since nuclear transport of doxorubicin was not evaluated, however, this possibility would still merit further investigation.

3. PRECLINICAL STUDIES

The solid scientific basis upon which combinations of a proteasome inhibitor and an anthracycline would seem to merit further investigation have led to studies along these lines, some of which have been performed in vitro with tumor cells; others have proceeded with in vivo xenograft studies.

3.1. Cell Line Studies

A variety of cell lines representing different tumor types have been used to investigate enhanced cytotoxicity with the combination of an anthracycline and a proteasome inhibitor. Yuan et al. *(45)*, for example, studied LNCap and Du-145 human prostate carcinoma cells and found that the proteasome inhibitors lactacystin and MG-132 increased doxorubicin cytotoxicity. In more mechanistically oriented studies, Lin et al. *(46)* found that brefeldin-induced activation of NF-κB resulted in resistance to the Top II-directed drug teniposide. They then used MG-132 to block nuclear translocation of NF-κB and found that this manipulation abrogated chemotherapy resistance *(46)*. Tabata et al. *(47)* have also noted that MG-132 enhanced apoptosis induced by etoposide, which, like teniposide and doxorubicin, targets Top II. Interestingly, based on studies with dominant-negative IκBα constructs, they concluded that this enhancement was not associated with inhibition of NF-κB, and occurred only if the proteasome inhibitor was added after the chemotherapeutic agent *(47)*. Brandes et al. *(48)*, in contrast, found that, in EMT6 mouse mammary carcinoma cells, blockade of NF-κB with dominant-negative IκBα was itself sufficient to enhance sensitivity to etoposide. These findings suggest that there may be some cell- and tumor-type specificity to the role of NF-κB inhibition in enhancing toxicity of Top II-directed agents.

The ability of proteasome inhibitors to inactivate signaling through p44/42 MAPK *(19)* has led us to be especially interested in the potential application of this class of agents to the therapy of breast cancer. Although activity of this pathway is associated with cellular proliferation and apoptosis in many cells *(20–22)*, signaling by the *erb*B receptor tyrosine kinase family, which occurs in part through p44/42 MAPK, has been implicated in the development and progression of breast cancer. High expression of *c-erb*B-2 (HER-2/neu) and the homologous epidermal growth factor (EGF) receptor (*c-erb*B-1) is a poor prognostic sign *(49)*. Indeed, elevated activity of p44/42 alone has been suggested to have prognostic significance for disease-free survival of breast cancer patients *(50)*. Finally, the ability of anthracyclines, which are already commonly used in patients with breast cancer, to stimulate antiapoptotic p44/42 MAPK, would seem to make an anthracycline/proteasome inhibitor regimen ideal for investigation in this population. Consistent with this possibility, studies with a variety of breast epithelial cell and carcinoma cell lines have shown that such a combination induced greater than additive induction of apoptosis, suggesting the possibility of a synergistic antitumor efficacy. Similar findings have been noted in cells derived from patients with hematologic malignancies (unpublished observations).

3.2. Xenograft Models

In addition to the apparent enhanced proapoptotic activity of anthracycline/proteasome inhibitor combinations in tissue culture, some reports have documented antitumor efforts in vivo. Using a Lewis lung carcinoma model system in C57BL mice, Teicher et al. *(51)*

showed that oral bortezomib given on d 4–18, in combination with intraperitoneal doxorubicin given on d 7–11, resulted in an at least additive tumor growth delay. When the presence of lung metastases was examined, a significant decrease was noted with this combination regimen as well *(51)*. Ogiso et al. *(38)* used a nude mouse xenograft model of HT-29 colon carcinoma cells and studied a combination of the proteasome inhibitor lactacystin, given at 25 mg/kg/d, with etoposide at 33 mg/kg/d. The latter, like doxorubicin, also targets topoisomerase II and is an agent with activity in several similar malignancies, including acute myelogenous leukemia and non-Hodgkin's lymphoma. Although lactacystin and etoposide each had some activity alone, use of the combination regimen resulted in enhanced antitumor effects *(38)*.

Given the previously noted rationale for targeting breast neoplasms with a doxorubicin/ proteasome inhibitor regimen, we have studied the combination of bortezomib and liposomal doxorubicin in a BT-474 xenograft model. Twice weekly therapy with the combination was superior with respect to antitumor activity compared with either agent alone, and increased apoptosis was induced in the tumor tissue itself (unpublished observations).

4. CLINICAL TRIALS

4.1. Doxorubicin and Bortezomib

The great potential of combinations of an anthracycline with a proteasome inhibitor have led to the initiation of two phase I clinical trials that will determine the maximum tolerated dose (MTD) and dose-limiting toxicity of these regimens. One such study, using doxorubicin and bortezomib, is ongoing at the University of Wisconsin Comprehensive Cancer Center. Patients with advanced solid tumors are being treated using a schedule in which bortezomib is administered on d 1, 4, 8, and 11 of each 3-wk cycle; doxorubicin is given on d 1 and 8. A preliminary report of the data presented to the American Society of Clinical Oncology has indicated that drug-related toxicities were generally mild, or grade I/II, including thrombocytopenia, fatigue, nausea, rash, and anorexia, as well as one injection site reaction, and an exacerbation of pre-existing neuropathic pain. More severe side effects, including one myocardial infarction, were not felt to be treatment-related. Of six patients who were evaluable for response, one with pulmonary metastases of hormone-refractory prostate cancer had been noted to have a partial response *(52)*.

4.2. Doxil® and Bortezomib

Bortezomib in combination with pegylated, liposomal doxorubicin (Doxil®) is being studied at the University of North Carolina at Chapel Hill's Lineberger Comprehensive Cancer Center. This formulation of doxorubicin was chosen because of its activity in a broad range of malignancies, including hematologic malignancies such as multiple myeloma and non-Hodgkin's lymphoma. It has also shown efficacy in solid tumors, including refractory ovarian and metastatic breast cancer, sometimes in the face of previous anthracycline-containing regimens *(53–55)*. Furthermore, the up to 80-h half-life *(56)* allows dosing once every 3 wk, and the liposomal formulation may decrease doxorubicin's cardiac toxicity *(57)*, which is one of the most notable complications of the use of this drug *(58)*. Because of the possibility, based on earlier studies, that patients with hematologic malignancies may tolerate lower doses of bortezomib than those with solid tumors, these two patient populations are being accrued along separate tracks that will allow for the definition of different MTDs.

Early results indicate that this combination was well tolerated by both groups of patients, with most of the drug-related toxicities being only grade I/II in intensity, including fatigue, nausea, thrombocytopenia, and sensory neuropathy. The one grade III event that has occurred was an episode of syncope, which occurred in a patient who also self-administered an excessive dose of narcotics. Because Doxil® (55) and bortezomib (59) have individually shown activity in patients with multiple myeloma, the combination would also be expected to be active in this population. Consistent with this possibility, several responses have already been seen in patients with myeloma on this study, including one complete response. Also of note, one patient with relapsed acute myelogenous leukemia has responded as well with a diminution in bone marrow blasts. These data, together with the demonstrated activity of Doxil® in patients with breast and ovarian carcinoma, as well as the available preclinical data in models of breast cancer, suggest that this regimen is worthy of further testing in phase II clinical studies. Once the MTD has been identified, therefore, that patient cohort will be expanded to determine better whether there is evidence of antitumor activity in these populations.

5. CONCLUSIONS

Regimens consisting of an anthracycline and bortezomib represent novel combinations of drugs that could have significantly enhanced antitumor efficacy compared with either agent alone, and possibly even compared with other drug regimens. The ability of proteasome inhibitors to block antiapoptotic pathways activated by anthracyclines, such as NF-κB and p44/42 MAPK, as well as their ability to overcome drug resistance mechanisms, such as P-glycoprotein-mediated drug efflux and hypoxia-induced downregulation of Top II, provides a strong scientific basis for this hypothesis. Early studies in both cell culture and xenograft models support the activity of this combination as well. Finally, patients in phase I clinical trials already under way, the primary endpoints of which are to identify appropriate drug dose levels, have tolerated the combination therapy and have shown preliminary evidence of antitumor activity. Although some important questions are still unanswered, such as the optimal anthracycline formulation to be used, these results strongly support formal efficacy testing in a phase II setting. Furthermore, they suggest the possibility that such combinations may prove to be significant advances in the care of a variety of tumor types for which patients currently have much more limited options. If this promise proves well founded, it will represent a true advance for translational medicine, and its attempt to use laboratory-based findings to make rational decisions about cancer therapy.

ACKNOWLEDGMENTS

The authors would like to acknowledge support from the Department of Defense Breast Cancer Research Program, BC991049, and the Leukemia and Lymphoma Society, R6206-02.

REFERENCES

1. Riggs CEJ. Antitumor antibiotics and related compounds. In: *The Chemotherapy Source Book.* (Perry MC, ed). Williams & Wilkins, Baltimore,1997:345–386.
2. Kiyomiya K, et al. Mechanism of specific nuclear transport of Adriamycin: the mode of nuclear translocation of Adriamycin-proteasome complex. *Cancer Res* 2001;61:2467–2471.

3. Kiyomiya K, et al. Proteasome is a carrier to translocate doxorubicin from cytoplasm into nucleus. *Life Sci* 1998;62:1853–1860.

4. Kumatori A, et al. Abnormally high expression of proteasomes in human leukemic cells. *Proc Natl Acad Sci USA* 1990;87:7071–7075.

5. Kanayama H, et al. Changes in expressions of proteasome and ubiquitin genes in human renal cancer cells. *Cancer Res* 1991;51:6677–6685.

6. Shimbara N, et al. Regulation of gene expression of proteasomes (multi-protease complexes) during growth and differentiation of human hematopoietic cells. *J Biol Chem* 1992;267:18100–18109.

7. Ciftci O, et al. Regulation of the nuclear proteasome activity in myelomonocytic human leukemia cells after Adriamycin treatment. *Blood* 2001;97:2830–2838.

8. Poizat C, et al. Proteasome-mediated degradation of the coactivator p300 impairs cardiac transcription. *Mol Cell Biol* 2000;20:8643–8654.

9. Isoe T, et al. Inhibition of different steps of the ubiquitin system by cisplatin and aclarubicin. *Biochim Biophys Acta* 1992;1117:131–135.

10. Figueiredo-Pereira ME, et al. The antitumor drug aclacinomycin A, which inhibits the degradation of ubiquitinated proteins, shows selectivity for the chymotrypsin-like activity of the bovine pituitary 20 S proteasome [published erratum appears in *J Biol Chem* 1996;271:23602]. *J Biol Chem* 1996;271:16455–16459.

11. Karanes C, et al. Phase I trial of aclacinomycin-A. A clinical and pharmacokinetic study. *Invest New Drugs* 1983;1:173–179.

12. Spataro V, et al. Resistance to diverse drugs and ultraviolet light conferred by overexpression of a novel human 26 S proteasome subunit. *J Biol Chem* 1997;272:30470–30475.

13. Baldwin AS. Control of oncogenesis and cancer therapy resistance by the transcription factor NF-kappaB. *J Clin Invest* 2001;107:241–246.

14. Wang CY, et al. Control of inducible chemoresistance: enhanced anti-tumor therapy through increased apoptosis by inhibition of NF-kappaB. *Nat Med* 1999;5:412–417.

15. Palombella VJ, et al. The ubiquitin-proteasome pathway is required for processing the NF-kappa B1 precursor protein and the activation of NF-kappa B. *Cell* 1994;78:773–785.

16. Cusack JC, Jr., et al. Enhanced chemosensitivity to CPT-11 with proteasome inhibitor PS-341: implications for systemic nuclear factor-kappaB inhibition. *Cancer Res* 2001;61:3535–3540.

17. Russo SM, et al. Enhancement of radiosensitivity by proteasome inhibition: implications for a role of NF-kappaB. *Int J Radiat Oncol Biol Phys* 2001;50:183–193.

18. Das KC, et al. Activation of NF-kappaB by antineoplastic agents. Role of protein kinase C. *J Biol Chem* 1997;272:14914–14920.

19. Orlowski RZ, et al. Evidence that inhibition of p44/42 mitogen activated protein kinase signaling is a factor in proteasome inhibitor-mediated apoptosis. *J Biol Chem* 2002;277:27864–27871.

20. Dent P, et al. The roles of signaling by the p42/p44 mitogen-activated protein (MAP) kinase pathway; a potential route to radio- and chemo-sensitization of tumor cells resulting in the induction of apoptosis and loss of clonogenicity. *Leukemia* 1998;12:1843–1850.

21. Schaeffer HJ, et al. Mitogen-activated protein kinases: specific messages from ubiquitous messengers. *Mol Cell Biol* 1999;19:2435–2444.

22. Cross TG, et al. Serine/threonine protein kinases and apoptosis. *Exp Cell Res* 2000;256:34–41.

23. Bonni A, et al. Cell survival promoted by the Ras-MAPK signaling pathway by transcription-dependent and -independent mechanisms [see comments]. *Science* 1999;286:1358–1362.

24. Fang X, et al. Regulation of BAD phosphorylation at serine 112 by the Ras-mitogen-activated protein kinase pathway. *Oncogene* 1999;18:6635–6640.

25. Jan MS, et al. Bad overexpression sensitizes NIH/3T3 cells to undergo apoptosis which involves caspase activation and ERK inactivation. *Biochem Biophys Res Commun* 1999;264:724–729.

26. Holmstrom TH, et al. MAPK/ERK signaling in activated T cells inhibits CD95/Fas-mediated apoptosis downstream of DISC assembly. *EMBO J* 2000;19:5418–5428.

27. Arai M, et al. Mechanism of doxorubicin-induced inhibition of sarcoplasmic reticulum Ca (2+)-ATPase gene transcription. *Circ Res* 2000;86:8–14.

28. Nielsen D, et al. Cellular resistance to anthracyclines. *Gen Pharmacol* 1996;27:251–255.

29. Robert J. Multidrug resistance in oncology: diagnostic and therapeutic approaches. *Eur J Clin Invest* 1999;29:536–545.

30. Bartlett NL, et al. Phase I trial of doxorubicin with cyclosporine as a modulator of multidrug resistance. *J Clin Oncol* 1994;12:835–842.

31. Warner E, et al. Phase II study of dexverapamil plus anthracycline in patients with metastatic breast cancer who have progressed on the same anthracycline regimen. *Clin Cancer Res* 1998;4:1451–1457.
32. Loo TW, et al. Superfolding of the partially unfolded core-glycosylated intermediate of human P-glycoprotein into the mature enzyme is promoted by substrate-induced transmembrane domain interactions. *J Biol Chem* 1998;273:14671–14674.
33. Loo TW, et al. The human multidrug resistance P-glycoprotein is inactive when its maturation is inhibited: potential for a role in cancer chemotherapy. *FASEB J* 1999;13:1724–1732.
34. Beck WT, et al. Mechanisms of resistance to drugs that inhibit DNA topoisomerases. *Semin Cancer Biol* 1991;2:235–244.
35. Tomida A, et al. Drug resistance mediated by cellular stress response to the microenvironment of solid tumors. *Anticancer Drug Des* 1999;14:169–177.
36. Nakajima T, et al. Degradation of topoisomerase IIalpha during adenovirus E1A-induced apoptosis is mediated by the activation of the ubiquitin proteolysis system. *J Biol Chem* 1996;271:24842–24849.
37. Kim HD, et al. Glucose-regulated stresses cause degradation of DNA topoisomerase IIalpha by inducing nuclear proteasome during G1 cell cycle arrest in cancer cells. *J Cell Physiol* 1999;180:97–104.
38. Ogiso Y, et al. Proteasome inhibition circumvents solid tumor resistance to topoisomerase II-directed drugs. *Cancer Res* 2000;60:2429–2434.
39. Smith PJ, et al. Multilevel therapeutic targeting by topoisomerase inhibitors. *Br J Cancer Suppl* 1994;23:S47–S51.
40. Mao Y, et al. 26 S proteasome-mediated degradation of topoisomerase II cleavable complexes. *J Biol Chem* 2001;276:40652–40658.
41. Laurent G, et al. Signaling pathways activated by daunorubicin. *Blood* 2001;98:913–924.
42. Meriin AB, et al. Proteasome inhibitors activate stress kinases and induce Hsp72. Diverse effects on apoptosis. *J Biol Chem* 1998;273:6373–6379.
43. Adams J, et al. Proteasome inhibitors: a novel class of potent and effective antitumor agents. *Cancer Res* 1999;59:2615–2622.
44. Fenteany G, et al. Lactacystin, proteasome function, and cell fate. *J Biol Chem* 1998;273:8545–8548
45. Yuan R, et al. P53-independent downregulation of p73 in human cancer cells treated with Adriamycin. *Cancer Chemother Pharmacol* 2001;47:161–169.
46. Lin ZP, et al. Prevention of brefeldin A-induced resistance to teniposide by the proteasome inhibitor MG-132: involvement of NF-kappaB activation in drug resistance. *Cancer Res* 1998;58:3059–3065.
47. Tabata M, et al. Roles of NF-kappaB and 26 S proteasome in apoptotic cell death induced by topoisomerase I and II poisons in human nonsmall cell lung carcinoma. *J Biol Chem* 2001;276:8029–8036.
48. Brandes LM, et al. Reversal of physiological stress-induced resistance to topoisomerase II inhibitors using an inducible phosphorylation site-deficient mutant of I kappa B alpha. *Mol Pharmacol* 2001;60:559–567.
49. Dickson RB, et al. Growth factors in breast cancer. *Endocr Rev* 1995;16:559–589.
50. Mueller H, et al. Potential prognostic value of mitogen-activated protein kinase activity for disease-free survival of primary breast cancer patients. *Int J Cancer* 2000;89:384–388.
51. Teicher BA, et al. The proteasome inhibitor PS-341 in cancer therapy. *Clin Cancer Res* 1999;5:2638–2645.
52. Thomas JP, et al. A phase I and pharmacodynamic study of the proteasome inhibitor PS-341 in combination with doxorubicin. In: *Proceedings of the American Society of Clinical Oncology*, Orlando, FL, 2002, vol 21.
53. Sparano JA, et al. Liposomal anthracyclines for breast cancer. *Semin Oncol* 2001;28:32–40.
54. Muggia F, et al. Phase III data on Caelyx in ovarian cancer. *Eur J Cancer* 2001;37(suppl 9):S15–S18
55. Muggia FM. Liposomal encapsulated anthracyclines: new therapeutic horizons. *Curr Oncol Rep* 2001;3:156–162.
56. Lyass O, et al. Correlation of toxicity with pharmacokinetics of pegylated liposomal doxorubicin (Doxil) in metastatic breast carcinoma. *Cancer* 2000;89:1037–1047.
57. Berry G, et al. The use of cardiac biopsy to demonstrate reduced cardiotoxicity in AIDS Kaposi's sarcoma patients treated with pegylated liposomal doxorubicin. *Ann Oncol* 1998;9:711–716.
58. Singal PK, et al. Doxorubicin-induced cardiomyopathy. *N Engl J Med* 1998;339:900–905.
59. Stinchcombe TE, et al. PS-341 is active in multiple myeloma: preliminary report of a phase I trial of the proteasome inhibitor PS-341 in patients with hematologic malignancies. In: *Proceedings of the American Society of Hematology*, San Francisco, CA, 2000, vol 96.

15 TNF-Related Apoptosis-Inducing Ligand (TRAIL)

Combination with Proteasome Inhibition for Anticancer Therapy?

Thomas J. Sayers

CONTENTS

INTRODUCTION
TRAIL AND ITS RECEPTORS
TRAIL SIGNALING AND APOPTOSIS
ANTICANCER PROPERTIES OF TRAIL
OUTSTANDING QUESTIONS

ABSTRACT

Tumor necrosis factor-related apoptosis-inducing ligand (Apo2L/TRAIL) is a protein of the tumor necrosis factor (TNF) family that has excited much recent interest as a potentially novel anticancer agent. TRAIL induces apoptosis in a wide variety of human and murine cancer cells, with no apparent apoptotic activity on normal nontransformed cells. Furthermore, TRAIL has also shown therapeutic efficacy when administered both to mice bearing various murine tumors and to immunodeficient mice bearing human tumor xenografts. Although some tumor cells are exquisitely sensitive to the proapoptotic effects of TRAIL, many tumor cells are only moderately sensitive to TRAIL as a single agent, and some remain highly resistant. The proteasome inhibitor bortezomib has also shown much initial promise as an anitcancer agent in vitro and in vivo. Treatment of tumor cells with bortezomib results in multiple biologic effects including inhibition of cell cycle, changes in adherence, inhibition of nuclear factor-κB, and increases in levels of apoptosis. Combinations of bortezomib and TRAIL synergistically interact to promote apoptosis of some tumor cells. The molecular mechanism(s) whereby bortezomib sensitizes tumor cells to apoptosis remains unclear. Nonetheless, a combination of these two novel agents may hold some promise for cancer therapy in the future.

From: *Cancer Drug Discovery and Development: Proteasome Inhibitors in Cancer Therapy*
Edited by: J. Adams © Humana Press Inc., Totowa, NJ

1. INTRODUCTION

Apoptosis has an essential role in embryogenesis, adult tissue homeostasis, and cellular responses to stressful stimuli *(1)*. Therefore, increased apoptosis is involved in the pathogenesis of various ischemic, degenerative, and immune disorders *(2)*. Conversely, genetic aberration that results in reduction or abolition of apoptosis can promote tumorigenesis and underlie the resistance of cancer cells to various genotoxic anticancer agents *(3)*. Therefore a detailed knowledge of the control of apoptotic pathways could aid in the rational design of effective therapeutics for a variety of human diseases including cancer. One major way to promote apoptosis involves signaling through members of the tumor necrosis factor (TNF) superfamily. On binding to their appropriate receptors, some TNF family members can promote caspase activation and apoptosis. Early studies on TNF indicated that a limited number of tumor cell lines could be induced to undergo apoptosis on exposure to TNF. Another member of the TNF family Fas ligand (FasL) is also known to induce apoptosis in a variety of tumor cells. Although TNF and FasL can efficiently induce apoptosis in a limited number of tumor cells, administration of either of these agents is associated with extreme toxicity. This toxicity has precluded further development of either TNF or FasL for cancer therapy. However, within the last 7 yr another member of the TNF family, TNF-related apoptosis-inducing ligand (TRAIL) has been characterized, which induces apoptosis of a wider range of cancer cells than either TNF or FasL *(4,5)*. Surprisingly, most normal nontransformed cells are quite resistant to the apoptotic effects of TRAIL. This selective toxicity for cancer cells is the basis for the current enthusiasm for TRAIL as a potential novel anticancer therapy.

2. TRAIL AND ITS RECEPTORS

TRAIL can induce apoptosis in a variety of tumor cells on binding to appropriate receptors. However, the interaction of TRAIL with cells is complex, because there are four well-defined receptors for TRAIL in humans, and a fifth protein capable of binding TRAIL has been identified.

TRAIL was discovered primarily through homology cloning. A conserved sequence present in many members of the TNF family was used to search expressed sequence tag (EST) databases. This resulted in the identification and cloning of a full-length cDNA for TRAIL *(4)*. Independently, TRAIL was isolated by another group that termed it APO2 ligand (APO2L) *(5)*. Northern blotting revealed the predominant 1.8–2.0-kb mRNA of TRAIL to be constitutively expressed in a wide variety of human tissues. Because TRAIL is widely expressed, most normal cells must be resistant to TRAIL-mediated apoptosis; however, the molecular basis for this resistance remains unclear. Analysis of the TRAIL sequence identified TRAIL as a type II membrane protein of 281 amino acids with its extracellular carboxyterminal domain showing considerable sequence similarity (up to 28% amino acid identity) to other members of the TNF superfamily. Also, in common with the members of the TNF family, TRAIL can exist as a membrane-bound protein or as a soluble protein generated through cysteine protease-mediated cleavage *(6)*. Several lines of evidence, including the resolution of TRAIL's crystal structure, indicate that TRAIL forms homotrimers in a similar manner to other TNF superfamily members *(7)*. This multimerization seems essential for the induction of apoptosis by TRAIL. A variety of TRAIL preparations have been engineered to enhance the biologic activity of TRAIL by promoting aggregation. These include a polyhistidine-tagged form (amino acids 114–281) *(5,8)*, a Flag epitope-tagged version (amino acids 95–281) *(4)*, and a TRAIL/leucine zipper fusion protein *(9)*. In addition, a recombinant soluble form devoid of foreign sequence has been developed. This version requires a central zinc ion to promote homotrimerization *(10)*. Mutations in residues that affect zinc binding to TRAIL result in loss of both trimer formation and apoptotic activity.

Shortly after the discovery of TRAIL, a similar strategy of searching EST databases using a highly conserved death domain motif from TNF receptor 1 (TNFR-1) resulted in identification of four TRAIL receptors. A TRAIL receptor termed death receptor 4 (DR4, TRAIL-R1) *(11)* and a second receptor molecule TRAIL-R2 (also TRICK, KILLER/DR5) *(12–16)* promoted apoptosis. Therefore, similar to other death receptors (such as Fas or TNFR1), overexpression of TRAIL-R1 and -R2 resulted in apoptosis in a caspase-dependent manner. Both these TRAIL receptors can also form heterotrimeric complexes. Because both TRAIL-R1 and -R2 as well as TRAIL itself were expressed in a variety of normal tissues, researchers could not account for the basis of TRAIL selectivity for inducing apoptosis in tumor cells.

The identification of two additional receptors termed TRAIL-R3 (TRID/DcR1/LIT) *(14–18)* and TRAIL-R4 (DcR2/TRUNDD) *(19–21)* offered a solution to this paradox. All four structurally related TRAIL receptors had similar extracellular domains, yet TRAIL-R3 and -R4 differ structurally from TRAIL-R1 and -R2 in the remaining portion of the molecule (Fig. 1). TRAIL-R3 lacked both a cytoplasmic domain and a transmembrane domain and was thus unable to transmit apoptotic death signals. Furthermore, this receptor was only linked to the cell surface via a glycosyl phosphatidylinositol anchor. TRAIL-R4 only contained a partial death domain, so was therefore also unable to trigger apoptotic cell death. Overexpression of TRAIL-R3 and -R4 provided protection from TRAIL-induced apoptosis. This led to the proposal that these decoy receptors could account for resistance to TRAIL. Indeed, expression of TRAIL-R3 and TRAIL-R4 was more prevalent in normal tissues than in most cancer cells. Recently the secreted protein osteoprotegrin (OPG) was identified as a protein that could bind to TRAIL *(22,23)*. Whether or not OPG plays a significant role in TRAIL-mediated cell death remains to be determined.

3. TRAIL SIGNALING AND APOPTOSIS

Binding of TRAIL to appropriate receptors containing the death domain motif (such as TRAIL-R1 and TRAIL-R2) can result in cellular apoptosis. As mentioned above, not all TRAIL receptors transmit this apoptotic signal. The death domain of TRAIL-R1 and TRAIL-R2 is essential for an apoptotic response, since it controls the recruitment of adapter proteins to the receptor complex that are critical for transmission of the apoptotic signal. In addition, the apoptotic signal can be inhibited by various proteins that block apoptotic signaling at proximal or distal sites on the signaling pathways.

Differential expression of functional (R1, R2) TRAIL as opposed to decoy (R3, R4) has long been considered the primary mechanisms controlling TRAIL sensitivity. How-

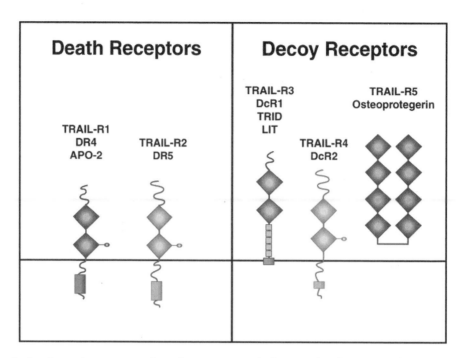

Fig. 1. A schematic representation of tumor necrosis factor-related apoptosis-inducing ligand (TRAIL) death receptors and decoy receptors. The intracellular death domain is depicted as a gray box. The boxes in the extracellular part represent homologous cysteine-rich domains that mediate ligand binding. The TRAIL decoy receptors TRAIL-R3 and TRAIL-R4 lack an intracellular domain or contain a nonfunctional death domain. TRAIL-R5 (osteoprotegrin) is secreted. Commonly used terms for the different death receptors are also given.

ever, a number of studies did not find a good correlation between decoy receptor expression and TRAIL sensitivity, suggesting that additional mechanisms are also involved in regulation TRAIL-mediated apoptosis *(24–26)*. In an analogous manner to Fas and TNF receptors, TRAIL receptors R1 and R2 use specific adaptor proteins for death signal transduction. On interaction with ligand, these receptors recruit specific adapter molecules such as FADD (Fas-associated death domain) *(27)*. The binding of adapter proteins such as FADD to the receptor complex then promotes the recruitment of procaspase 8 *(28,29)* through homotypic interactions between a second protein motif, the death effector domain (DED). This complex of proteins has been called the death-inducing signaling complex (DISC) *(30)*. Both FADD and procaspase 8 contain these DEDs, and it is likely that aggregation of procaspase 8 molecules results in enzymatic conversion to active caspase 8 and further activation of the caspase cascade of enzymes *(31)*. The recruitment of caspase 8 can be inhibited by another DED-containing protein called FADD-like IL-1β-converting enzyme (FLICE) inhibitory protein (c-FLIP) *(32–35)*. FLIP was originally described as a viral protein (v-FLIP) that prevented death receptor-induced apoptosis *(36)*. The cellular homolog c-FLIP can also inhibit apoptosis by preventing the recruitment and activation of proximal caspases (Fig. 2). High levels of endogenous c-FLIP often correlate with resistance of cells to TRAIL-mediated apoptosis. However, in a similar manner to receptor heterogeneity, a direct correlation between high c-FLIP levels and TRAIL resistance does not always apply *(25)*.

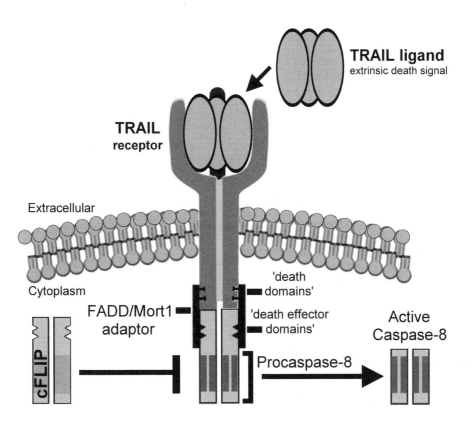

Fig.2. Control of tumor necrosis factor-related apoptosis-inducing ligand (TRAIL) signaling. The extrinsic cell death pathway is triggered by binding of death-receptor ligands that causes recruitment adapter proteins, such as Fas-associated death domain (FADD)/Mort1 to the receptor. Subsequent binding and oligomerization of caspase 8 results in a proximity-induced autoproteolytic activation. Activation is regulated by decoy receptors (*see* Fig. 1) or dominant-negative pseudo-caspases such as FADD-like IL-1β-converting enzyme (FLICE) inhibitory protein (c-FLIP), which prevent recruitment of the caspase-8 proenzyme into the receptor complex (Adapted from Nicholson D. *Nature* 2001;407.)

If a productive signal occurs from the DISC, many data suggest that the induction of caspase of activity is crucial for apoptosis to occur in most cells. For Fas-mediated signaling, it is generally believed that caspase 8 may either induce apoptosis in the absence of mitochondrial involvement, or alternatively cleave the proapoptotic Bcl-2 family protein Bid, which induces apoptosis by promoting changes in mitochondrial homeostasis culminating in the release of cytochrome c *(37)*. Which of these pathways is more important for TRAIL-mediated apoptosis? The answer probably involves cell type-specific differences in TRAIL-mediated apoptotic signaling (Fig. 3). Recent evidence suggests that the proapoptotic proteins Bax and Bak may be crucially involved in TRAIL-mediated apoptosis in some cells *(38)*.

In addition to its ability to initiate cell death, TRAIL has also been shown to activate nuclear factor-κB (NF-κB), which is known to suppress cytokine production and induce apoptosis-suppressing genes. TRAIL receptors 1, 2, and 4 can activate NF-κB under certain conditions *(19,39,40)*. Although activation of NF-κB is often associated with cell

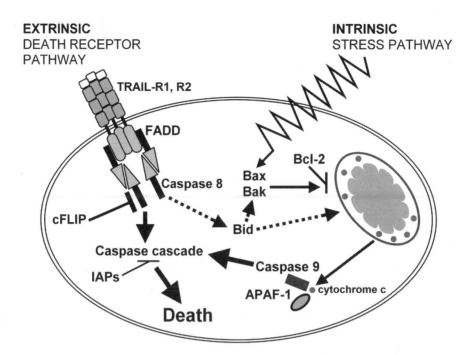

Fig. 3. Apoptosis mediated by tumor necrosis factor-related apoptosis-inducing ligand (TRAIL). In some cells the death receptor pathway involves direct activation of the caspase cascade by activation of proximal caspases such as caspase 8. Alternatively, in other cells there may be involvement of Bcl-2 family members, whereby caspase cleavage of proapoptotic Bid (probably also involving interaction with Bax and/or Bak) results in a linkage to the stress pathway, mitochondrial perturbation, and subsequent apoptosis. These pathways are controlled by the inhibitors c-FLIP, antiapoptotic Bcl-2 family members, or inhibitors of apoptosis proteins (IAPs). APAF-1, apoptotic protease-activating factor 1; c-FLIP, FADD-like IL-1β-converting enzyme (FLICE) inhibitory protein; FADD, Fas ligand death domain.

survival signals, under some circumstances NF-κB can trigger cell death *(41–43)*. Differential use of the adapter proteins FADD and TNF receptor-associated death domain (TRADD) may be the molecular switch that determines whether proximal caspase (i.e., apoptosis and death) or NF-κB (i.e., cell survival) pathways become activated. Activation of the c-Jun N-terminal kinase (JNK) by TRAIL has also been demonstrated. However, JNK activity alone appears to be insufficient to elicit apoptosis; it may contribute to the induction of cell death following cellular stress by activating the expression of cell death-promoting proteins.

4. ANTICANCER PROPERTIES OF TRAIL

The fact that TRAIL potently induces rapid apoptosis in a wide spectrum of tumor cell lines, whereas it lacks cytotoxicity toward many normal cells suggests it could have application as a novel biologic anticancer therapeutic *(4)*. In athymic nude mice or severe combined immunodeficiency disease (SCID) mice carrying human tumor xenografts, TRAIL treatment substantially inhibited tumor progression in a variety of human tumors including a human mammary adenocarcinoma (MDA-231) and two colon carcinomas (COLO-205 and HCT-15) *(9,10)*. TRAIL treatment also provided benefit when administered by locoregional injection into human U87MG glioma xenografts growing intrac-ranially in althymic mice *(44)*.

4.1. Trail as a Tumor Suppressor

Recently the first evidence that TRAIL plays a role in tumor suppression in vivo has been reported. Takeda and colleagues *(45)* noted that TRAIL expression in the liver played a significant role in limiting the development of experimental liver metastases. This conclusion was based on a substantial increase in experimental liver metastases in three murine tumor models (L929, Renca, and LB27.4) after administration of a neutral-izing antibody to mouse TRAIL. Natural killer (NK) cells were proposed as the most likely source of TRAIL in the liver, since depletion of NK cells enhanced the number of metastases, and NK cells were the only liver cells to express cell surface TRAIL by fluorescence-activated cell sorting analysis *(45,46)*. In an extension of this work, it has recently been reported that administration of neutralizing antibodies to TRAIL increased spontaneous tumor incidence in wild-type as well as p53 ± mice treated with the carcino-gen methyl cholanthrene *(47)*. Furthermore, mice gene-targeted for TRAIL (TRAIL –/ –) developed more experimental liver metastases following injection of a murine renal carcinoma (Renca), as well as more spontaneous liver metastases from a mammary carcinoma (4T1) *(48)*. Taken together, these data provide strong evidence that TRAIL is an effector molecule that suppresses developing tumors. Another interesting observation from these studies was that although TRAIL played an important role in limiting liver metastasis, it had no obvious role in controlling metastasis development in the lungs.

4.2. TRAIL in Combination with Radiation and Chemotherapy

Because TRAIL alone has exhibited significant therapeutic benefit as a single agent in various animal tumor models, it has also been used in combination with commonly used therapies such as chemotherapy or irradiation. Ionizing radiation can sensitize breast cancer cells to TRAIL-induced apoptosis *(49)*. This synergistic effect was shown to be p53-dependent and may involve radiation-induced upregulation of TRAIL-R2. Radia-tion also enhanced the efficacy of TRAIL-induced apoptosis of breast cancer cells in vivo. Therefore further studies on combinations of radiotherapy and TRAIL are required. Also, the combination of TRAIL with chemotherapeutics such as doxorubicin, 5-fluo-rouracil, etoposide, CPT-11, actinomycin D, and camptothecin has been shown to en-hance TRAIL-mediated apoptosis significantly in a variety of human tumor cell lines *(50–55)*. However, if the basis of synergy between chemotherapy and TRAIL is depen-dent on p53 activity, this may pose a serious limitation on a successful combination of these agents, since inactivating p53 mutations are present in about 50% of human malig-nancies.

4.3. TRAIL in Combination with Proteasome Inhibition

The proteasome inhibitor bortezomib (Velcade™; formerly known as PS-341) has shown initial promise as an anticancer agent both in vitro and in vivo. Treatment of tumor cells with bortezomib results in multiple biologic effects including inhibition of the cell cycle, inhibition of NF-κB activation, changes in cell adherence, and increased apoptosis *(56–58)*. Because of the pivotal role the proteasome plays in apoptosis, inhibitors of this enzyme, such as bortezomib, provide an opportunity to explore synergy between proteasome inhibition and other apoptosis-inducing agents. One of the major effects of proteasome inhibition in many cells is the inhibition of NF-κB activation. Because TRAIL binding to its receptors activates NF-κB (which can result in the induction of apoptosis-suppressing genes), it is tempting to speculate that proteasome inhibition may enhance TRAIL-mediated apoptosis by blocking NF-κB. Blocking of NF-κB using either degradation-resistant inhibitor κB (IκB) constructs *(59,60)* or proteasome inhibition *(60,61)* has been demonstrated to increase the sensitivity of a variety of tumor cells to TRAIL-mediated apoptosis. Evidence suggests that bortezomib, in combination with TRAIL, enhances apoptosis of some human multiple myeloma cells in vitro *(62)*. However, NF-κB activation does not protect all cells from TRAIL-mediated apoptosis *(63,64)*.

Interestingly, we have observed that bortezomib can sensitize a murine myeloid leukemia to TRAIL apoptosis independent of any effects on NF-κB activation. Sensitization appears to involve decreases in levels of the antiapoptotic protein c-FLIP *(65)*. Reduction in c-FLIP has also been noted on sensitization of human multiple myeloma cells to TRAIL-mediated lysis *(66)*. Interestingly, T-cells synchronized in various stages of the cell cycle show high levels of c-FLIP in G_1, with subsequent decreases at later stages (S, G_2M) *(67)*. Because bortezomib can arrest many tumor cells in the G_2-M phase of the cell cycle, the involvement of cell cycle arrest in the reduction of c-FLIP and the resultant TRAIL sensitization is worthy of further investigation. Other studies have noted that proteasome inhibition can modulate the balance between pro and antiapoptotic members of the Bcl-2 family, resulting in accumulation of the proapoptotic protein Bik *(68)*. Additionally, proteasome inhibition is also reported to promote activation of proapoptotic caspases such as caspase 3 *(69)*. Clearly proteasome inhibition may sensitize cells to TRAIL apoptosis by modification of both NF-κB-dependent and -independent pathways. Because some tumor cells are only moderately sensitive or are completely resistant to the apoptotic effects of TRAIL, a combination of TRAIL with enhancers of its activity (such as proteasome inhibitors) may be required for optimal therapeutic effects in vivo.

5. OUTSTANDING QUESTIONS

Although much knowledge has been made gathered TRAIL and its signaling pathways, the physiologic role of TRAIL remains unknown. Mice gene targeted for TRAIL show no obvious phenotype, in contrast to Fas- or FasL-defective mice. Some studies suggest that TRAIL may play some role in inhibiting the progression of autoimmune disease *(70)* or may function as an antiviral effector molecule *(71)*. The TRAIL –/– mice should prove to be important tools in dissecting out the physiologic role(s) of TRAIL. So far the major in vivo role demonstrated for TRAIL has been the limitation of tumor metastases, as mentioned previously.

Although TRAIL expression has been demonstrated at the mRNA level in many organs, little information is available on the expression of either the TRAIL protein or its receptors in vivo. The availability of better technology may hopefully improve the detection of TRAIL and its receptors in vivo at the protein level. Furthermore, scant information is available on what modifies the expression of TRAIL or its receptors in a variety of cell types. From the standpoint of using TRAIL as an antitumor agent, it is important to know whether tumor cells can be sensitized to TRAIL-mediated apoptosis. Some experiments have suggested that chemotherapy and radiation therapy can be combined with TRAIL to enhance tumor cell death. Nonetheless, more information on the TRAIL signaling pathways could allow for a more rational design of agents to augment TRAIL's apoptotic activity.

The initial promise of TRAIL as an anticancer agent lay in its ability to be selectively toxic for cancer cells. However, a number of recent reports have questioned the resistance of some normal cells to TRAIL-mediated apoptosis. Toxicity of TRAIL to human hepatocytes *(72)* and neuronal cells *(73)* has been reported, but, it must be borne in mind that a number of different TRAIL preparations are being used in these studies. Recent evidence indicates that this observed toxicity may depend on the particular TRAIL preparation that was used, with the preparation lacking an additional modification and trimerized by Zn being less toxic to normal cells *(74)*. Little toxicity was observed in mice and chimpanzees after administration of this unmodified TRAIL *(75)*. However, care is clearly warranted prior to administration of TRAIL to patients. The potency of death ligands such as TRAIL to kill cancer cells is impressive, but the dangers of eliciting deleterious systemic toxicity cannot be neglected. Studies currently under way in cancer patients should hopefully define an optimal dose of TRAIL and a safe therapeutic window. Optimism remains that apoptosis by death ligands can be modulated, and a clearer understanding of signaling cascades may define target proteins that protect or specifically sensitize cancer cells to TRAIL-mediated apoptosis.

ACKNOWLEDGMENTS

Thanks to Mr. Alan Brooks for his assistance with the artwork.

REFERENCES

1. Steller H. Mechanisms and genes of cellular suicide. *Science* 1995;267:1445–1449.
2. Thompson CB. Apoptosis in the pathogenesis and treatment of disease. *Science* 1995;267:1456–1462.
3. Vaux DL, et al. Bcl-2 gene promotes haemopoietic cell survival and cooperates with c-myc to immortalize pre-B cells. *Nature* 1988;335:440–442.
4. Wiley SR, et al. Identification and characterization of a new member of the TNF family that induces apoptosis. *Immunity* 1995;3:673–682.
5. Pitti RM, et al. Induction of apoptosis by Apo-2 ligand, a new member of the tumor necrosis factor cytokine family. *J Biol Chem* 1996;271:12687–12690.
6. Mariani SM, et al. Differential regulation of TRAIL and CD95 ligand in transformed cells of the T and B lymphocyte lineage. *Eur J Immunol* 1998;28:973–982.
7. Hymowitz SG, et al. A unique zinc-binding site revealed by a high-resolution X-ray structure of homotrimeric Apo2L/TRAIL. *Biochemistry* 2000;39:633–640.
8. Marsters SA, et al. Activation of apoptosis by Apo-2 ligand is independent of FADD but blocked by CrmA. *Curr Biol* 1996;6:750–752.
9. Walczak H, et al. Tumoricidal activity of tumor necrosis factor-related apoptosis- inducing ligand in vivo. *Nat Med* 1999;5:157–163.
10. Ashkenazi A, et al. Safety and antitumor activity of recombinant soluble Apo2 ligand. *J Clin Invest* 1999;104:155–162.
11. Pan G, et al. The receptor for the cytotoxic ligand TRAIL. *Science* 1997;276:111–113.
12. Walczak H, et al. TRAIL-R2: a novel apoptosis-mediating receptor for TRAIL. *EMBO J* 1997;16:5386–5397.
13. Wu GS, et al. KILLER/DR5 is a DNA damage-inducible p53-regulated death receptor gene. *Nat Genet* 1997;17:141–143.
14. MacFarlane M, et al. Identification and molecular cloning of two novel receptors for the cytotoxic ligand TRAIL. *J Biol Chem* 1997;272:25417–25420.
15. Pan G, et al. An antagonist decoy receptor and a death domain-containing receptor for TRAIL. *Science* 1997;277:815–818.

16. Sheridan JP, et al. Control of TRAIL-induced apoptosis by a family of signaling and decoy receptors. *Science* 1997;277:818–821.
17. Schneider P, et al. Characterization of two receptors for TRAIL. *FEBS Lett* 1997;416:329–334.
18. Mongkolsapaya J, et al. Lymphocyte inhibitor of TRAIL (TNF-related apoptosis-inducing ligand): a new receptor protecting lymphocytes from the death ligand TRAIL. *J Immunol* 1998;160:3–6.
19. Degli-Esposti MA, et al. The novel receptor TRAIL-R4 induces NF-kappaB and protects against TRAIL-mediated apoptosis, yet retains an incomplete death domain. *Immunity* 1997;7:813–820.
20. Pan G, et al. TRUNDD, a new member of the TRAIL receptor family that antagonizes TRAIL signalling. *FEBS Lett* 1998;424:41–45.
21. Marsters SA, et al. A novel receptor for Apo2L/TRAIL contains a truncated death domain. *Curr Biol* 1997;7:1003–1006.
22. Emery JG, et al. Osteoprotegerin is a receptor for the cytotoxic ligand TRAIL. *J Biol Chem* 1998;273:14363–14367.
23. Lacey DL, et al. Osteoprotegerin ligand is a cytokine that regulates osteoclast differentiation and activation. *Cell* 1998;93:165–176.
24. Griffith TS, et al. TRAIL: a molecule with multiple receptors and control mechanisms. *Curr Opin Immunol* 1998;10:559–563.
25. Zhang XD, et al. Relation of TNF-related apoptosis-inducing ligand (TRAIL) receptor and FLICE-inhibitory protein expression to TRAIL-induced apoptosis of melanoma. *Cancer Res* 1999;59:2747–2753.
26. Leverkus M, et al. Regulation of tumor necrosis factor-related apoptosis-inducing ligand sensitivity in primary and transformed human keratinocytes. *Cancer Res* 2000;60:553–559.
27. Chinnaiyan AM, et al. FADD/MORT1 is a common mediator of CD95 (Fas/APO-1) and tumor necrosis factor receptor-induced apoptosis. *J Biol Chem* 1996;271:4961–4965.
28. Boldin MP, et al. Involvement of MACH, a novel MORT/FADD-interacting protease, in Fas/APO-1- and TNF receptor-induced cell death. *Cell* 1996;85:803–815.
29. Muzio M, et al. FLICE, a novel FADD-homologous ICE/CED-3-like protease, is recruited to the CD95 (Fas/APO-1) death-inducing complex. *Cell* 1996;85:817–827.
30. Kischkel FC, et al. Cytotoxicity-dependent APO-1 (Fas/CD95)-associated proteins form a death-inducing signaling complex (DISC) with the receptor. *EMBO J* 1995;14:5579–5588.
31. Salvesen GS, et al. Caspases: intracellular signaling by proteolysis. *Cell* 1997;91:443–446.
32. Goltsev YV, et al. CASH, a novel caspase homologue with death effector domains. *J Biol Chem* 1997;272:19641–19644.
33. Shu HB, et al. Casper is a FADD and caspase homologue with death effector domians. *Immunity* 1997;6:751–763.
34. Srinivasula SM, et al. FLAME-1, a novel FADD-like anti-apoptotic molecule that regulates Fas/TNFR1-induced apoptosis. *J Biol Chem* 1997;272:18542–18545.
35. Irmler M, et al. Inhibition of death receptor signals by cellular FLIP. *Nature* 1997;388:190–195.
36. Thome M, et al. Viral FLICE-inhibitory proteins (FLIPs) prevent apoptosis induced by death receptors. *Nature* 1997;386:517–521.
37. Li H, et al. Cleavage of BID by caspase 8 mediates the mitochondrial damage in the Fas pathway of apoptosis. *Cell* 1998;94:491–501.
38. LeBlanc H, et al. Tumor-cell resistance to death receptor-induced apoptosis through mutational inactivation of the proapoptotic Bcl-2 homolog Bax. *Nat Med* 2002;8:274–281.
39. Schneider P, et al. TRAIL receptors 1 (DR4) and 2 (DR5) signal FADD-dependent apoptosis and activate NF-kappaB. *Immunity* 1997;7:831–836.
40. Chaudhary PM, et al. Death receptor 5, a new member of the TNFR family, and DR4 induce FADD-dependent apoptosis and activate the NF-kappaB pathway. *Immunity* 1997;7:821–830.
41. Schneider A, et al. NF-kappaB is activated and promotes cell death in focal cerebral ischemia. *Nat Med* 1999;5:554–559.
42. Baichwal VR, et al. Activate NF-kappa B or die? *Curr Biol* 1997;7:R94–R96.
43. Ryan KM, et al. Role of NF-kappaB in p53-mediated programmed cell death. Nature 2000;404:892–897.
44. Roth W, et al. Locoregional Apo2L/TRAIL eradicates intracranial human malignant glioma xenografts in athymic mice in the absence of neurotoxicity. *Biochem Biophys Res Commun* 1999;265:479–483.
45. Takeda K, et al. Involvement of tumor necrosis factor-related apoptosis-inducing ligand in surveillance of tumor metastasis by liver natural killer cells. *Nat Med* 2001;7:94–100.
46. Smyth MJ, et al. Tumor necrosis factor-related apoptosis-inducing ligand (TRAIL) contributes to interferon gamma-dependent natural killer cell protection from tumor metastasis. *J Exp Med* 2001;193:661–670.
47. Takeda K, et al. Critical role for tumor necrosis factor-related apoptosis-inducing ligand in immune surveillance against tumor development. *J Exp Med* 2002;195:161–169.

48. Cretney E, et al. Increased susceptibility to tumor initiation and metastasis in TNF-related apoptosis-inducing ligand-deficient mice. *J Immunol* 2002;168:1356–1361.
49. Chinnaiyan AM, et al. Combined effect of tumor necrosis factor-related apoptosis-inducing ligand and ionizing radiation in breast cancer therapy. *Proc Natl Acad Sci USA* 2000;97:1754–1759.
50. Kim K, et al. Molecular determinants of response to TRAIL in killing of normal and cancer cells. *Clin Cancer Res* 2000;6:335–346.
51. Keane MM, et al. Chemotherapy augments TRAIL-induced apoptosis in breast cell lines. *Cancer Res* 1999;59:734–741.
52. Nagane M, et al. Increased death receptor 5 expression by chemotherapeutic agents in human gliomas causes synergistic cytotoxicity with tumor necrosis factor-related apoptosis-inducing ligand in vitro and in vivo. *Cancer Res* 2000;60:847–853.
53. Gibson SB, et al. Increased expression of death receptors 4 and 5 synergizes the apoptosis response to combined treatment with etoposide and TRAIL. *Mol Cell Biol* 2000;20:205–212.
54. Gliniak B, et al. Tumor necrosis factor-related apoptosis-inducing ligand's antitumor activity in vivo is enhanced by the chemotherapeutic agent CPT-11. *Cancer Res* 1999;59:6153–6158.
55. Yamanaka T, et al. Chemotherapeutic agents augment TRAIL-induced apoptosis in human hepatocellular carcinoma cell lines. *Hepatology* 2000;32:482–490.
56. Adams J, et al. Proteasome inhibitors: a novel class of potent and effective antitumor agents. *Cancer Res* 1999;59:2615–2622.
57. Adams J. Proteasome inhibition in cancer: development of PS-341. *Semin Oncol* 2001;28:613–619.
58. Elliott PJ, et al. The proteasome: a new target for novel drug therapies. *Am J Clin Pathol* 2001;116:637–646.
59. Keane MM, et al. Inhibition of NF-kappaB activity enhances TRAIL mediated apoptosis in breast cancer cell lines. *Breast Cancer Res Treat* 2000;64:211–219.
60. Jeremias I, et al. Inhibition of nuclear factor kappaB activation attenuates apoptosis resistance in lymphoid cells. *Blood* 1998;91:4624–4631.
61. Franco AV, et al. The role of NF-kappa B in TNF-related apoptosis-inducing ligand (TRAIL)-induced apoptosis of melanoma cells. *J Immunol* 2001;166:5337–5345.
62. Mitsiades CS, et al. TRAIL/Apo2L ligand selectively induces apoptosis and overcomes drug resistance in multiple myeloma: therapeutic applications. *Blood* 2001;98:795–804.
63. Pawlowski JE, et al. NF-kappa B does not modulate sensitivity of renal carcinoma cells to TNF alpha-related apoptosis-inducing ligand (TRAIL). *Anticancer Res* 2000;20:4243–4255.
64. Hu WH, et al. Tumor necrosis factor-related apoptosis-inducing ligand receptors signal NF-kappaB and JNK activation and apoptosis through distinct pathways. *J Biol Chem* 1999;274:30603–30610.
65. Sayers TJ, et al. The proteasome inhibitor PS-341 sensitizes neoplastic cells to TRAIL-mediated apoptosis by reducing levels of c-FLIP. *Blood* 2003;102:303–310.
66. Mitsiades N, et al. Intracellular regulation of tumor necrosis factor-related apoptosis-inducing ligand-induced apoptosis in human multiple myeloma cells. *Blood* 2002;99:2162–2171.
67. Algeciras-Schimnich A, et al. Cell cycle-dependent regulation of FLIP levels and susceptibility to Fas-mediated apoptosis. *J Immunol* 1999;162:5205–5211.
68. Marshansky V, et al. Proteasomes modulate balance among proapoptotic and antiapoptotic Bcl-2 family members and compromise functioning of the electron transport chain in leukemic cells. *J Immunol* 2001;166:3130–3142.
69. Zhang XM, et al. Inhibition of ubiquitin-proteasome pathway activates a caspase-3-like protease and induces Bcl-2 cleavage in human M-07e leukaemic cells. *Biochem J* 1999;340:127–133.
70. Song K, et al. Tumor necrosis factor-related apoptosis-inducing ligand (TRAIL) is an inhibitor of autoimmune inflammation and cell cycle progression. *J Exp Med* 2000;191:1095–1104.
71. Sedger LM, et al. IFN-gamma mediates a novel antiviral activity through dynamic modulation of TRAIL and TRAIL receptor expression. *J Immunol* 1999;163:920–926.
72. Jo M, et al. Apoptosis induced in normal human hepatocytes by tumor necrosis factor-related apoptosis-inducing ligand. *Nat Med* 2000;6:564–567.
73. Nitsch R, et al. Human brain-cell death induced by tumour-necrosis-factor-related apoptosis-inducing ligand (TRAIL). *Lancet* 2000;356:827–828
74. Lawrence D, et al. Differential hepatocyte toxicity of recombinant Apo2L/TRAIL versions. *Nat Med* 2001;7:383–385.
75. Kelley SK, et al. Preclinical studies to predict the disposition of Apo2L/tumor necrosis factor-related apoptosis-inducing ligand in humans: characterization of in vivo efficacy, pharmacokinetics, and safety. *J Pharmacol Exp Ther* 2001;299:31–38.

16 Rationale for Combining the Proteasome Inhibitor Bortezomib with Cisplatin

Edward G. Mimnaugh and Leonard M. Neckers

ABSTRACT

The proteasome inhibitor bortezomib is currently undergoing advanced clinical evaluation as a new anticancer drug. Found to be highly effective against multiple myeloma, bortezomib will soon be tested with first-line anticancer drugs against a broad range of human malignancies, including solid tumors. Preclinical studies indicate that proteasome inhibition potentiates the activity of several conventional antitumor agents. Here we offer a rationale for combining bortezomib with the DNA-targeting drug cisplatin. First, the removal of cisplatin covalent adducts from DNA by nucleotide excision repair is greatly diminished by proteasome inhibition, and second, induction of the crucial DNA-repair enzyme excision repair cross-complementation group 1 (ERCC-1) by cisplatin is prevented by proteasome inhibitor pretreatment. Both of these pharmacologic events have been linked to proteasome inhibitor-caused de-ubiquitination of nucleosomal core histones H2A and H2B, which is associated with chromatin condensation and transcriptional inhibition. Thus, bortezomib has the potential to simultaneously enhance the anticancer efficacy of cisplatin and to prevent the emergence of ERCC-1-dependent cisplatin resistance.

KEY WORDS

Bortezomib, chromatin, cisplatin, DNA adducts, ERCC-1, histones, nucleotide excision repair, proteasomes, ubiquitin.

From: *Cancer Drug Discovery and Development: Proteasome Inhibitors in Cancer Therapy*
Edited by: J. Adams © Humana Press Inc., Totowa, NJ

1. INTRODUCTION

1.1. Traditional Anticancer Drug Combinations

Multidrug combination chemotherapy has been one of the most effective strategies in the clinical management of human cancers, reducing the incidence of metastatic disease as well as primary tumor burden and dramatically improving patient prognosis. Initially, multidrug combinations were selected because different drugs had different mechanisms of action and minimal overlapping host toxicities (1,2). As new anticancer agents became available over the decades, these were frequently incorporated into pre-existing multidrug regimens, often with little, if any, pharmacologic or biochemical rationale. Serendipity, rather than sound pharmacologic considerations of new drug combinations, occasionally yielded a beneficial clinical response. Eventually, designers of combination chemotherapeutic regimens took into consideration such factors as cell cycle kinetics, drug pharmacology and pharmacokinetics, and unfavorable drug–drug interactions, and anticancer drug combinations were sometimes supplemented with agents having the potential to reverse drug resistance (3–5).

Today's medical literature is replete with descriptions of multidrug permutations including essentially every clinically useful anticancer agent. Although modern combination chemotherapy has improved the quality of life and extended the life spans of thousands of cancer patients, unfortunately, most human cancers become refractory to chemotherapy, and disease recurrence remains a significant clinical problem. Both basic and clinical research on multidrug anticancer combination therapy must therefore extend beyond disease palliation toward the ultimate goal of providing a rationally designed curative chemotherapy.

1.2. New Anticancer Drug Combination

A possible novel drug combination just over the clinical horizon is the DNA-targeting chemotherapeutic agent cis-diamminedichloro-platinum II (CDDP; hereafter called cisplatin) paired with a new drug, bortezomib, a potent and highly selective inhibitor of the multicatalytic 26S proteasome (see structures in Fig. 1). Bortezomib (Velcade™; formerly called PS-341) is currently undergoing multicenter clinical evaluation in a variety of advanced solid tumor malignancies (6,7). Preclinical studies have indicated that proteasome inhibitors like bortezomib can potentiate the antiproliferative activity of several standard, first-line anticancer drugs, including cisplatin (8–10). Additional investigations hint that cotreatment with proteasome inhibitors might circumvent the development of acquired resistance to cisplatin, a major limitation of cisplatin chemotherapy (11–13). In this chapter, we critically evaluate the preclinical experimental evidence and describe prospectively biochemical and pharmacologic rationales for combining cisplatin—or a second-generation analog like carboplatin or oxaliplatin—with bortezomib for the treatment of human cancers.

2. CISPLATIN-DNA ADDUCTS AND DNA REPAIR IN CANCER TREATMENT

Cisplatin and its congeners have been recognized and well documented (a PubMed search lists 26,443 citations) as effective agents for treating malignant disease for nearly 25 years (14,15). These drugs are among the most effective in the oncologist's armamen-

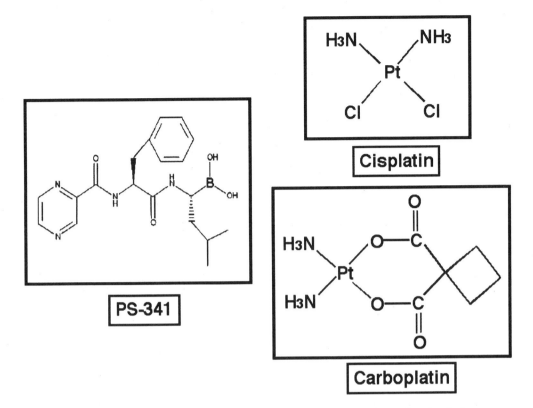

Fig. 1. Chemical structures of bortezomib (PS-341), cisplatin, and carboplatin.

tarium today. Cisplatin-based chemotherapeutic combinations have significant antitumor activity against solid tumors arising from the testis, ovaries, bladder, and lung, as well as head and neck neoplasms; cisplatin has poor activity against breast and colorectal cancers (for recent reviews, see refs. *16–18*). It is generally accepted that the antineoplastic activity of cisplatin can be attributed to its intracellular activation to an aquated electrophilic species that forms bifunctional covalent attachments to DNA *(14,19,20)*. Cisplatin forms predominantly 1,2-intrastrand DNA crosslinks between adjacent guanine–guanine residues (N-7 position) or between guanine–adenine residues, with far lesser amounts of interstrand crosslinks, monofunctional adducts, and protein–drug–DNA complexes *(21,22)*. These bulky cisplatin–DNA crosslinks and adducts significantly distort the conformation of DNA to the extent that it strongly interferes with replication and transcription, ultimately inhibiting cell proliferation and triggering tumor cells to undergo apoptosis *(23,24)*. Unfortunately, many human tumors have the capability to resolve cisplatin–DNA lesions by either an intrinsic or acquired highly efficient nucleotide excision repair (NER) mechanism *(16,25,26)*, one of several types of DNA repair used by eukaryotic cells *(27)*. Human tumor cells with intrinsic cisplatin resistance usually have significantly elevated NER activity *(25,28)*, whereas cells possessing a NER deficiency phenotype, such as those collected from patients suffering from the hereditary disease xeroderma pigmentosum or from human testicular tumors are hypersensitive to cisplatin cytotoxicity *(16,18,29)*. Of course, drug resistance mechanisms are usually multifactorial and include enhanced efflux, glutathione-S-transferase-dependent inactivation of cisplatin by thiols like glutathione and metallothionein, oncogene overexpression, and a poorly understood tumor cell tolerance to cisplatin–DNA adducts, all of which contribute to cisplatin resistance by tumors *(30–32)*. Because there is no evidence that these particular mechanisms are likely to be influenced by proteasome inhibition, they are not addressed here.

3. THE PROTEASOME INHIBITOR BORTEZOMIB AS AN INVESTIGATIONAL ANTICANCER AGENT

The boronated dipeptide, originally designated as PS-341 (see structure in Fig. 1) is a new (only 41 PubMed citations) investigational anticancer agent specifically designed to target the proteosome (Fig. 2A) (for recent reviews, see refs. *7, 9, 10, 33,* and *34*). Although all cells rely on the multicatalytic proteasome to degrade short-lived regulatory proteins as well as the bulk of damaged or otherwise misfolded cellular proteins numbering in the thousands *(35,36)*, nevertheless, tumor cells seem to be more sensitive to proteasome inhibitors than cells from normal tissues *(9)*. For example, myeloma cells, usually refractory to chemotherapy, were much more sensitive to bortezomib-induced apoptosis compared with isolated normal bone marrow stromal cells when tested in vitro *(13)*. Likewise, the peptide aldehyde proteasome inhibitor Z-Ile-Glu(O-t-But)-Ala-leucinal (PSI) was more effective against chronic myelogenous leukemic cells than normal hematopoietic progenitor cells *(37)*. A nonreversible natural product proteasome inhibitor, lactacystin, induces more apoptosis in malignant lymphocytes isolated from chronic lymphocytic leukemia patients than in normal peripheral lymphocytes collected from healthy individuals *(38,39)*. In addition to inhibiting the proliferation of a variety of tumor cell lines in culture [arresting the cell cycle at G1/S *(40)*, G2/M *(6,41)*, or both], bortezomib limited the growth of human tumor xenografts grown in rodents *(6,8,42)*.

The selectivity of proteasome inhibitors for tumor cells most likely results from the deregulation of multiple proteins that are particularly important for regulating cell proliferation *(10,43)*, such as several cyclins *(41)* and cyclin-dependent kinases *(44)*. Alternative proapoptotic mechanisms that selectively increase tumor cell susceptibility to proteasome inhibitors compared with nonneoplastic cells may include the stabilization and accumulation of the p53 tumor suppressor *(45)*, preventing the degradation of the inhibitor κB (IκB) of nuclear factor-κB (NF-κB) transcription factor activation *(46)* and stabilization of the short-lived cyclin-dependent kinase inhibitors p21[WAF1] *(47)* and p27[KIP1] *(36)*, all of which are known proteasome substrates. Thus, proteasome inhibitors, including bortezomib, simultaneously, but indirectly, interfere with the functions of multiple cell cycle-regulatory and checkpoint pathways, tumor suppressor proteins, and transcription factors that are critically important for the rapid and sustained growth of human tumors, making the proteasome an attractive molecular target for chemotherapy by bortezomib *(9,48,49)*.

3.1. Preliminary Reports from Ongoing Clinical Studies of Bortezomib

Early results from phase I and II clinical trials of bortezomib in patients with tumors insensitive to conventional antineoplastic agents have clearly demonstrated that bortezomib possesses antitumor activity against several types of neoplasia *(7,9)*. These included trials in patients with prostate and non-small-cell lung solid tumors *(9)*, melanoma lung metastases, and, especially, refractory multiple myeloma, in which approx

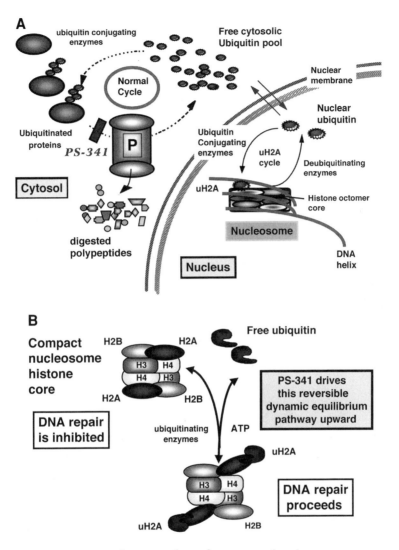

Fig. 2. Diagram showing that proteasome inhibitors cause protein ubiquitination, consumption of unconjugated ubiquitin, nucleosomal ubiquinitated (u)H2A de-ubiquitination, and nucleosome condensation. (**A**) The left side depicts ubiquitin-proteasome protein degradation *(92–95)*. P, the 26S proteasome, the specific target for bortezomib (PS-341). When proteasome inhibitors like bortezomib block the proteasome, high-molecular-weight polyubiquitinated proteins accumulate, and the cytosolic pool of free ubiquitin is depleted. In the nucleus, the constitutive level of free ubiquitin is extremely low, with essentially all the nuclear ubiquitin conjugated to histones H2A and H2B. Histone ubiquitination or de-ubiquitination status depends on an enzyme-catalyzed "dynamic equilibrium," which is regulated, in part, by the availability of free ubiquitin. Depletion of cytosolic free ubiquitin by bortezomib-caused protein ubiquitination upsets the dynamic equilibrium and promotes the enzymatic de-ubiquitination of uH2A *(53)*, which, in turn, initiates the condensation of nucleosomes and tight packing of chromatin. (**B**) Interplay between nucleosomal histone tail ubiquitination and the reversible nucleosomal octameric histone core that undergoes structural modification during the normal uH2A-H2A cycle.

50% of 202 patients had a marked or partial decline in circulating M-protein, a marker monoclonal antibody produced by myeloma cells *(50)*. Based on these early trials, the National Cancer Institute is sponsoring additional bortezomib trials through the Cancer Therapy Evaluation Program (CTEP, NCI, on line at: http//ctep.cancer.gov) that will target chronic lymphocytic leukemia and chronic myeloid leukemia and a broad range of advanced, drug-resistant solid tumors in combination with established anticancer drugs. Host toxicities in bortezomib-treated patients were low grade, reversible, and generally managable *(7,9)*. Importantly, these patients experienced no host toxicities that would potentially overlap with cisplatin, with the possible exception of an infrequently occurring peripheral neuropathy, a side effect with the potential to enhance cisplatin ototoxicity; notably, bortezomib did not cause hematologic toxicity or renal toxicity, the usual dose-limiting side effect of cisplatin and its congeners *(9)*.

4. INDICATIONS THAT CISPLATIN PLUS BORTEZOMIB MIGHT BE AN EFFECTIVE COMBINATION

In perhaps the first preclinical study undertaken to investigate broadly the potential antitumor properties of bortezomib, Teicher et al. *(8)* found that bortezomib potently inhibited the proliferation of carcinoma cells in culture and diminished the growth of solid tumors in mice. They further reported that bortezomib combined with cisplatin was additive in decreasing the growth of Lewis lung carcinoma, and, importantly, the two drugs markedly decreased the number and size of pulmonary metastases *(8)*. Unfortunately, additional forthcoming preclinical studies of the bortezomib/cisplatin drug combination have not yet been published; however, several groups have studied the antitumor properties of other proteasome inhibitors combined with cisplatin.

PSI, a peptidyl aldehyde proteasome inhibitor, is potently cytotoxic to a number of myeloid leukemia cells lines carrying the BCR-ABL fusion protein, which generates an abnormally active signaling tyrosine kinase *(37)*. PSI also sensitizes HL60 leukemia cells to cisplatin, and the dual drug treatment result in synergistic cytotoxicity by apoptosis, compared with either drug alone. We *(11)* and others *(51,52)* have reported that the proteasome inhibitors *N*-acetyl-leucyl-leucyl-norleucinal (ALLnL) and lactacystin (LC) potentiate cisplatin-induced apoptosis of both cisplatin-sensitive A2780 and cisplatin–resistant A2780/CP70 ovarian carcinoma cells by inhibiting the NER-dependent repair of cisplatin-DNA adducts *(11,52)*. Two probable mechanisms explain how proteasome inhibition is linked to NER-dependent removal of cisplatin adducts from DNA. The first is based on proteasome inhibitor-caused depletion of ubiquitinated histone H2A (uH2A) in nucleosomes *(53)*, which promotes chromatin condensation *(54–56)* and possibly interferes with the function of DNA damage recognition and repair enzymes. The alternative mechanism is that proteasome inhibitors diminish the excision repair cross-complementation group 1 (ERCC-1) response to cisplatin *(11,12)*, perhaps secondary to changes in chromatin structure that interfere with transcription of the *ERCC-1* gene *(11,53)*.

4.1. Role of Histone De-ubiquitination and Chromatin Structure

Normally when the ubiquitin polypeptide is conjugated to proteins, it targets them for rapid degradation by the proteasome; however, mono-ubiquitination of nucleosomal histones H2A and H2B in chromatin instead plays a regulatory role *(57,58)* (Fig. 2B). uH2A is predominantly localized in transcriptionally active regions of chromatin *(59–61)*, and this particular histone tail modification is thought to loosen the conformation of nucleosomes, open the structure of chromatin, and facilitate access of transcription activation complexes to gene promoter sites (54,55). Nucleosome unfolding occurs during DNA repair (55), and, interestingly, the human homologs of the yeast Rad6 postreplication DNA repair proteins, hHR6A and hHR6B (62) have E2 ubiquitin-conjugating activity toward histones (63,64). uH2A and uH2B are enzymatically de-ubiquitinated concomitant with chromatin condensation when proliferating cells enter metaphase and chromatin condenses into chromosomes (65); histones become re-ubiquitinated as cells return to anaphase (66), when chromatin decondenses and becomes transcriptionally active again. In temperature-sensitive cells that harbor a thermolabile E1 ubiquitin activating enzyme, de-ubiquitination of uH2A and uH2B occurs at the restrictive temperature (53). De-ubiquitination of uH2A also occurs during apoptosis induced by a variety of apoptogenic agents (67,68), including proteasome inhibitors (38,43,69). De-ubiquitination of uH2A takes place downstream of caspase activation and may be related to the accumulation of high-molecular-weight ubiquitinated proteins that depletes unconjugated ubiquitin in the nucleus (69). Additionally, we have observed that proteasome inhibition by either ALLnL or LC decreases DNA replication and transcription of mRNA by more than 50%, in a process that closely tracks with uH2A de-ubiquitination (53). We have presented evidence that unscheduled condensation of chromatin into a highly ordered structure as a direct consequence of histone de-ubiquitination induced by proteasome inhibitors prevents the recognition of cisplatin–DNA adducts and blocks their removal by the activation of NER (11,53). Although we have not examined the specific ability of bortezomib to interfere with NER of cisplatin-damaged DNA, we have observed that bortezomib promoted the accumulation of high-molecular-weight ubiquitinated proteins and caused uH2A de-ubiquitination in ovarian and breast carcinoma cells within hours (unpublished observations). By extrapolation, one would expect bortezomib, like ALLnL and LC, to interfere with NER of cisplatin–DNA adducts by unbalancing histone ubiquitination dynamics and tightening chromatin structure.

4.2. Role of ERCC-1 in Cisplatin Action and Sensitivity

Perhaps the most critical determinant of the efficiency of NER-dependent repair of cisplatin–DNA adducts in human tumor cells is the *ERCC-1* gene product (70,71). Overexpression of the ERCC-1 endonuclease, which in cooperation with other DNA damage recognition and DNA repair proteins initiates the cleavage of cisplatin-damaged nucleotides from genomic DNA (27,72,73), is associated with especially efficient repair of cisplatin-damaged DNA (74) and confers tumor cell resistance to cisplatin (28,32,75,76). Conversely, the level of expression of *ERCC-1* mRNA in cisplatin-hypersensitive cells may be as much as 30–50-fold lower than that measured in cisplatin-resistant cells (77). Supporting this concept convincingly, testicular tumor cells have recently been found to have unusually low levels of the ERCC-1-XPF endonuclease complex compared with normal tissues (78), suggesting that the exceptional sensitivity of testicular tumors to cisplatin-based chemotherapy (a 90% cure rate) may be linked to the inability of these cells to repair cisplatin cross-linked DNA (18). Furthermore, cultured human A2780/CP70 ovarian tumor cells induce their level of ERCC-1 mRNA expression as much as sixfold in response to cisplatin exposure, and this response correlates with both a higher level of DNA repair and acquired resistance to cisplatin (79,80).

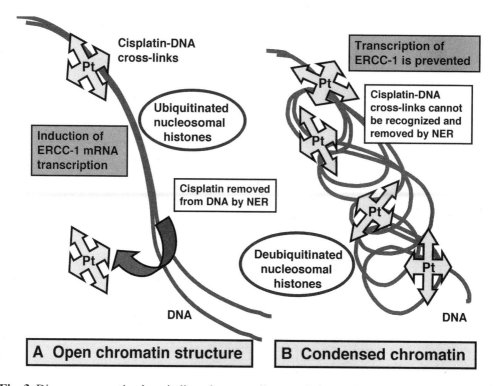

Fig. 3. Diagram suggesting how indirect bortezomib-caused chromatin structural changes could prevent the induction of excision repair cross-complementation group 1 (ERCC-1) and inhibit nucleotide excision repair (NER) of cisplatin-DNA lesions. **(A)** With an open chromatin structure, most of the cisplatin-DNA crosslinks are efficiently removed by NER through the action of ERCC-1, the excision nuclease that cleaves cisplatin-damaged DNA strands from chromatin. ERCC-1 mRNA is induced by cisplatin in tumor cells, possibly contributing to development of a drug-resistant phenotype. **(B)** Proteasome inhibitor-driven, histone de-ubiquitination–linked chromatin condensation would be expected to interfere with NER by obscuring cisplatin-DNA lesions from DNA damage recognition proteins and DNA repair enzymes and simultaneously preventing upregulation of ERCC-1 expression.

We have recently reported that the proteasome inhibitors ALLnL and LC greatly decrease the constitutive level and suppress the induction of ERCC-1 mRNA in A2780/CP70 ovarian tumor cells cotreated with cisplatin *(11,12)*, possibly by inducing condensation of nucleosomes (Fig. 3). Without the ability to remove cisplatin–DNA adducts by NER and without the compensatory ERCC-1 response, tumor cells succumb to the cisplatin–proteasome inhibitor combination *(11,52)*. Based on these observations, we predict that bortezomib would also diminish ERCC-1–dependent NER of cisplatin–DNA lesions by a similar mechanism in human solid tumors and show at least additive antitumor activity, as has been demonstrated in EMT-6 tumors in mice *(8)*. Particularly important is the possibility that bortezomib treatment might circumvent the emergence of acquired cisplatin resistance in human tumors if bortezomib is capable of preventing induction of ERCC-1 expression by cisplatin.

It should be mentioned that ALLnL pretreatment of A2780/CP70 ovarian tumor cells increases cisplatin accumulation by approx 50% over the cisplatin level measured in non-pretreated cells 1 h after cisplatin exposure *(11)*. The mechanism of this small, but consistent, proteasome inhibitor-caused increase in cell-associated cisplatin is unknown, but if it occurs in human tumors, it could sensitize those tumors to cisplatin.

5. BORTEZOMIB BLOCKS I-κB DEGRADATION AND PREVENTS NF-κB ACTIVATION

Although proteasome inhibition stabilizes many cell cycle-regulating proteins, signal-transducing kinases, and multiple transcription factors, the focus of current thinking about the antitumor mechanism of bortezomib is that its ability to block activation of the key transcription factor, NF-κB, may be very important *(9,34)*. This pathway is activated by proteasome-dependent degradation of ubiquitinated IκB *(81–84)*, which is normally complexed with the two NF-κB subunits and restricts their localization to the cytosol *(85)*. The activation process is initiated by the phosphorylation and ubiquitination of IκB *(86)*. Subsequent to the degradation of ubiquitinated IκB by the proteasome, NF-κB freely translocates to the nucleus, where it activates the expression of a diversity of genes controlling cell–cell interactions, cell cycle progression, and anti-apoptosis cell survival programs *(85,87)*. These various NF-κB–dependent gene products include cytokines and growth factors, several cell adhesion molecules, stress response enzymes, the Bcl-2 antiapoptotic protein, and inhibitors of apoptosis (IAPs) *(9,34,87)*. Therefore, blocking the expression of cytoprotective NF-κB–responsive genes by preventing the proteasome-mediated degradation of its inhibitor protein, IκB, greatly amplifies the number of target molecules that are potentially disabled by bortezomib well beyond the proteasome alone. Recently, bortezomib has been shown to inhibit the activation of NF-κB and block proliferation of various tumor cell lines in vitro, inhibit squamous cell carcinoma growth, and prevent angiogenesis in mice *(42)*. The simultaneous inactivation of the many NF-κB–dependent survival pathways is probably a major mechanism by which bortezomib may cause the demise of tumors.

6. CISPLATIN AND NF-κB

However, what about NF-κB and cisplatin? In macrophages, cisplatin transiently increases the cellular level and nuclear translocation of NF-κB within minutes of exposure *(88)*, and gel shift assays of HeLa cell extracts reveal that cisplatin indeed increases the DNA-binding capability of NF-κB *(89)*. HeLa cells made resistant to cisplatin by fractionated γ-irradiation have an elevated NF-κB level, but blocking IκB degradation with the proteasome inhibitor PSI to prevent activation of NF-κB induced more cell death in the parental cells than the cisplatin-resistant HeLa cells *(90)*. In another study, overexpression of a transfected, mutant, nondegradable IκB gene inhibited NF-κB activation and sensitized head and UM-SCC-9 neck squamous carcinoma cells to radiation, but not to cisplatin, raising the question of whether NF-κB activation really influences cisplatin sensitivity *(91)*. Finally, Li and Reed *(79)* reported that the induction of *ERCC-1* mRNA by cisplatin in A2780/CP70 ovarian tumor cells is preceded by a four- to five-fold increase in *c-fos* and *c-jun* mRNA expression and increased nuclear extract binding to the activator protein-1 (AP-1)-like site of the *ERCC-1* gene. The induction of AP-1 binding activity in cisplatin-treated cells was selective, as the DNA binding activities for NF-κB and CREB were unaltered by cisplatin *(79)*. At this time there is simply insufficient experimental evidence to propose that NF-κB might be a shared molecular target that is subject to modulation by both cisplatin and bortezomib. On the other hand, cisplatin and bortezomib could very well interact with different target molecules and still generate additive or synergistic antitumor activity.

7. CONCLUSIONS

In the early phase I and phase II clinical trials with bortezomib, the potent proteasome inhibitor has shown promise in the treatment of several types of solid tumors and hematologic malignancies. There is enthusiastic support for extending those trials to include combinations of bortezomib with standard anticancer drugs. As described very recently by the Cancer Therapy Evaluation Program of the National Cancer Institute, bortezomib is slated to be combined in separate trials with carboplatin against ovarian cancer and with paclitaxel and carboplatin against advanced, drug-resistant solid tumors. We hope that our preclinical experiments with cisplatin and proteasome inhibitors have contributed in some small way to the decision to conduct these trials, and we wish the greatest success to the oncologists and protocol nurses who will manage those trials and those cancer patients who might benefit from this novel drug combination.

REFERENCES

1. DeVita VT, et al. Current chemotherapeutic combinations. *Ser Haematol* 1973;6:182–195.
2. DeVita VT, et al. Combination versus single agent chemotherapy: a review of the basis for selection of drug treatment of cancer. *Cancer* 1975;35:98–110.
3. Chabner BA. The role of drugs in cancer treatment. In: *Pharmacologic Principles of Cancer Treatment.* (Chabner BA, ed). Philadelphia: WB Saunders, 1982:3–14.
4. Schabel FM, et al. Increasing therapeutic response rates to anticancer drugs by applying the basic principles of pharmacology. *Pharmacol Ther* 1983;20:283–305.
5. Creaven PJ. Rationale for chemotherapeutic approaches to prostate cancer. *Prostate* 1984;5:63–74.
6. Adams J, et al. Proteasome inhibitors: a novel class of potent and effective antitumor agents. *Cancer Res* 1999;59:2615–2622.
7. Adams J, et al. New agents in cancer clinical trials. *Oncogene* 2000;19:6687–6692.
8. Teicher BA, et al. The proteasome inhibitor PS-341 in cancer therapy. *Clin Cancer Res* 1999;5:2638–2645.
9. Adams J. Proteasome inhibition: a novel approach to cancer therapy. *Trends Mol Med* 2002;8:S49–S54.
10. Almond JB, et al. The proteasome: a novel target for cancer chemotherapy. *Leukemia* 2002;16:433–443.
11. Mimnaugh EG, et al. Prevention of cisplatin-DNA adduct repair and potentiation of cisplatin-induced apoptosis in ovarian carcinoma cells by proteasome inhibitors. *Biochem Pharmacol* 2000;60:1343–1354.
12. Li QQ, et al. Proteasome inhibition suppresses cisplatin-dependent ERCC-1 mRNA expression in human ovarian tumor cells. *Res Commun Mol Pathol Pharmacol* 2000;107:387–396.
13. Hideshima T, et al. The proteasome inhibitor PS-341 inhibits growth, induces apoptosis, and overcomes drug resistance in human multiple myeloma cells. *Cancer Res* 2001;61:3071–3076.
14. Rosenberg B. Anticancer activity of cis-dichlorodiammineplatinum (II) and some relevant chemistry. *Cancer Treat Rep* 1979;63:1433–1444.
15. Rozencweig M, et al. Cisplatin: impact of a new anticancer agent on current therapeutic strategies. *Anticancer Res* 1981;1:199–204.
16. Zamble DB, et al. Cisplatin and DNA repair in cancer chemotherapy. *Trends Biol Sci* 1995;20:435–439.
17. Dabholkar M, et al. Cisplatin. In: *Cancer Chemotherapy and Biological Response Modifiers Annual 16* (Pinedo HM, Longo DL, Chabner BA, eds). New York: Elsevier Science, 1996:88–110.
18. Trimmer EE, et al. *Essays Biochem* 1999;34:191–211.
19. Zwelling LA, et al. Mechanism of action of cis-dichlorodiammineplatinum(II). *Cancer Treat Rep* 1979;63:1439–1444.
20. Reed E, et al. Quantitation of platinum-DNA binding in human tissues following therapeutic levels of drug exposure—a novel use of graphite furnace spectrometry. *Atomic Spectroscopy* 1988;9:93–95.

21. Lippard SJ, et al. Binding of cis- and trans-dichlorodiammineplatinum(II) to the nucleosome core. *Proc Natl Acad Sci USA* 1979;76:6091–6095.

22. Zwelling LA, et al. DNA-protein and DNA interstrand cross-linking by cis- and trans-platinum(II) diamminedichloride in L1210 mouse leukemia cells and relation to cytotoxicity. *Cancer Res* 1979;39:365–369.

23. Eastman A. Activation of programmed cell death by anticancer agents: cisplatin as a model system. *Cancer Cells* 1990;2:275–280.

24. Henkels KM, et al. Induction of apoptosis in cisplatin-sensitive and -resistant human ovarian cancer cell lines. *Cancer Res* 1997;57:4488–4492.

25. Chu G. Cellular responses to cisplatin. The roles of DNA-binding proteins and DNA repair. *J Biol Chem* 1994;269:787–790.

26. Friedberg EC. How nucleotide excision repair protects against cancer. *Nat Rev Cancer* 2001;1:22–33.

27. Sancar A. Mechanisms of DNA excision repair. *Science* 1994;266:1954–1956.

28. Parker RJ, et al. Acquired cisplatin resistance in human ovarian cancer cells is associated with enhanced repair of cisplatin-DNA lesions and reduced drug accumulation. *J Clin Invest* 1991;87:772–777.

29. Sancar A. DNA excision repair. In: *Annual Review of Biochemistry*, vol 65. (Richardson CC, Abelson JN, Raetz CRH, eds). Palo Alto: Annual Reviews, 1996:48–81.

30. Gosland M, et al. Insights into mechanisms of cisplatin resistance and potential for its clinical reversal. *Pharmacotherapy* 1996;16:16–39.

31. Johnson SW, et al. Increased platinum-DNA damage tolerance is associated with cisplatin resistance and cross-resistance to various chemotherapeutic agents in unrealed human ovarian cancer cell lines. *Cancer Res* 1997;57.

32. Kartalou M, et al. Mechanisms of resistance to cisplatin. *Mutat Res* 2001;478:23–43.

33. Adams J, et al. Potent and selective inhibitors of the proteasome: dipeptidyl boronic acids. *Bioorg Med Chem Lett* 1998;8:333–338.

34. Adams J. Development of the proteasome inhibitor PS-341. *Oncologist* 2002;7:9–16.

35. Rock KL, et al. Inhibitors of the proteasome block the degradation of most cell proteins and the generation of peptides presented on MHC class 1 molecules. *Cell* 1994;78:761–771.

36. Pagano M, et al. Role of the ubiquitin-proteasome pathway in regulating abundance of the cyclin-dependent kinase inhibitor p27. *Science* 1995;269:682–685.

37. Soligo D, et al. The apoptogenic response of human myeloid leukaemia cell lines and of normal and malignant haematopoietic progenitor cells to the proteasome inhibitor PSI. *Br J Haematol* 2001;113:126–135.

38. Delic J, et al. The proteasome inhibitor lactacystin induces apoptosis and sensitizes chemo- and radioresistant human chronic lymphocytic leukaemia lymphocytes to TNF-alpha-initiated apoptosis. *Br J Cancer* 1998;77:1103–1107.

39. Masdehors P, et al. Increased sensitivity of CLL-derived lymphocytes to apoptotic death activation by the proteasome-specific inhibitor lactacystin. *Br J Haematol* 1999;105:752–757.

40. Shah SA, et al. 26S proteasome inhibition induces apoptosis and limits growth of human pancreatic cancer. *J Cell Biochem* 2001;82:110–122.

41. Pagano M. Cell cycle regulation by the ubiquitin pathway. *FASEB J* 1997;11:1067–1075.

42. Sunwoo JB, et al. Novel proteasome inhibitor PS-341 inhibits activation of nuclear factor- kappa B, cell survival, tumor growth, and angiogenesis in squamous cell carcinoma. *Clin Cancer Res* 2001;7:1419–1428.

43. Orlowski RZ. The role of the ubiquitin-proteasome pathway in apoptosis. *Cell Death Differ* 1999;6:303–313.

44. Koepp DM, et al. How the cyclin became a cyclin: regulated proteolysis in the cell cycle. *Cell* 1999;97:431–434.

45. Maki CG, et al. In vivo ubiquitination and proteasome-mediated degradation of p53. *Cancer Res* 1996;56:2649–2654.

46. Chen Z, et al. Signal-induced site-specific phosphorylation targets IκBα to the ubiquitin-proteasome pathway. *Genes Dev* 1995;9:1586–1597.

47. Blagosklonny MV, et al. Proteasome-dependent regulation of p21WAF1/CIP1 expression. *Biochem Biophys Res Commun* 1996;227:564–569.

48. Hershko A, et al. The ubiquitin system. *Annu Rev Biochem* 1998;67:425–479.

49. Shah SA, et al. Ubiquitin proteasome pathway: implications and advances in cancer therapy. *Surg Oncol* 2001;10:43–52.

50. Richardson PG, et al. A phase 2 study of bortezomib in relapsed, refractory myeloma. *N Engl J Med* 2003;348:2609–2617.

51. Li QQ, et al. Lactacystin enhances cisplatin sensitivity in resistant human ovarian cancer cell lines via inhibition of DNA repair and ERCC-1 expression. *Cell Mol Biol (Noisy-le-grand)* 2001;47:OL61–OL72.

52. Yunmbam MK, et al. Effect of the proteasome inhibitor ALLnL on cisplatin sensitivity in human ovarian tumor cells. *Int J Oncol* 2001;19:741–748.

53. Mimnaugh EG, et al. Rapid deubiquitination of nucleosomal histones in human tumor cells caused by proteasome inhibitors and stress response inducers: effects on replication, transcription, translation, and the cellular stress response. *Biochemistry* 1997;36:14418–14429.

54. Van Holde KE, et al. What happens to nucleosomes during transcription? *J Biol Chem* 1992;267:2837–2840.

55. Davie JR. Histone modifications, chromatin structure and the nuclear matrix. *J Cell Biochem* 1996;62:149–157.

56. Wolffe AP, et al. Chromatin disruption and modification. *Nucleic Acids Res* 1999;27:711–720.

57. Seale R. Rapid turnover of the histone-ubiquitin conjugate, protein A24. *Nucleic Acids Res* 1981;9:3151–3158.

58. Wu RS, et al. Metabolism of ubiquitinated histones. *J Biol Chem* 1981;256:5916–5920.

59. Nickel BE, et al. Ubiquitinated histone H2B is preferentially located in transcriptionally active chromatin. *Biochemistry* 1989;28:958–963.

60. Davie JR, et al. Level of ubiquitinated histone H2B in chromatin is coupled to ongoing transcription. *Biochemistry* 1990;29:4752–4757.

61. Hansen JC, et al. A role for histones H2A/H2B in chromatin folding and transcriptional repression. *Proc Natl Acad Sci USA* 1994;91:2339–2343.

62. Jentsch S, et al. The yeast DNA repair gene *RAD6* encodes a ubiquitin-conjugating enzyme. *Nature* 1987;329:131–134.

63. Koken MH, et al. Structural and functional conservation of two human homologs of the yeast DNA repair gene *RAD6*. *Proc Natl Acad Sci* USA 1991;88:8865–8869

64. Koken MHM, et al. Expression of the ubiquitin-conjugating DNA repair enzymes HHR6A and B suggests a role in spermatogenesis and chromatin modification. *Dev Biol* 1996;173:119–132.

65. Matsui S, et al. Disappearance of a structural chromatin protein A24 in mitosis: implications for molecular basis of chromatin condensation. *Proc Natl Acad Sci USA* 1979;76:6386–6390.

66. Mueller RD, et al. Identification of ubiquitinated histones 2A and 2B in *Physarum polycephalum*. *J Biol Chem* 1985;260:5147–5153.

67. Marushige Y, et al. Disappearance of ubiquitinated histone H2A during chromatin condensation in TGFB1-induced apoptosis. *Anticancer Res* 1995;15:267–272.

68. Tanimoto Y, et al. Peptidyl aldehyde inhibitors of proteasome induce apoptosis rapidly in mouse lymphoma RVC cells. *J Biochem* 1997;121:542–549.

69. Mimnaugh EG, et al. Caspase-dependent deubiquitination of monoubiquitinated nucleosomal histone H2A induced by diverse apoptogenic stimuli. *Cell Death Differ* 2001;8:1182–1196.

70. Van Duin M, et al. Genomic characterization of the human DNA excision repair gene ERCC-1. *Nucleic Acids Res* 1987;15:9195–9213.

71. Weeda G, et al. Disruption of mouse ERCC1 results in a novel repair syndrome with growth failure, nuclear abnormalities and senescence. *Curr Biol* 1997;7:427–439.

72. Johnson SW, Swiggard PA, Handel LM, et al. Relationship between platinum-DNA adduct formation and removal and cisplatin cytotoxicity in cisplatin-sensitive and -resistant human ovarian cancer cells. *Cancer Res* 1994;54:5911–5916.

73. Wood RD. DNA repair in eukaryotes. *Annu Rev Biochem* 1996;65:135–167.

74. Lee KB, et al. Cisplatin sensitivity/resistance in UV repair-deficient Chinese hamster ovary cells of complementation groups 1 and 3. *Carcinogenesis* 1993;14:2177–2180.

75. Parker RJ, et al. Platinum-DNA damage in leukocyte DNA of patients receiving carboplatin and cisplatin chemotherapy, measured by atomic absorption spectrometry. *Carcinogenesis* 1991;12:1253–1258.

76. Dabholkar M, et al. Messenger RNA levels of XPAC and ERCC1 in ovarian cancer tissue correlate with response to platinum-based chemotherapy. *J Clin Invest* 1994;94:703–708.

77. Taverna P, et al. Gene expression in X-irradiated human tumour cell lines expressing cisplatin resistance and altered DNA repair capacity. *Carcinogenesis* 1994;15:2053–2056.

78. Koberle B, et al. Defective repair of cisplatin-induced DNA damage caused by reduced XPA protein in testicular germ cell tumours. *Curr Biol* 1999;9:273–276.

79. Li Q, et al. Cisplatin induction of *ERCC-1* mRNA expression in A2780/CP70 human ovarian cancer cells. *J Biol Chem* 1998;273:23419–23425.

80. Li Q, et al. Cisplatin and phorbol ester independently induce ERCC1 protein in human ovarian tumor cells. *Int J Oncol* 1998;13:987–992.
81. Palombella VJ, et al. The ubiquitin-proteasome pathway is required for processing the NF-κB1 precursor protein and the activation of NF-κB. *Cell* 1994;78:773–785.
82. Lin YC, et al. Activation of NF-kB requires proteolysis of the inhibitor IkB-alpha: signal-induced phosphorylation of IkB-alpha alone does not release active NF-kB. *Proc Natl Acad Sci USA* 1995;92:552–556.
83. Scherer DC, et al. Signal-induced degradation of IkB alpha requires site-specific ubiquitination. *Proc Natl Acad Sci USA* 1995;92:11259–11263.
84. Roff M, et al. Role of IκBα ubiquitination in signal-induced activation of NF-κB *in vivo*. *J Biol Chem* 1996;271:7844–7850.
85. May MJ, et al. Signal transduction through NF-kB. *Immunol Today* 1998;19:80–88.
86. Alkalay I, et al. Stimulation-dependent IkBa phosphorylation marks the NF-kB inhibitor for degradation via the ubiquitin-proteasome pathway. *Proc Natl Acad Sci USA* 1995;92:10599–10603.
87. Rothwarf DM, et al. The NF-kB activation pathway: a paradigm in information transfer from membrane to nucleus. *Science's Signal Transduction Knowledge Environment* 1999;5:1–16.
88. Sodhi A, et al. Mechanism of NF-kB translocation in macrophages treated in vitro with cisplatin. *Immunol Lett* 1998;63:9–17.
89. Maldonado V, et al. Modulation of NF-kB, and Bcl-2 in apoptosis induced by cisplatin in HeLa cells. *Mutat Res* 1997;381:67–75.
90. Eichholtz-Wirth H, et al. IkB/NF-kB mediated cisplatin resistance in HeLa cells after low-dose gamma-irradiation is associated with altered SODD expression. *Apoptosis* 2000;5:255–263.
91. Kato T, et al. Cisplatin and radiation sensitivity in human head and neck squamous carcinomas are independently modulated by glutathione and transcription factor NF-kB. *Head Neck* 2000;22:748–759.
92. Hershko A, et al. The ubiquitin system for protein degradation. *Annu Rev Biochem* 1992;61:761–807.
93. Ciechanover A. The ubiquitin-proteasome proteolytic pathway. *Cell* 1994;79:13–21.
94. Hochstrasser M. Ubiquitin-dependent protein degradation. *Annu Rev Genet* 1996;30:405–439.
95. Pickart CM. Mechanisms underlying ubiquitination. *Annu Rev Biochem* 2001;70:503–533.

17 Effects of the HIV-1 Protease Inhibitor Ritonavir on Proteasome Activity and Antigen Presentation

Marcus Groettrup, Rita de Giuli, and Gunter Schmidtke

CONTENTS

ABSTRACT

Ritonavir is a potent inhibitor of the protease encoded by the human immunodeficiency virus (HIV)-1 and is clinically applied to suppress HIV-1 replication in AIDS patients. When following up clinical hints pointing at a virus-independent effect of ritonavir on the cytotoxic immune response, we found that ritonavir is a modulator of proteasome activity. It competitively inhibits the chymotrypsin-like activity of the proteasome while the trypsin-like activity is markedly enhanced. Kinetic inhibitor studies revealed that the latter effect is due to binding of ritonavir to a non-catalytic modifier site. In this review we summarize the effects of ritonavir and other proteasome inhibitors on antigen presentation and the antiviral immune response. Moreover, we review experiments which show that selective proteasome inhibitors can serve as immune modulators, a function that could be exploited for the treatment of autoimmune diseases.

From: *Cancer Drug Discovery and Development: Proteasome Inhibitors in Cancer Therapy*
Edited by: J. Adams © Humana Press Inc., Totowa, NJ

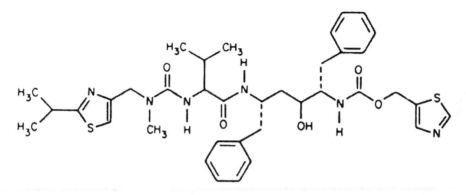

Fig. 1. Structure of ritonavir (ABT-538). Ritonavir was designed as a peptide analogon that mimics the transition state of a Phe-Pro peptide bond frequently found at the cleavage sites of the HIV-1 protease in the gag-pol polyprotein of HIV-1. It does not have a *chemical warhead* that could covalently modify the active center, but it competes with the viral substrate for binding to the substrate binding site.

KEY WORDS

Proteasome; HIV-1; inhibitor; antigen presentation; autoimmunity.

1. INTRODUCTION

For several years AIDS patients have been successfully treated with a regime called *highly active antiretroviral therapy* (HAART), which includes nucleoside analogs as inhibitors of HIV-1 reverse transcriptase and inhibitors of the HIV-1 protease *(1)*. Ritonavir is one of the protease inhibitors applied in AIDS therapy (ABT-538, produced by Abbott Laboratories under the trade name Norvir®). It potently inhibits the HIV-1 protease in a competitive and reversible manner *(2)* (Fig. 1). Depending on the virus isolate and the cell culture system used, the concentration required to inhibit 50% of viral replication varies between 22 and 130 n*M (2)*. The protease encoded by HIV-1 is an appropriate target for antiviral drugs because its activity is required for productive replication of the virus *(3)*. HIV-1 protease is an aspartic protease that is in charge of the post-translational processing of the gag and gag-pol polyproteins into enzymes and structural proteins of the viral core. Inhibition of the HIV-1 protease leads to the accumulation of the polyprotein precursors Pr55gag and Pr160gag-pol and results in the production of noninfectious viral particles.

A milestone for the rational design of HIV-1 protease inhibitors was the determination of its three-dimensional structure by X-ray crystallography in 1989 *(4,5)*. The HIV-1 protease differs structurally from other human aspartic proteases like renin, pepsin, or cathepsin D and E in that the HIV-1 protease is a homodimer, whereas the endogenous human proteases are formed from a single polypeptide chain. In addition, the cleavage specificity of HIV-1 protease differs from that of other human proteases because the HIV-1 protease cleaves the gag-pol polyprotein between phenylalanine (or tyrosine) and proline. A cleavage at the N-terminus of the amino acid proline cannot be performed by most endogenous human proteases, and therefore HIV-1 protease inhibitors are designed as peptide analogs that mimic the transition state of the Phe-Pro peptide bond during the cleavage reaction (Fig. 1). An exception to this rule is the proteasome for which the capability to cleave N-terminal of proline residues has been described in several studies *(6–9)*.

At first sight the reader may find it peculiar that a chapter about an HIV-1 protease inhibitor is included in a book on the clinical effects of proteasome inhibitors. We too were surprised when we found that the HIV-1 protease inhibitor ritonavir can also function as a modulator of proteasome activity. The mechanistic investigation of how ritonavir affects proteasome activity led us to interesting and novel insights as to how effectors of proteasome activity can operate and how such modulators of proteasome activity can be used to influence antigen presentation and the cytotoxic immune response.

2. EFFECTS OF RITONAVIR ON THE CYTOTOXIC IMMUNE RESPONSE IN A MOUSE MODEL OF VIRAL INFECTION

The incentive to investigate the effect of ritonavir on the immune response in a defined model system was given by clinical observations suggesting that ritonavir may have a direct effect on the immune response that is unrelated to the suppression of HIV-1 replication *(10,11)*. Therefore we examined whether the oral administration of ritonavir to mice in therapeutically relevant concentrations would affect the cytotoxic T-lymphocyte (CTL) response against a model virus, the lymphocytic choriomeningitis virus (LCMV). (For a scheme of MHC class I-restricted antigen presentation to CTLs *see* Fig. 2.) Surprisingly, a striking suppression of the CTL response against LCMV was observed in ritonavir-treated mice *(12)*. The expansion of $CD8^+$ T-lymphocytes in the spleen that is normally observed on d 8 after LCMV infection was barely apparent in ritonavir-treated mice, and the generation of CTLs specific for the LCMV T-cell epitopes GP33 and NP396 was markedly reduced. This reduction was not caused by inhibition of LCMV replication because the virus load remained higher throughout the course of the infection in ritonavir-treated compared with control mice, and there was no effect of ritonavir on LCMV replication in vitro. A negative effect of ritonavir on the general survival and proliferation of T-cells was also unlikely because ritonavir treatment did not lead to a change in the number and distribution of $CD4^+$ and $CD8^+$ T-lymphocytes in the spleen and lymph nodes of uninfected mice. Also the humoral immune response to LCMV (IgM and IgG) was not affected in ritonavir-treated mice.

Therefore, we searched for an alternative rationale and tested whether the generation and MHC class I-restricted presentation of LCMV epitopes was altered by ritonavir. Interestingly, the treatment of LCMV-infected cells with 7 μM ritonavir (corresponding to the peak serum levels reached in patients; *2*) led to a significant reduction in the MHC class I-restricted presentation of the LCMV epitopes GP33 and NP396. This finding led us to hypothesize that a reduction in LCMV epitope generation and/or presentation may at least in part account for the attenuated CTL response to LCMV in vivo *(12)*.

3. HOW RITONAVIR AFFECTS PROTEASOME ACTIVITY

Since peptide epitopes presented by MHC class I molecules to CTLs on the cell surface are generated through the intracellular degradation of protein antigens by the proteasome, we hypothesized that proteasome activity may be perturbed by ritonavir, thus leading to a change in antigen processing. As shown in Fig. 3, this was indeed the case. Ritonavir inhibited the chymotrypsin-like activity of the proteasome (i.e., cleavage after hydropho-

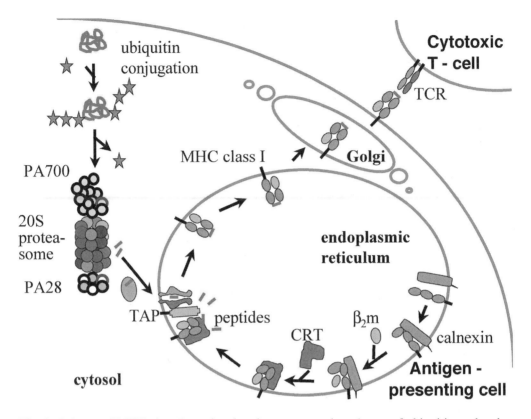

Fig. 2. Scheme of MHC class I-restricted antigen presentation. A tree of ubiquitin molecules, assembled by an enzymatic cascade onto a virus-derived protein, targets it to the proteasome in the form of a so-called *hybrid proteasome* (consisting of PA700/20S proteasome/PA28 α/β) in which the protein becomes degraded to peptides while the ubiquitin moieties are cleaved off and recycled. The peptides are transported via the transporter associated with antigen processing (TAP) into the lumen of the endoplasmic reticulum, where they can bind to nascent MHC class I molecules associated with β_2-microglobulin (β_2m). Peptide binding induces a conformational change so that the trimeric class I complex consisting of class I heavy chain, β_2m, and peptide can leave the endoplasmic reticulum and migrate to the cell surface, where it can be recognized by the antigen receptor of cytotoxic T-cells (TCR). If a cytotoxic T-cell with specificity for a virus-derived epitope, recognizes its epitope, it will be activated, kill the infected cell, and thus prevent spread of the virus.

bic amino acids) with a median inhibitory concentration (IC_{50}) of 5 μM, which was comparable to inhibition by the fairly potent but rather nonselective proteasome inhibitor *N*-acetyl-leucyl-leucyl-norleucinal (LLnL). Consistent with an almost complete inhibition of the chymotrypsin-like activity at a concentration of 50 μM ritonavir, we found that at such a dose polyubiquitinylated proteins were accumulating in treated cells and the degradation of inhibitor κB (IκB) was slowed down. Computer modeling predicted that ritonavir would fit well into the substrate binding pocket of the β5 subunit of the yeast 20S proteasome to which the chymotrypsin-like activity has been assigned *(14)*. In accordance with this prediction, ritonavir selectively protected the β5 subunit of the proteasome but not the other two active site subunits β1 and β2, from covalent modification with a radiolabeled vinyl sulfone inhibitor *(13)*.

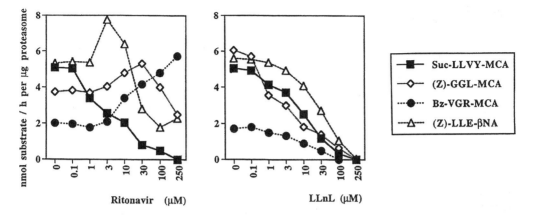

Fig. 3. The effect of ritonavir and N-acetyl-leucyl-leucyl-norleucinal (LLnL) on the hydrolysis of four fluorogenic substrates by the proteasome. The cleavage activity of isolated 20S proteasomes from murine B8 fibroblast cells is plotted against the concentration of inhibitors. The concentrations of fluorogenic substrates were left constant: 100 μM (Z)-GGL-MCA, 100 μM Suc-LLVY-MCA (chymotrypsin-like activity), 400 μM Bz-VGR-MCA (trypsin-like activity), and 200 μM (Z)-LLE-βNA (caspase-like activity). Activities were calculated from fluorescence of the MCA leaving group 60 min after initiation of digests when the reaction was in linear progression with 500 ng of 20S proteasome in a final volume of 100 μL. (Reprinted with permission from Schmidtke G, Holzhütter H, Bogyo M, et al. How an inhibitor of the HIV-1 protease modulates proteasome activity. *J Biol Chem* 1999;274:35734–35740.)

However, in contrast to LLnL, which inhibited all peptidolytic activities of the proteasome to a comparable extent, ritonavir consistently induced a marked enhancement of the proteasomal trypsin-like activity (i.e., cleavage after basic amino acids) *(13)*. It hence appeared that ritonavir functioned as a genuine modulator of proteasome activity in that it simultaneously enhanced one but suppressed another peptidolytic activity. How ritonavir may accomplish such a complex and unprecedented effect was subsequently addressed experimentally.

4. HOW PEPTIDE MODIFIERS CAN MODULATE PROTEASOME ACTIVITY: A NOVEL MECHANISM

An obvious hypothesis was that binding of ritonavir to the β5 active site would cause an allosteric activation of the trypsin-like activity that has been assigned to the β2 subunit in both the yeast *(14)* and mammalian proteasome *(15)*. This scenario seemed likely in particular because an allosteric regulation between the active sites of the β5 and β1 subunits was proposed for the proteasome *(16)*. However, when we monitored the trypsin-like activity in the presence of increasing concentration of a peptide substrate for the chymotrypsin-like activity, we could not find evidence for an allosteric regulation between these two activities. Furthermore, we could show that activation of the trypsin-like activity through ritonavir persisted in the presence of lactacystin, an inhibitor that completely and selectively blocked chymotrypsin-like activity at the concentration used (1 μM) *(17)*. Also, inhibition of the caspase-like activity of the proteasome (i.e., cleavage after acidic amino acids accomplished by the β1 subunit) did not interfere with enhancement of the trypsin-like activity through ritonavir. We concluded from these experiments

notation: $\left(\begin{array}{cc}\text{ligand at} & \text{ligand at}\\ \text{modifier site} & \text{active site}\end{array}\right)$

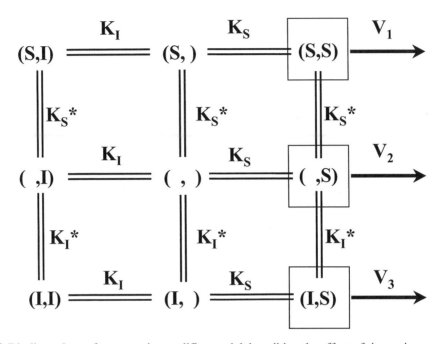

Fig. 4. Binding scheme for a two-site modifier model describing the effect of ritonavir on peptide hydrolysis by the proteasome. Both a peptide substrate and an effector (ritonavir) may competitively bind to a modifier site (left) or the active site (right). The dissociation constants for binding of the peptide and the effector are denoted as K_S* and K_I* for binding to the modifier site and as K_S and K_I for binding to the active site. Depending on the occupation of the modifier site, the cleavage rates are denoted V_1, V_2, or V_3. (Reprinted with permission from Schmidtke G, Emch S, Groettrup M, Holzhütter HG. Evidence for the existence of a non-catalytic modifier site of peptide hydrolysis by the 20S proteasome. *J Biol Chem* 2000;275:22056–22063.)

that ritonavir enhances the trypsin-like activity by binding to a noncatalytic site. We designed a two-site modifier model (Fig. 4) in which one site is a peptidolytically active site and the other is a noncatalytic binding site for an effector. Our kinetic model could describe the observed experimental kinetics adequately, suggesting that this is a valid model for the effect of ritonavir on proteasome activity.

The existence of one or more noncatalytic modifier binding sites in the proteasome was further corroborated when we demonstrated that strong enhancement of the caspase-like activity mediated by peptide substrates of the chymotrypsin-like activity, as described by Kisselev et al. *(16)*, is not a true allosterism between two active sites, as proposed in their *bite-chew model*. Instead, we showed that a noncatalytic binding site for the peptide substrate must account for the observed phenomenon because—in this case also—inhibitors of the involved active sites did not interfere with the regulatory effect *(17,18)*. It therefore appears that the study of ritonavir as a modifier of proteasome activity has revealed a new paradigm for the control of proteasome activity through noncatalytic modifier sites. Where in the proteasome such sites may be located remains to be elucidated. In collaboration with the Huber group in Munich, we tried to identify such sites by soaking proteasome crystals with ritonavir *(19)*, but we failed to identify these sites, most likely because ritonavir binds with much lower affinity to the yeast proteasome compared with the mammalian complex (G. Schmidtke and M. Groll, unpublished data).

5. IMPACT OF RITONAVIR ON THE IMMUNE RESPONSE: EVIDENCE FOR MODES OF ACTION NOT RELATED TO THE MODULATION OF PROTEASOME ACTIVITY

A cardinal question that remains to be clarified is whether the impressive dampening of the CTL response in the presence of ritonavir is indeed caused by the modulation of proteasome activity observed in vitro. Although the peak plasma level reached under therapy with ritonavir (7 μM) is sufficient to suppress the chymotrypsin-like activity of the purified proteasome by 50% in vitro, we cannot be sure whether this concentration is reached in the cytoplasm because ritonavir is easily bound and absorbed by proteins in the serum. Recently, it was reported that the susceptibility of peripheral blood mononuclear cells (PBMCs) or CD4+ T-helper cells to spontaneous or CD95-triggered apoptosis in vitro was greatly reduced in the presence of 10–500 nM ritonavir, a concentration range at which the peptidolytic activity of the proteasome is barely affected *(20–22)*. Moreover, the secretion of tumor necrosis factor (TNF)-α by PBMCs after anti-CD3 activation was dramatically reduced by 100 nM ritonavir. It was suggested that ritonavir may counteract the increased susceptibility of CD4+ T-cells to apoptotic cell death in HIV-1–infected patients and by this means rescue T-helper cells in patients even if the virus becomes resistant to the protease inhibitor. Several mechanisms have been proposed to explain the reduced propensity to apoptosis, including reduction in caspase-1 expression *(22)*, downregulation of Fas ligand *(23)*, or interference with a loss of mitochondrial transmembrane potential *(24)*.

We do not yet know to what degree the described effects of ritonavir on TNF-α secretion and apoptosis contributed to the marked reduction in the CTL response against LCMV. Protease inhibitors like indinavir and nelfinavir, which did not show a significant effect on proteasome activity at therapeutically relevant concentrations, also did not affect the CTL response against LCMV in our mouse model of viral infection *(12)* and in experimental autoimminue encephalomyelitis (EAE) *(25)*, but this is merely a correlation and not a proof. Also, for some of the numerous other pathways that were influenced by ritonavir (for instance, lipoprotein metabolism *[26,27]*, adipocyte differentiation *[28,29]*, ATP-dependent drug export *[30]*, and dendritic cell function *[31]*), the proteasome has been discussed as a potential target underlying the effects, but direct evidence is scarce and a discussion of these data is beyond the scope of our review.

6. USE OF SELECTIVE PROTEASOME INHIBITORS TO CONTROL ANTIGEN PROCESSING AND PRESENTATION

The finding that the proteasome modifier ritonavir had such prominent effects on antigen presentation and on the CTL response against LCMV and the notion that not all targets of ritonavir have been characterized to date encouraged us to explore whether intensively studied and specific proteasome inhibitors could be used to control antigen presentation systematically. We chose the inhibitors lactacystin *(32)* and epoxomicin

(33) because, like ritonavir, both of them are selective for the chymotrypsin-like activity of the proteasome, at least when used in low concentrations, which do not interfere with the housekeeping functions of the proteasome. We have generated T-cell hybridomas for three LCMV epitopes (GP33, GP276, and NP118) and against the $pp89_{168-176}$ epitope of mouse cytomegalovirus (MCMV) *(34)* and used these hybridomas to evaluate the presentation of these epitopes quantitatively in the presence of titrated amounts of proteasome inhibitors *(35)*. At high inhibitor concentrations, which interfered with cellular proliferation, the presentation of all four epitopes tested was blocked, indicating that they were generated in a proteasome-dependent manner. Interestingly, whereas the presentation of epitopes GP33, NP118, and $pp89_{168-176}$ was diminished at low inhibitor concentrations, the presentation of GP276 was markedly enhanced with both lactacystin and epoxomicin. We think that this is a proof of principle that the selective and partial inhibition of a certain peptidolytic activity of the proteasome can be a means either to enhance or to reduce the production of an epitope.

It is known that the proteasome can destroy T-cell epitopes in the cell and in vitro by cleaving within or close to the sequence of a particular epitope *(36–38)*. It was initially assumed that in such a case, epitope production was achieved by proteases other than the proteasome and that the proteasome destroyed the respective epitopes *(39)*. In our situation, however, it seems that a change in the fragmentation mode through selective and partial inhibition of one of the active sites results in the production of different kinds of peptides. Low inhibitor concentrations sufficed to change the fragmentation of precursor polypeptides by the 20S proteasome in vitro, and the relative amount of a *bona fide* GP276 precursor peptide was actually enhanced in the presence of lactacystin *(35)*. Given that proteasome inhibitors are now in development for clinical application as chemotherapeutics, it would be interesting to test in animal experiments whether the administration of low doses of proteasome inhibitors could actually be used in vivo to change the hierarchy of T-cell epitopes. If this was the case, further clinical applications of proteasome inhibitors as therapeutics in autoimmune disease may be a promising approach, taking into account that tissue damage in numerous autoimmune diseases occurs because cells that present autoantigens are destroyed by epitope-specific CTLs.

When we observed the strong effects of ritonavir on the CTL response in LCMV-infected mice in 1998, we reasoned that ritonavir deserves to be tested as a potential therapeutic in an animal model of autoimmune disease. In the meantime, Lotteau and co-workers *(25)* have examined the impact of ritonavir on the severity of EAE, an experimental model of multiple sclerosis in Lewis rats and SJL mice. Intriguingly, they found that daily treatment with ritonavir effectively prevented the clinical symptoms of EAE in a dose-dependent manner. The protection was accompanied by the inhibition of the mononuclear cell infiltration into the central nervous system that is usually observed in EAE. It seems, therefore, that the use of proteasome inhibitors as immunomodulators may hold potential for reducing the severity of autoimmune assaults.

7. CONCLUSIONS

Ritonavir is a potent inhibitor of the protease encoded by HIV-1 and is clinically applied to suppress HIV-1 replication in AIDS patients. When following up clinical hints pointing at a virus-independent effect of ritonavir on the cytotoxic immune response, we found that ritonavir is a modulator of proteasome activity. It competitively inhibits the chymotrypsin-like activity of the proteasome and markedly enhances the trypsin-like activity. Kinetic inhibitor studies revealed that the latter effect is caused by binding of ritonavir to a noncatalytic modifier site. In this review we summarize the effects of ritonavir and other proteasome inhibitors on antigen presentation and the antiviral immune response. Moreover, we review experiments showing that selective proteasome inhibitors can serve as immune modulators, a function that could be exploited for the treatment of autoimmune diseases.

ACKNOWLEDGMENTS

The work in our laboratory on ritonavir was funded by the Swiss National Science Foundation (grant 32-53674.98/1), the Roche Foundation, the Novartis Foundation, and Rentenanstalt Jubiläumsstiftung.

REFERENCES

1. Moyle G, et al. Current knowledge and future prospects for the use of HIV protease inhibitors. *Drugs* 1996;51:701–712.
2. Kempf DJ, et al. ABT-538 is a potent inhibitor of human immunodeficiency virus protease and has high oral bioavailability in humans. *Proc Natl Acad Sci USA* 1995;92:2484–2488.
3. Kohl NE, et al. Active human immunodeficiency virus protease is required for viral infectivity. *Proc Natl Acad Sci USA* 1988;85:4686–4690.
4. Wlodawer A, et al. Conserved folding in retroviral proteases: crystal structure of a synthetic HIV-1 protease. *Science* 1989;245:616–621.
5. Navia MA, et al. Three-dimensional structure of aspartyl protease from human immunodeficieny virus HIV-1. *Nature* 1989;337:615–620.
6. Groettrup M, et al. The interferon-γ-inducible 11S regulator (PA28) and the LMP2/LMP7 subunits govern the peptide production by the 20S proteasome in vitro. *J Biol Chem* 1995;270:23808–23815.
7. Niedermann G, et al. Contribution of proteasome-mediated proteolysis to the hierarchy of epitopes presented by major histocompatibility complex class I molecules. *Immunity* 1995;2:289–299.
8. Nussbaum AK, et al. Cleavage motifs of the yeast 20S proteasome beta subunits deduced from digests of enolase 1. *Proc Natl Acad Sci USA* 1998;95:12504–12509.
9. Dick TP, et al. Contribution of proteasomal beta-subunits to the cleavage of peptide substrates analyzed with yeast mutants. *J Biol Chem* 1998;273:25637–25646.
10. Perrin L, et al. HIV treatment failure: testing for HIV resistance in clinical practice. *Science* 1998;280:1871–1873.
11. Tovo PA. Highly active antiretroviral therapy inhibits cytokine production in HIV-uninfected subjects. *AIDS* 2000;14:743–744.
12. André P, et al. An inhibitor of HIV-1 protease modulates proteasome activity, antigen presentation, and T cell responses. *Proc Natl Acad Sci USA* 1998;95:13120–13124.
13. Schmidtke G, et al. How an inhibitor of the HIV-1 protease modulates proteasome activity. *J Biol Chem* 1999;274:35734–35740.
14. Heinemeyer W, et al. The active sites of the eukaryotic 20 S proteasome and their involvement in subunit precursor processing. *J Biol Chem* 1997;272:25200–25209.
15. Salzmann U, et al. Mutational analysis of subunit i beta 2 (MECL-1) demonstrates conservation of cleavage specificity between yeast and mammalian proteasomes. *FEBS Lett* 1999;454:11–15.
16. Kisselev AF, et al. Proteasome active sites allosterically regulate each other, suggesting a cyclical bite-chew mechanism for protein breakdown. *Mol Cell* 1999;4:395–402.
17. Schmidtke G, et al. Evidence for the existence of a non-catalytic modifier site of peptide hydrolysis by the 20S proteasome. *J Biol Chem* 2000;275:22056–22063.
18. Myung J, et al. Lack of proteasome active site allostery as revealed by subunit- specific inhibitors. *Mol Cell* 2001;7:411–420.
19. Groll M, et al. Structure of 20 S proteasome from yeast at 2.4A resolution. *Nature* 1997;386:463–471.
20. Johnson N, et al. Anti-retroviral therapy reverses HIV-associated abnormalities in lymphocyte apoptosis. *Clin Exp Immunol* 1998;113:229–234.

21. Weichold FF, et al. HIV-1 protease inhibitor Ritonavir modulates susceptibility to apoptosis of uninfected T cells. *J Hum Virol* 1999;2:261–269.
22. Sloand EM, et al. Human immunodeficiency virus type 1 protease inhibitor modulates activation of peripheral blood CD4+ T cells and decreases their susceptibility to apoptosis in vitro and in vivo. *Blood* 1999;94:1021–1027.
23. Böhler T, et al. Downregulation of increased CD95 (APO-1/Fas) ligand in T cells from human immunodeficiency virus-type 1-infected children after antiretroviral therapy. *Blood* 1997;90:886–898.
24. Phenix BN, et al. Antiapoptotic mechanism of HIV protease inhibitors: preventing mitochondrial transmembrane potential loss. *Blood* 2001;98:1078–1085.
25. Hosseini H, et al. Protection against experimental autoimmune encephalomyelitis by a proteasome modulator. *J Neuroimmunol* 2001;118:233–244.
26. Berthold HK, et al. Influence of protease inhibitor therapy on lipoprotein metabolism. *J Intern Med* 1999;246:567–575.
27. Liang J, et al. HIV protease inhibitors protect apolipoprotein B from degradation by the proteasome: a potential mechanism for protease inhibitor-induced hyperlipidemia. *Nat Med* 2001;7:1327–1331.
28. Gagnon AM, et al. Protease inhibitors and adipocyte differentiation in cell culture. *Lancet* 1998;352:1032.
29. Zhang B, et al. Inhibition of adipocyte differentiation by HIV protease inhibitors. *J Clin Endocrinol Metab* 1999;84:4274–4277.
30. Gutmann H, et al. Interactions of HIV protease inhibitors with ATP-dependent drug export proteins. *Mol Pharmacol* 1999;56:383–389.
31. Gruber A, et al. Differential effects of HIV-1 protease inhibitors on dendritic cell immunophenotype and function. *J Biol Chem* 2001;276:47840–47843.
32. Fenteany G, et al. Inhibition of proteasome activities and subunit-specific amino-terminal threonine modification by lactacystin. *Science* 1995;268:726–731.
33. Meng L, et al. Epoxomicin, a potent and selective proteasome inhibitor, exhibits in vivo antiinflammatory activity. *Proc Natl Acad Sci USA* 1999;96:10403–10408.
34. Schwarz K, et al. The use of LCMV-specific T cell hybridomas for the quantitative analysis of MHC class I restricted antigen presentation. *J Immunol Methods* 2000;237:199–202.
35. Schwarz K, et al. The selective proteasome inhibitors lactacystin and expoxomicin can be used to either up- or downregulate antigen presentation at non-toxic doses. *J Immunol* 2000;164:6147–6157.
36. Ossendorp F, et al. A single residue exchange within a viral CTL epitope alters proteasome-mediated degradation resulting in lack of antigen presentation. *Immunity* 1996;5:115–124.
37. Theobald M, et al. The sequence alteration associated with a mutational hotspot in p53 protects cells from lysis by cytotoxic T lymphocytes specific for a flanking peptide epitope. *J Exp Med* 1998;188:1017–1028.
38. Valmori D, et al. Modulation of proteasomal activity required for the generation of a cytotoxic T lymphocyte-defined peptide derived from the tumor antigen MAGE-3. *J Exp Med* 1999;189:895–905.
39. Vinitsky A, et al. The generation of MHC class I-associated peptides is only partially inhibited by proteasome inhibitors: involvement of nonproteasomal cytosolic proteases in antigen processing? *J Immunol* 1997;159:554–564.

18 Function(s) of the Ubiquitin–Proteasome System in Retrovirus Budding

Ulrich Schubert

CONTENTS

ABSTRACT

Several retroviruses contain mono-ubiquitinylated Gag protein, which is modified adjacent to the viral late asembly domain (L, a sequence required for efficient virus release). Furthermore, it has been demonstrated for HIV that inhibition of proteasome activity blocks virus budding and processing of the virus Gag polyproteins without direct inhibition of viral protease. Two mutually exclusive hypotheses have been investigated, that proteasome inhibition acts by causing (1) depletion of free ubiquitin and thus preventing mono-ubiquitinylation of the L-domain containing Gag proteins, or (2) accumulation of defective, possibly misfolded Gag proteins that interfere with assembly, budding, and maturation of progeny virions. The ubiquitin-depletion hypothesis originates from the observation that extended proteasome inhibition significantly reduces the levels of free ubiquitin in HIV-1–infected cells and prevents the mono-ubiquitinylation of Gag proteins. A potential role of ubiquitin in virus budding is, however, inconsistent with the finding that mutants of HIV-1 carrying mutations of ubiquitin acceptor sites in Gag exhibit wild-type replication and maintain sensitivity to proteasome inhibitors. In contrast, the defective Gag hypothesis originates from the finding that poly-ubiquitinylated and misfolded forms of defective ribosomal products (DRiPs) of HIV-1 Gag accumulate immediately following proteasome inhibition and that such Gag-DRiPs ultimately inter-

From: *Cancer Drug Discovery and Development: Proteasome Inhibitors in Cancer Therapy*
Edited by: J. Adams © Humana Press Inc., Totowa, NJ

fere with the folding and processing of viral structure proteins. Regardless of the mechanism, the phenomenon suggests a novel pharmaceutical strategy for interfering with retrovirus replication.

KEY WORDS

Ubiquitin, proteasome, proteasome inhibitors, mono-ubiquitinylation, HIV, virus budding and assembly, late assembly domain, defective ribosomal products (DRiPs), antiretroviral therapy.

1. INTRODUCTION

In December 2001, approx 20 years after the first clinical evidence of acquired immunodeficiency syndrome (AIDS) was reported, the United Nations estimated that more than 22 million people had died from infection with human immunodeficiency viruses (HIVs) and that 40 million living individuals were infected with HIV. Such infection remains the most devastating disease humankind has ever faced. Unfortunately, there is little hope that an effective vaccine will be developed soon. Current anti-retroviral treatment is based on drugs that target either the viral protease or reverse transcriptase. A drawback to these treatments is that with HIV's high mutation rate, drug-resistant mutants are evolving, particularly when antiretroviral treatment suppresses virus replication to only marginal levels. Cellular genes have much lower mutation rates, and a potential solution to this problem is to target cellular factors required for HIV replication.

2. THE HIV REPLICATION CYCLE

As do other retroviruses, the HIV replication cycle begins with virus attachment and penetration through the plasma membrane. After reverse transcription, viral DNA is transported to the nucleus, where it is integrated into chromosomes. Upon activation of integrated provirus, viral RNAs are processed and transported into the cytosol for translation into structural proteins that assemble at the plasma membrane into budding particles. The main structural components of retrovirus particles are synthesized as three polyproteins that produce either the inner virion interior (Gag), the viral enzymes (Pol), or the glycoproteins of the virion envelope (Env). The processing of the HIV-1 Gag polyprotein Pr55 by the viral protease (PR) generates the matrix (MA), capsid (CA), nucleocapsid (NC), and p6^{Gag} proteins. Gag proteins of different retroviruses exhibit a certain structural and functional similarity: MA mediates the plasma membrane targeting of the Gag polyprotein and lines the inner shell of the mature virus particle, CA regulates assembly of Gag and forms the core shell of the infectious virus, and NC regulates packaging and condensation of the viral genome. In addition to those canonical mature retrovirus proteins, other Gag domains have been described, like the HIV-1 p6^{Gag} region that functions in virus budding and encapsidation of the lentiviral regulator protein Vpr (1–4). A summary of the virus replication cycle and the HIV-1 gene products is shown in Fig. 1.

HIV particles bud from the plasma membrane as immature noninfectious viruses consisting predominantly of uncleaved polyproteins. Subsequently and in concert with PR activation, processing of Gag polyproteins and condensation of the inner core structure occurs, resulting in the formation of mature infectious viruses (1) (Fig. 1). Besides PR and Env, at least two other viral factors are known to promote efficient virus release: the HIV-1–specific accessory protein Vpu (5) and the p6^{Gag} domain (6). Whereas Vpu

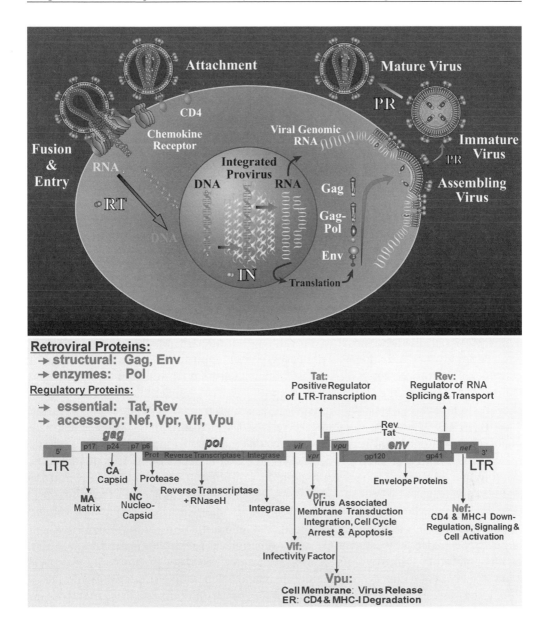

Fig. 1. The HIV-1 replication cycle, HIV-1 genes, and the functions of their products. The HIV replication cycle begins with virus attachment, followed by membrane fusion and uncoating of the incoming virus. Upon reverse transcription (RT), viral DNA as part of the preintegration complex is transported to the nucleus, where it is integrated into chromosomes. Following proviral activation, late steps of the replication cycle are initiated. These involve transcription, transport, and splicing of viral RNAs, as well as translation and transport of *de novo* synthesized viral proteins to the plasma membrane, where assembly, budding, and proteolytic maturation of progeny virions occur. Beside the canonical retroviral genes (*gag* for virus core, *env* for envelope, and *pol* for viral enzymes), HIV-1 also encodes six regulatory proteins: Tat and Rev are essential for virus replication, and Vif, Nef, Vpr, and Vpu are nonessential for virus replication in certain tissue culture systems but govern accessory functions in vivo. LTR, long terminal repeat. (Courtesy of Louis E. Henderson, SAIC-Frederick, NCI, Frederick, MD.)

supports virus release by an ion channel activity, p6^{Gag} contains the late assembly (L) domain that is required for efficient separation of assembled virions from the cell surface by a mechanism that has not been clearly defined *(2–4,6)*.

From entry to release and maturation into infectious progeny virions, each individual step in the HIV replication cycle exploits cellular pathways. Well-characterized examples are the virus receptors (CD4 and chemokine receptors), which enable virus entry into specific host cells, the role of the chromatin-remodeling system *(7)* and the HMG I family proteins *(8)* for proviral DNA integration, and the requirement of different factors of the endosomal protein trafficking and ubiquitinylation systems for virus release *(2–4)*. The latter phenomenon was discovered recently while our group was studying the degradation of the virus receptor CD4 mediated by the HIV-1–specific regulatory protein Vpu *(9)*. In the course of these studies, we serendipitously found that inhibitors of the proteasome specifically interfere with late steps within the replication cycle, the assembly, budding, and maturation of HIV-1 and HIV-2 virions *(10)*.

3. THE UBIQUITIN–PROTEASOME SYSTEM

More than a quarter of a century ago it was discovered that mammalian cells harbor a highly sophisticated proteolytic system, now known as the ubiquitin–proteasome system (UPS) *(11)*. Unlike lysosomal proteases (the other major proteolytic system in eukaryotic cells), which, like most proteases, do not require an energy source, the ATP-dependent UPS is not membrane-enclosed but is distributed throughout the cytosol and nucleus *(12)*. Proteasomes are plentiful (approx 0.5% of total cellular protein) multienzyme complexes that digest damaged or unwanted proteins into peptides ranging from 4 to 30 residues. Many substrates are targeted for destruction by the covalent attachment of ubiquitin, a small, highly conserved 76-residue protein that is abundant in eukaryotic cells and is conjugated to the ε-amino group of Lys residues by its COOH terminus, creating the "isopeptide" bond. An internal Lys of ubiquitin is used for conjugation to another ubiquitin, and when the "tree" reaches four ubiquitin molecules, the substrate is targeted to proteasomes. Cells also use ubiquitin in other ways, and addition of a single ubiquitin to proteins (mono-ubiquitylation), even at multiple sites in the protein, does not target the protein to proteasomes, but rather functions as a regulator in activity, location, and assembly of various cellular and viral proteins. To date, mono-ubiquitylation is known to be involved in distinct cellular mechanisms including transcriptional regulation, virus assembly, and membrane trafficking, particularly internalization and degradation of plasma membrane proteins *(13)*.

As might be expected, regulation of conjugation and turnover of ubiquitin is highly sophisticated, and a number of factors have been proposed to control the UPS *(12)*. The 26S proteasome consists of a 20S catalytic cylindrical particle with 19S regulatory subunits attached to either end. The 19S subunit recognizes tetra (or higher) ubiquitin trees, removes ubiquitin (for reuse), unfolds the substrate, and feeds it into the narrow opening of the 20S subunit. Proteasomes are involved in cell division and cell death and numerous processes in between. They are essential for cell viability in yeast and, despite a report to the contrary *(14)*, also in mammalian cells *(15)*.

4. PROTEASOME INHIBITORS INTERFERE WITH HIV BUDDING

The introduction of low-molecular-weight, membrane-permeable proteasome inhibitors opened up an important avenue for studying the function of the UPS in cell culture and living organisms. Several groups of proteasome inhibitors have been developed and are now extensively used to study the biologic function of the UPS. Two of the most specific proteasome inhibitors, the β-lactone derivative lactacystin *(16)* and the epoxyketone derivative epoxomicin *(17)*, are natural products of microorganisms, demonstrating that certain antibiotics also target the vital function of the 26S proteasome. Synthetic inhibitors have been described as chemically modified peptide aldehydes, peptide-vinyl-sulfones, or peptide boronic acid derivatives *(18)*. Since different inhibitors possess different specificities for blocking the proteasomes, it is important to demonstrate that chemically distinct inhibitors exhibit comparable effects in similar experimental setups.

We did this by showing that various classes of reversibly as well as irreversibly acting proteasome inhibitors severely retarded budding, maturation, and infectivity of both HIV-1 and HIV-2 *(10)*. Steady-state and pulse-chase analyses in various epithelial and lymphoid cells indicate that the detrimental effects of different proteasome inhibitors on HIV replication involve the processing of Gag polyprotein by the viral PR without affecting the activity of PR itself. Although processing of the Env glycoproteins was not changed, accumulation of Gag-processing intermediates and decreased levels of intracellular and virus-associated $p24^{CA}$ was observed (Fig. 2). Furthermore, this block in Gag processing caused almost complete loss of infectivity for HIV-1 virions released from cells with inactivated proteasomes (Fig. 3). The block of virus release could be indirectly linked to defects in Gag processing as inhibitors do not affect release of HIV-1 $Pr55^{Gag}$ virus-like particles expressed from HIV-1 PR mutants *(10)*. However, this detrimental effect on Gag processing could not be attributed to direct inhibition of HIV-1 PR, which is highly resistant to proteasome inhibitors, as demonstrated by in vitro processing studies of HIV-1 Gag *(10)*. Furthermore, this effect occurs independently of the virus release function of the HIV-1 accessory protein Vpu and is not limited to HIV-1, as proteasome inhibitors also reduce virus release and Pr58 Gag processing of HIV-2 (Fig. 2). Electron microscopy analysis of inhibitor-treated cells revealed retarded virus budding structures reminiscent of HIV-1 L-domain mutants in $p6^{Gag}$ (Fig. 4).

In an attempt to unravel the underlying mechanism(s) of those phenomena, two major hypothesis have been proposed to explain the impact of proteasome inhibition on HIV budding, that proteasome inhibition acts by causing (1) depletion of free ubiquitin, thus preventing mono-ubiquitinylation of L-domain–containing Gag proteins; or (2) accumulation of defective, possibly misfolded Gag proteins that interfere with assembly, budding, and maturation of progeny virions.

5. HYPOTHESIS 1: MONO-UBIQUITINYLATED GAG PROTEINS FUNCTION IN HIV BUDDING

The first hypothesis involves the effects of proteasome inhibitors on ubiquitin conjugation to Gag. More than a decade ago it was discovered that free ubiquitin is present in avian leukosis virions at concentrations up to fivefold higher than in the cytosol *(19)*. Although the function of free ubiquitin in retroviruses remains enigmatic, unconjugated ubiquitin was also found to be incorporated into virus particles of HIV-1, simian immunodeficiency virus (SIV), Moloney murine leukemia virus (Mo-MuLV), and equine infectious anemia virus (EIAV). In those later studies the presence of mono-ubiquitinylated forms of retroviral Gag proteins in virions, specifically mono-ubiquitinylation of the C-terminal $p6^{Gag}$ regions of HIV-1 and SIV Gag proteins, the p12 region of Mo-MuLV Gag,

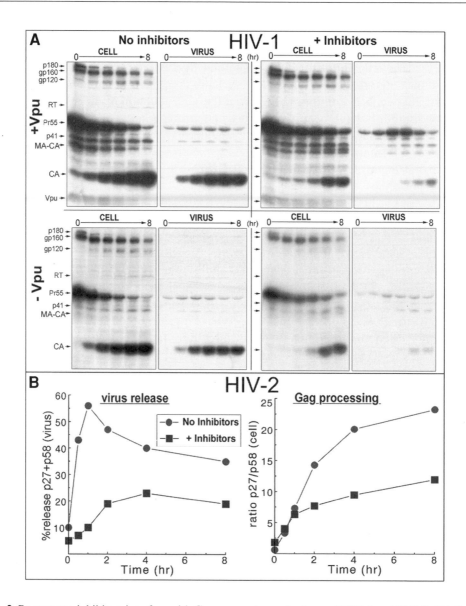

Fig. 2. Proteasome inhibitors interfere with Gag processing and release of HIV-1 and HIV-2. **(A)** Cells of the human CD4+ T-cell line A3.01 were infected with HIV-1$_{NL4-3}$ (+Vpu) or a mutant deficient for the HIV-1–specific virus release factor Vpu (–Vpu). **(B)** Cells of the human fibroblast cell line HeLa were transfected with HIV-2 proviral DNA. Parallel cultures of HIV-1– or HIV-2–expressing cells were incubated in the presence or absence of proteasome inhibitors (10 μM each of MG132 and lactacystin) and subjected to pulse-chase experiments as described *(10)*. Using patient serum, viral proteins were immunoprecipitated from the cell lysates and pelleted as virions. AIDs was separated by SDS-PAGE and analyzed by fluorography. The HIV-2 Gag precursor Pr58 and the major processing product p27^{CA} collected by immunoprecipitation were quantitated, and the time-course of particle release and efficiency of intracellular Gag processing was calculated. Virus release kinetics were calculated as the percent of Gag (Pr58 and CA) present in the virus pellet relative to the total amount of Gag detected intra- and extracellularly. The rate of Pr58 processing was estimated by calculating the ratio of CA vs Pr58 detected intracellularly at different time points.

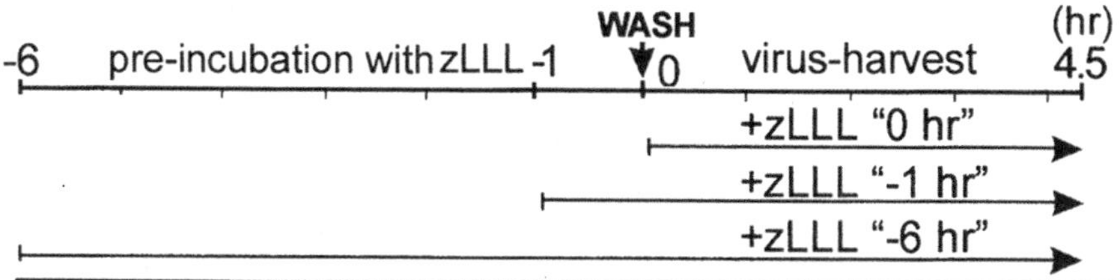

Treatment	virus release in ng p24^{CA} / ml	TC$_{ID50}$ virus titer / ml	infectivity = titer / ng p24^{CA}	infectivity in % of "no zLLL"
No zLLL	263	1.9×10^{7}	7.2×10^{4}	100
+zLLL, "0 hr"	122	1.2×10^{6}	1.0×10^{4}	14
+ zLLL, "-1 hr"	88	4.4×10^{5}	5.0×10^{3}	7
+zLLL, "-6 hr"	26	3.8×10^{4}	1.5×10^{3}	2

Fig. 3. Proteasome inhibitors decrease virus infectivity. Parallel cultures of HIV-1$_{NL4-3}$ infected A3.01 cells were either left untreated or were incubated with 40 μM zLLL for 1 or 6 h. Cells were washed, and incubation in the presence or absence of the reversibly acting proteasome inhibitor MG-132 was continued for another 4.5 h, as indicated in the time scheme on top. Virus-containing medium was collected, and the amount of p24^{CA} antigen was quantitated by enzyme-linked immunosorbent assay. Virus titer was determined by endpoint dilution on human CD4^{+} T-cells as described *(10)*. Specific infectivity was calculated as infectious titer per ng capsid (CA) and expressed in percent of the untreated sample.

and the p9Gag region of EIAV Gag, was also reported *(20,21)*. Interestingly, Gag proteins that become mono-ubiquitinylated harbor a so-called late (or L) domain, a proline-rich sequence that is required for late steps in virion budding, in which the membrane of the nascent virus particle has to be pinched off from the host cell membrane *(3,4,6)*.

   Three different types of proline-containing sequences have been shown to possess L-domain function among different retroviruses: PPPY, found in Rous sarcoma virus (RSV) and murine leukemia virus (MuLV); PTAP, found in HIV-1 [presumably P(T/S)AP for HIV-2 and simian immunodeficiency virus]; and YXDL, found in equine infectious anemia virus (EIAV) *(2–4)*. The term *L-domain* for describing fission of nascent virions from the cell membrane was first introduced while budding of the avian oncoretrovirus RSV was being studied *(2,4)*. The function of various L-domains appears to be conserved among different virus genera; even Ebola virus (a filovirus) was shown to possess an L-domain that could functionally substitute for that of HIV-1 p6^{Gag} in promoting budding *(22)*. Because L-domains act in a position-independent manner within viral structural proteins, it was hypothesized that those motifs function primarily as docking sites to engage cellular factors during Gag assembly. This hypothesis received support in a number of reports that demonstrated a functional relationship between L-domains with the host ubiquitinylation machinery. For instance, L-domains of RSV, HIV-1, and Ebola virus were found to induce ubiquitinylation of HIV-1 Gag in retrovirus-like particles, most probably by directing the interaction of Gag with cellular ubiquitin ligases *(23,24)*.

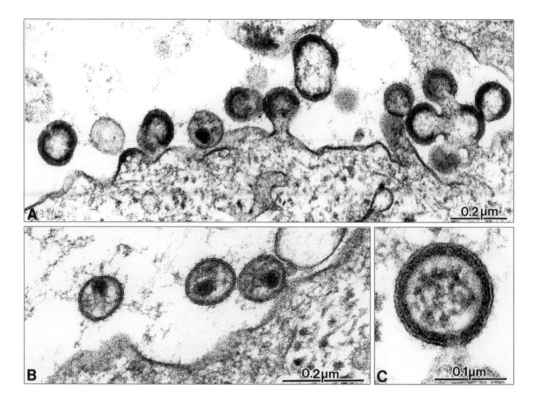

Fig. 4. Electron microscopy analysis of proteasome inhibitor-treated HIV-1–infected cells. HIV-1–infected cells of the human CD4⁺ T-cell line MT-4 were treated with 50 μ*M* MG-132 for 5 h and fixed for thin-section electron microscopy as described *(10)*. (**A**) Overview of infected cells with budding structures and immature virus. (**B**) Mature extracellular HIV-1 particles. (**C**) Higher magnification view of an immature virus particle still connected to the cellular membrane by formation of a membranous stalk. This late-stage budding arrest is reminiscent of L-domain mutants in HIV-1 p6^Gag.

Retroviral L-domains are generally known to interact with a variety of cellular proteins. The PPPY motif interacts with WW domain proteins, an extensive family with a variety of functions *(25)*. The YXDL motif of EIAV interacts with the activation protein-2 (AP-2) adaptor protein complex, which is involved in clathrin-mediated endocytosis. Finally, the PTAPP motif interacts with Tsg101, a homolog of an ubiquitin ligase involved in protein trafficking *(2,22,26,27)*. Mammalian Tsg101 and its yeast homolog Vps23p (a vacuolar protein sorting [Vps] factor) participate as part of the endosomal multivesicular body system in protein trafficking between the *trans*-Golgi network, the lysosome, and the plasma membrane. Both Tsg101 and Vps23p sort ubiquitinylated proteins (presumably by acting as ubiquitin receptors) into inward-budding vesicles in late endosomes, which give rise to multivesicular bodies *(28)*. This provides an intriguing connection to L-domain function if one considers the formation of virions and multivesicular bodies as similar budding processes on cellular membranes. Furthermore, in a search for host-cell proteins governing L-domain function, another constituent of the Vps pathway, Vps4, was identified as PTAP-interacting factor *(27)*.

In vitro studies demonstrated that mono-ubiquitinylation of HIV-1 p6^{Gag} increases the affinity of Tsg101 for Gag. Furthermore, reduction of Tsg101 expression or activity by treating cells with small interfering RNAs [siRNA] or expressing a dominant-negative form of Tsg101 obliterated HIV-1 budding *(2,27)*. Notably, Ebola virus matrix (EbVp40) L-domain recruits Tsg101 to virus particle assembly sites at the plasma membrane, and this intracellular redistribution of Tsg101 can restore budding of L-domain–deficient HIV-1 *(22)*. Direct evidence that ubiquitin-conjugating activities are part of the retroviral budding machinery was provided for RSV: either overexpression of ubiquitin or genetic fusion of ubiquitin onto RSV Gag restored budding from cells treated with proteasome inhibitors *(29)*. In addition, the RSV L-domain was shown in vitro to interact with both the ubiquitin ligase Nedd4 and a related enzyme termed LDI-1, although no role in virus budding was provided *(30)*. Given that mono-ubiquitinylation can be regulated by phosphorylation of the target protein, the recent characterization of HIV-1 p6^{Gag} as a highly phosphorylated virus protein *(31)* awaits further investigation of its potential role in the L-domain-UPS puzzle. Similarly, preliminary data indicate that at least one of the highly conserved lysine residues (although dispensable for virus replication *[21]*) in HIV-1 p6^{Gag} can be modified by the ubiquitin-like protein SUMO-2/3 *(39)*.

What are the role(s) of ubiquitin in L-domain function? A major consequence of proteasome inhibition is to alter the dynamics of ubiquitin level and turnover, resulting in an accumulation of poly-ubiquitinylated proteins and a reduction in the amount of free ubiquitin available for conjugation, and as a consequence for the de-ubiquitinylation of cellular proteins *(32)*. Indeed, we found that treatment with proteasome inhibitors for an extended period (36 h) significantly reduced the levels of free ubiquitin in HIV-1 infected T-cells and prevented the mono-ubiquitinylation of p6^{Gag} *(10)*. This, and our observation that variants of HIV-1 that either do not express p6^{Gag} or possess mutations within the L-domain of p6^{Gag} are insensitive to proteasome inhibitors suggested that virus release and proteolytic maturation require mono-ubiquitylation of p6^{Gag} *(10)*. Consistent with this hypothesis, in-frame fusion of ubiquitin to RSV Gag ameliorated the effect of proteasome inhibitors on virus assembly *(29)*. Taken together, these findings suggest that proteasome inhibitors act on HIV assembly by interfering with mono-ubiquitinylation of Gag.

A potential role of ubiquitin in L-domain function is, however, inconsistent with our finding that mutants of HIV-1 carrying Arg for Lys exchanges in ubiquitin acceptor sites, (positions 27 and 33) in HIV-1 p6^{Gag} were completely deficient in mono-ubiquitinylation of Gag, exhibited wild-type replication in cell culture, displayed "normal" levels of free ubiquitin in virus particles, and maintained sensitivity to proteasome inhibitors *(21)*. Similar to HIV-1, dispensability of ubiquitin for virus replication was also observed for another retrovirus: mono-ubiquitinylation of MuLV p12^{Gag} is not required for virus replication in tissue culture *(21)*. Furthermore, the negative impact of proteasome inhibition on HIV-1 Gag processing occurs within minutes, whereas the decline in free ubiquitin (as well as de-ubiquitinylation of mono-ubiquitinylated histones) occurs only after 2–4 h of treatment with proteasome inhibitors in a cell type-dependent fashion *(39)*.

6. HYPOTHESIS 2: DEFECTIVE GAG MOLECULES INTERFERE WITH VIRUS BUDDING

As an alternative mechanism for the adverse effect of proteasome inhibition on virus budding, we proposed that the accumulation of defective Gag translation products that otherwise would be rapidly turned over by the UPS interferes in a *trans*-dominant–negative manner with highly organized processes that regulate virus assembly and release. Considering the inherent intermolecular protein–protein interaction of Gag, one could assume that even a few misfolded Gag molecules would have a detrimental impact on virus budding. This hypothesis originates from our recent finding that poly-ubiquitinylated and misfolded forms of defective ribosomal products (DRiPs) of HIV-1 Gag accumulate immediately following proteasome inhibition *(33)*. DRiPs in general are short-lived polypeptides that never attain their native structure due to errors in translation or immediate post-translational processes necessary for proper protein folding *(34)* (Fig. 5). Gag-DRiPs may be sufficiently folded to assemble with normal Gag and interfere with its processing by PR, or they may act as competitive noncleavable substrate inhibitors of the viral protease. This process would be particularly driven by the inherent propensity of Gag molecules for self-assembly during the process of virus budding. In support of this pathway it was observed that HIV-1 Gag molecules isolated from proteasome inhibitor-treated cells interfere with Pr55 processing by recombinant HIV-1 PR in vitro *(39)*. Therefore, our experimental evidence obtained so far favors the hypothesis that the negative impact of proteasome inhibitors on virus maturation is, at least partially, a consequence of the accumulation of Gag-DRiPs being coassembled with native Gag into virus particles, resulting in retarded Gag processing and virion release.

On the other hand, the Gag-DRiP hypothesis is somewhat inconsistent with the recent observation that among all retroviruses tested, at least one, EIAV, is relatively insensitive to proteasome inhibition *(35,36)*. Despite the fact that, similar to HIV-1, EIAV virions contained mono-ubiquitinylated p9Gag, in addition to free ubiquitin, proteasome inhibition exhibited only a subtle, at most twofold inhibitory effect on virus release, whereas there was no appreciable effect on EIAV Gag processing. Similar results obtained by Patnaik and co-workers *(36)* were further supported by the finding that a region of p9Gag, when placed in the context of RSV Gag, can overcome the effect of proteasome inhibitors on RSV Gag release. Besides known differences in the assembly and budding strategies between pgGag EIAV and lentiviruses like HIV, it can be anticipated that certain activities in p9Gag from EIAV (that was predicted to be structural and functional similar to ubiquitin *[36]*) support protein folding similar to the "chaperonic" function previously suggested for ubiquitin when it is covalently fused onto other proteins *(37)*.

7. OUTLOOK: DEVELOPMENT OF PROTEASOME INHIBITORS FOR ANTIRETROVIRAL THERAPY

Regardless of the underlying mechanism(s), certain proteasome inhibitors have the potential to be developed as novel anti-retroviral drugs. Obviously, this strategy suffers from the essential nature of proteasomes in cellular function. Nevertheless, proteasome inhibitors like the highly potent and reversibly acting peptide boronate bortezomib (Velcade™; formerly known as PS-341) developed by Millennium Pharmaceuticals (Cambridge, MA) have given promising results as anticancer agents *(38)*. The key issue is whether there is a therapeutic window in which the inhibitors can systematically interfere with virus replication without deploying significant adverse effects on uninfected cells. If such a window exists, it offers the possibility of a highly mutation-resistant target for anti-retroviral therapy that may serve as a useful adjunct in combination with other drugs currently used in the therapy of HIV infection. Considering the extreme, up to a

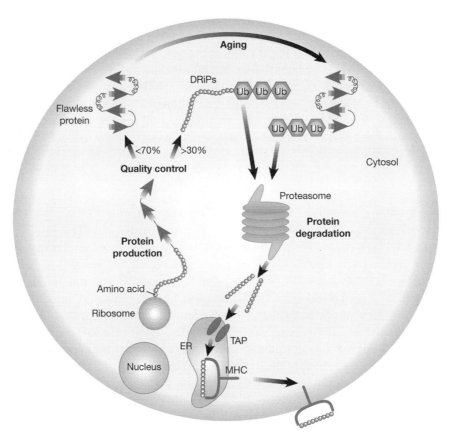

Fig. 5. Defective ribosomal product (DRiP) pathway. All *de novo* synthesized proteins pass through a so far undefined quality control system instantaneously after or even cotranslationally with protein synthesis. A certain percentage (up to 30% in *ex vivo* lymph node cells *[33]*) of all original translation products do not fulfill the quality criteria and will recycled immediately through the UPS. The residual proteins will follow the standard route of folding and aging; and eventually, after a relatively long period of life time, they will be recycled through the same pathway. Given the universal function of the UPS in cell biology, the DRiP pathway may be involved in various cellular mechanisms that are different from antigen processing and virus assembly. For example, recent reports have demonstrated the importance of DRiPs in MHC class I antigen presentation *(40)* and in regulation of protein degradation of dendritic cells upon inflammatory stimulation *(41)*. These data support our hypothesis that DRiPs provide a shortcut for antigen processing by guaranteeing rapid and efficient generation of class I peptides of otherwise "normally" folded and fully functional proteins with long half-lives. (From ref. *42*, courtesy of Hansjoerg Schild and Hans-Georg Rammensee, Tuebingen, Germany.)

million times higher evolution rate of HIV compared with DNA replication of higher eucaryotes, the design of pharmaceuticals that target cell processes involved in virus replication represents an attractive alternative approach to current anti-retroviral treatment targeting mutation-prone viral proteins. As an alternative to broadly acting proteasome inhibitors, the development of small molecule inhibitors specifically intervening with cellular factors that govern ubiquitinylation and/or de-ubiquitinylation of HIV proteins may open new directions for anti-HIV–based therapies.

Note added in proof: After acceptance of the manuscript in 2002, important observations were published in the field of virus budding. Among those is the finding that components of the multivesicular body (MVB) and the endosomal sorting complex required for transport (ESCRT) machineries that in the cell regulate sorting of cell-surface receptors are also involved in L-domain dependent budding of HIV and other enveloped RNA viruses *(43–47)*. Furthermore, it was shown that independent of the presence of mono-ubiquitinylated Gag in virions and the site of virus assembly but dependent on the type of L-domain, retroviruses have differing requirements for proteasome function in the budding process *(50–52)*.

ACKNOWLEDGMENTS

I am grateful to the members of the laboratories at the Heinrich Pette Institute (HPI; Hamburg, Germany) and the Laboratory of Viral Diseases (LVD), NIAID, NIH (Bethesda, MD), particularly Uwe Tessmer, Reinhold Welker, Heinz Hohenberg, Felicita Hornung, Luis C. Anton, Michael Princiotta, James Gibbs, and Shubing Qian, as well as David Ott (NCI, Frederick, MD), John W. Wills (Hershey, PA), and Julian Adams, Michael Kauffman, and Nadine Weich (Millennium Pharmaceuticals) for our year-long successful collaboration and helpful discussions. I am exceptionally grateful to Jonathan W. Yewdell and Jack R. Bennink (LVD, NIAID, NIH) as well Hans-Georg Kraeusslich and Hans Will (HPI) for their continuous and generous support during studies summarized in this review. I am thankful to Jonathan W. Yewdell for comments on the manuscript, and I thank Louis E. Henderson for help with graphic work.

REFERENCES

1. Swanstrom R, Wills J. In: *Retroviruses* (Coffin J, Hughes S, Varmus H, eds). Cold Spring Harbor Press, Plainview, NY, 1997:263–334.
2. Perez OD, et al. Resistance is futile: assimilation of cellular machinery by HIV-1. *Immunity* 2001;15:687–690.
3. Vogt VM. Ubiquitin in retrovirus assembly: actor or bystander? *Proc Natl Acad Sci USA* 2000;97:12945–12947.
4. Luban J. HIV-1 and Ebola virus: the getaway driver nabbed. *Nat Med* 2001;12:1278–1280.
5. Strebel K, et al. A novel gene of HIV-1, vpu, and its 16-kilodalton product. *Science* 1988;241:1221–1223.
6. Goettlinger HG, et al. Effect of mutations affecting the p6 gag protein on human immunodeficiency virus particle release. *Proc Natl Acad Sci USA* 1991;88:3195–3199.
7. Yung E, et al. Inhibition of HIV-1 virion production by a transdominant mutant of integrase interactor 1. *Nat Med* 2001;8:920–926.
8. Farnet, CM, et al. HIV-1 cDNA integration: requirement of HMG I(Y) protein for function of preintegration complexes in vitro. *Cell* 199788:483–492.
9. Schubert U, et al. CD4 glycoprotein degradation induced by human immunodeficiency virus type 1 Vpu protein requires the function of proteasomes and the ubiquitin-conjugating pathway. *J Virol* 1998;72:2280–2288.
10. Schubert U, et al. Proteasome inhibition interferes with gag polyprotein processing, release, and maturation of HIV-1 and HIV-2. *Proc Natl Acad Sci USA* 2000;97:13057–13062.
11. Etlinger JD, et al. A soluble ATP-dependent proteolytic system responsible for the degradation of abnormal proteins in reticulocytes. *Proc Natl Acad Sci USA* 1977;1:54–58.
12. Hershko A, et al. The ubiquitin system. *Annu Rev Biochem* 1998;67:425–479.
13. Hicke L. Gettin' down with ubiquitin: turning off cell-surface receptors, transporters and channels. *Trends Cell Biol* 1999;9:107–112.
14. Glas R, et al. A proteolytic sysytem that compensates for loss of proteasome function. *Nature* 1998;392:618–622.

15. Princiotta MF, et al. Cells adapted to the proteasome inhibitor 4-hydroxy- 5-iodo-3- nitrophenylacetyl-Leu-Leu-leucinal-vinyl sulfone require enzymatically active proteasomes for continued survival. *Proc Natl Acad Sci USA* 2001;98:513–518.
16. Fenteany G, et al. Inhibition of proteasome activities and subunit-specific amino-terminal threonine modification by lactacystin. *Science* 1995;268:726–731.
17. Meng L, et al. Epoxomicin, a potent and selective proteasome inhibitor, exhibits in vivo antiinflammatory activity. *Proc Natl Acad Sci USA* 1999;96:10403–10408.
18. Goldberg AL, et al. Not just research tools-proteasome inhibitors offer therapeutic promise. *Nat Med* 2002;4:338–340.
19. Putterman D, et al. Ubiquitin in avian leukosis virus particles. *Virology* 1990;176:633–637.
20. Ott DE, et al. Ubiquitin is covalently attached to the p6Gag proteins of human immunodeficiency virus type 1 and simian immunodeficiency virus and to the p12Gag protein of Moloney murine leukemia virus. *J Virol* 1998;72:2962–2968.
21. Ott DE, et al. Ubiquitination of HIV-1 and MuLV Gag. *Virology* 2000;278:111–121.
22. Martin-Serrano J, et al. HIV-1 and Ebola virus encode small peptide motifs that recruit Tsg101 to sites of particle assembly to facilitate egress. *Nat Med* 2001;7:1313–1319.
23. Strack B, et al. A role for ubiquitin ligase recruitment in retrovirus release. *Proc Natl Acad Sci USA* 2000;97:13063–13068.
24. Harty RN, et al. A PPxY motif within the VP40 protein of Ebola virus interacts physically and functionally with a ubiquitin ligase: implications for filovirus budding. *Proc Natl Acad Sci USA* 2000;97:13871–13876.
25. Garnier L, et al. WW domains and retrovirus budding. *Nature* 1996;381:744–745.
26. VerPlank L, et al. Tsg101, a homologue of ubiquitin-conjugating (E2) enzymes, binds the L domain in HIV type 1 Pr55(Gag). *Proc Natl Acad Sci USA* 2001;98:7724–7729.
27. Garrus JE, et al. Tsg101 and the vacuolar protein sorting pathway are essential for HIV-1 budding. *Cell* 2001;107:55–65.
28. Dupre S, et al. Membrane transport: ubiquitylation in endosomal sorting. *Curr Biol* 2001;11:932‹934.
29. Patnaik A, et al. Ubiquitin is part of the retrovirus budding machinery. *Proc Natl Acad Sci USA* 2000;97:13069–13074.
30. Kikonyogo A, et al. Proteins related to the Nedd4 family of ubiquitin protein ligases interact with the L domain of Rous sarcoma virus and are required for gag budding from cells. *Proc Natl Acad Sci USA* 2001;98:11199–11204.
31. Muller B, et al. The late-domain-containing protein p6 is the predominant phosphoprotein of human immunodeficiency virus type 1 particles. *J Virol* 2002;76:1015–1024.
32. Mimnaugh EG, et al. Rapid deubiquitination of nucleosomal histones in human tumor cells caused by proteasome inhibitors and stress response inducers: effects on replication, transcription, translation, and the cellular stress response. *Biochemistry* 1997;36:14418–14429.
33. Schubert U, et al. Rapid degradation of a large fraction of newly synthesized proteins by proteasomes. *Nature* 2000;404:770–774.
34. Yewdell JW, et al. Defective ribosomal products (DRiPs): a major source of antigenic peptides for MHC class I molecules? *J Immunol* 1996;157:1823–1826.
35. Ott DE, et al. Equine infectious anemia virus and the ubiquitin-proteasome system. *J Virol* 2002;76:3038–3044.
36. Patnaik A, et al. Budding of equine infectious anemia virus is insensitive to proteasome inhibitors. *J Virol* 2002;76:2641–2647.
37. Finley D, et al. The tails of ubiquitin precursors are ribosomal proteins whose fusion to ubiquitin facilitates ribosome biogenesis. *Nature* 1989;338:394–401.
38. Adams J. Development of the proteasome inhibitor PS-341. *Oncologist* 2002;7:9–16.
39. Ott DE, et al. Unpublished observations.
40. Reits EA, et al. The major substrates for TAP in vivo are derived from newly synthesized proteins. *Nature* 2000;404:774–778.
41. Lelouard H, et al. Transient aggregation of ubiquitinated proteins during dendritic cell maturation. *Nature* 2002;417:177–182.
42. Schild H, et al. Perfect use of imperfection. *Nature* 2000;404:709–710.
43. Martin-Serrano J, et al. Role of ESCRT-I in retroviral budding. *J Virol* 2003;77:4794–4804.

44. Martin-Serrano J, et al. Divergent retroviral late-budding domains recruit vacuolar protein sorting factors by using alternative adaptor proteins. *Proc Natl Acad Sci USA* 2003;100:12414–12419.
45. Martin-Serrano J, Bieniasz PD. A bipartite late-budding domain in human immunodeficiency virus type 1. *J Virol* 2003;77:12373–12377.
46. von Schwedler U, et al. The protein network of HIV budding. *Cell* 2003;114:701–713.
47. Pelchen-Matthews A, et al. Infectious HIV-1 assembles in late endosomes in primary macrophages. *J Cell Biol* 2003;162:443–455.
48. Pornillos O. Mechanisms of enveloped RNA virus budding. *Trends Cell Biol* 2002;12:569–579.
49. Strack B. AIP1/ALIX is a binding partner for HIV-1 p6 and EIAV p9 functioning in virus budding. *Cell* 2003;114:689–699.
50. Shehu-Xhilaga M. Late domain-dependent inhibition of equine infectious anemia virus budding. *J Virol* 2004;78:724–732.
51. Gottwein E. The Mason-Pfizer monkey virus PPPY and PSAP motifs both contribute to virus release. *J Virol* 2003;77:9474–9485.
52. Ott DE. Retroviruses have differing requirements for proteasome function in the budding process. *J Virol* 2003;77:3384–3393.

IV CLINICAL TRIALS

19 Preclinical Development of Bortezomib (VELCADE™)

Rationale for Clinical Studies

Julian Adams, Peter J. Elliott, and Page Bouchard

ABSTRACT

The first three clinical studies of bortezomib tested regimens of differing dose-intensities: once weekly for 4 wk on a 6 wk cycle (least intensive), twice weekly for 2 wk of a 3 wk cycle, and twice weekly for 4 wk of a 6 wk cycle (most intensive). From these studies, the intermediate-intensity regimen has been advanced, because it is the best tolerated but still achieves a high level of proteasome activity. Patients on this regimen treated with $1.0–1.50$ mg/m^2 bortezomib had a reduction in proteasome activity to about 40% of baseline but recovered most activity within the 72 h period between doses. Dose-limiting toxicities for this regimen were peripheral sensory neuropathy (PSN) and diarrhea. Patients with preexisting damage from prior neurotoxic chemotherapy may be more likely to develop PSN, and this possibility is being investigated in ongoing trials. Diarrhea is also adequately managed with loperamide. Notably, hematologic events in the early phase I trials were uncommon—thrombocytopenia was not dose-limiting; febrile neutropenia was rare; and hepatic, renal, and cardiotoxicity have not been noted. Given this favorable side effect profile, bortezomib may be particularly effective in combination-treatment regimens. In preclinical studies, bortezomib has shown at least an additive effect with CPT-11, gemcitabine, and docetaxel, and trials are in progress to determine the optimum dosing schedules for these combinations. In these ongoing trials, no unexpected or additive toxicities have been observed yet.

From: *Cancer Drug Discovery and Development: Proteasome Inhibitors in Cancer Therapy*
Edited by: J. Adams © Humana Press Inc., Totowa, NJ

KEY WORDS

Bortezomib, hematologic malignancies, solid tumors, phase I studies, proteasome, proteasome inhibitors

1. INTRODUCTION

Preclinical studies, carried out in both cell culture and animal models of cancer, provide evidence that proteasome inhibitors have antitumor activity. In addition to arresting cell cycle regulation and inducing apoptosis in tumor cells, proteasome inhibitors appear to have antiangiogenic effects toward tumors. Proteasome inhibition may also attenuate the protective interactions between cancer cells and their microenvironment by affecting the expression of cell adhesion molecules, growth factors, and cytokines. Furthermore, as discussed in previous chapters, proteasome inhibition enhances the sensitivity of cancer cells to both chemotherapy and radiotherapy.

This chapter reviews the preclinical studies of proteasome inhibition in laboratory models of cancer, with particular attention given to the dipeptidyl boronate bortezomib (Velcade™; formerly known as PS-341, LDP-341, and MLN341), the first proteasome inhibitor to be examined in human clinical trials.

2. SUSCEPTIBILITY OF CANCER CELLS TO PROTEASOME INHIBITION

Proteasome inhibition interferes with fundamental metabolic activities within the cell that can result in cell growth arrest and apoptosis. Importantly, however, research has shown that cancer cells may be significantly more sensitive to the effects of proteasome inhibition than are normal cells (Table 1). For example, multiple myeloma cell lines are considerably more sensitive to the proapoptotic effects of bortezomib-induced proteasome inhibition than are bone marrow cells or peripheral blood mononuclear cells from healthy individuals (1,2). The fungal product-derived proteasome inhibitor lactacystin induced apoptosis in chronic lymphocytic leukemia (CLL) cells at concentrations that were not cytotoxic to normal human lymphocytes (3,4). Moreover, the peptide aldehyde inhibitor Z-LLF-CHO induced apoptosis in transformed fibroblasts at concentrations that were up to 40-fold lower than those needed in primary rodent fibroblasts or immortalized, nontransformed human lymphoblasts (5).

It has also been noted that actively dividing cells are considerably more sensitive to proteasome inhibition than are quiescent or differentiated cells. Proteasome inhibitor (PI)-induced apoptosis in murine mammary epithelial cells appears to be dependent on active cell cycle progression in some systems (6). Quiescent bovine and vascular human endothelial cells are considerably less susceptible to PI-induced apoptosis than are proliferating cells (7). Research has suggested that dividing cells may take up or inactivate the drugs at different rates, or that apoptosis may occur secondary to cell cycle arrest (8). However, slowly growing spheroid cultures of DU-145 prostate cancer cells that have a very low growth fraction are highly sensitive to PI-induced apoptosis by bortezomib (9), which suggests that an accelerated growth rate is unnecessary for PI-induced apoptosis. Similarly, Almond et al. (10) demonstrated that slow-growing B-CLL cells, isolated from patients, were sensitive to lactacystin and MG-132–induced apoptosis; thus, quiescence could not account for the reduced sensitivity for proteasome inhibition that normal cells have compared with cancer cells.

Table 1
Cancer Cells With Constitutive NF-κB Activation

Tumors and/or cells	Reference
Hematologic	
Hodgkin's lymphoma	Bargou et al. *(72)*
Activated B-cell-like diffuse large B-cell lymphoma (patient sample)	Davis et al. *(73)*
B-cell lymphoma	Kurland and Meyn *(49)*
Burkitt's lymphoma Daudi cell line	Rath and Aggarwal *(74)*
Myeloma J558L	Wolchok et al. *(75)*
Myeloma U-266, JJN-3	Borset et al. *(76)*
Myeloma ARP-1, RPMI 8226, ARH-77	Feinman et al. *(77)*
Adult T-cell leukemia (patient sample)	Mori et al. *(78)*
ALL	Kordes et al. *(79)*
CLL (patient sample B-cell)	Furman et al. *(80)*
CLL (B-cell)	Munzert et al. *(81)*
AML (patient sample)	Guzman et al. *(82)*
Prostate	
PC-3 high invasive	Lindholm et al. *(83)*
Androgen-independent DU145, PC-3, JCA1, CL2 derived from LNCaP	Gasparian et al. *(84)*
Breast	
Estrogen-receptor-negative MDA-MB-231 and MDA-MB-435	Nakshatri et al. *(85)*
Estrogen-dependent MCF7, estrogen-receptor-negative 578T	Sovak et al. *(86)*
Estrogen receptor-negative	Palayoor et al. *(87)*
Ovarian	
OVCAR-3	Bours et al. *(88)*
OV-MZ-6	Reuning et al. *(89)*
EFO-21, EFO-27	Grundker et al. *(90)*
Colon	
Metastatic HTM-29	Bours et al. *(88)*
SW48	Lind et al. *(91)*
Pancreatic	
MDA Panc-3, MDA Panc-28, MDA Panc-48, ASPC-1, BXPC-3, Capan-1, Capan-2, CFPAC-1, Hs766T, MiaCaPa-2	Wang et al. *(92)*
A818-4 and PancTu-1	Arlt et al. *(93)*
Lung	
Non-small cell patient samples and 13 NSCLC cell lines	Mukhopadhyay et al. *(94)*

ALL, acute lymphocytic leukemia; AML, acute myeloid leukemia; CLL, chronic lymphocytic leukemia; NF-κB, nuclear factor-κB.

[a]PubMed search terms: "NF-kappaB constitutive [cancer type]").

Another hypothesis regarding the differential sensitivity of cells to proteasome inhibition is that cancer cells require a higher rate of protein turnover than do normal cells and may therefore be more susceptible to losing proteasome function. Proteasome levels are abnormally high in cancer cells and in bone marrow isolated from patients with a variety of hematologic malignancies, compared with resting peripheral lymphocytes and monocytes from healthy volunteers *(11)*. Moreover, when Palermo et al. *(12)* measured the expression of proteasome subunits in normal and tumor tissues, they found that some tumors demonstrated higher proteasome activity and expression, suggesting that certain tumors may be more dependent on proteasome function for survival than others. This finding was further supported by a recent study performed by LeBlanc et al. *(13)*, which demonstrated the in vivo antitumor activity of bortezomib toward human myeloma xenografted tumors in mice. Using an ex vivo proteasome inhibition assay, the degree of proteasome inhibition caused by bortezomib treatment was measured in normal liver, spleen, and red blood cells, as well as in tumor tissues. Even though the normal tissues had a greater degree of proteasome inhibition than the myeloma tumor cells, bortezomib treatment resulted in tumor regression and tumor cell death without extreme toxicity in the test animals. Thus, these in vivo results are in concordance with findings suggesting that tumors express more proteasomal proteins than normal cells, yet demonstrate a higher level of sensitivity to proteasome-inhibiting drugs.

However, there have been reports in two different primary cell types—terminally differentiated thymocytes and neurons—of proteasome inhibition blocking the cell death pathway *(14,15)*. Taken together, these results suggest that proteasome function may be necessary for apoptosis to occur in normal cells, whereas in cancer cells, it is only sufficient. Nonetheless, additional studies will be necessary to determine the precise mechanism for cancer cell hypersensitivity to proteasome inhibition.

Interestingly, there is one protein—nuclear factor-κB (NF-κB)—whose activity appears to be repressed by proteasome inhibition, which may be related to preferential cancer cell sensitivity to such agents. It seems that many tumor cell types have constitutively active NF-κB (*see* Table 1 in Chap. 6 and Table 1 in this chapter). Under normal circumstances, NF-κB is sequestered in the cytoplasm and rendered inactive by the inhibitor protein inhibitor κB (IκB). In times of cell stress, however, IκB is degraded by the proteasome, and NF-κB translocates to the nucleus. NF-κB promotes cell survival by initiating the transcription of genes encoding stress response enzymes, including cell adhesion molecules *(16)* and antiapoptotic proteins such as Bcl-2, cellular inhibitor of apoptosis protein 1 (cIAP1), and cIAP2 *(17,18)*. NF-κB is also important in the transcriptional activation of many growth factors including interleukin-6 (IL-6), IL-8, and vascular endothelial growth factor (VEGF) *(19,20)*. Thus, the inhibition of NF-κB may play an important role in PI-induced apoptosis in cancer cells.

3. ACTIVITY OF PROTEASOME INHIBITORS AGAINST CANCER CELLS

Several types of PIs have been demonstrated to induce apoptosis in a variety of cancer cell types. Lactacystin and MG-132 potently induce apoptosis in B-cells isolated from patients with B-CLL *(10)*, in cultured p53-defective leukemic cells *(21)*, and in several malignant glioma cell lines *(22)*. Similarly, MG-132 has been shown to induce apoptosis in Hodgkin's lymphoma cells and in gastric cancer cells with and without functional p53

(23). However, a lack of enzyme specificity complicates the use of such agents in differentiating the effects of proteasome inhibition from other cellular proteases.

In contrast to other proteasome inhibitors, bortezomib exhibits enzyme specificity as well as metabolic stability. It binds to the proteasomal chymotrypsin-like active site with high affinity ($K_i = 0.6$ nM), exhibiting 600 times more specificity for the site than does the cellular protease chymotrypsin *(24)*. Interest in dipeptidyl boronates and bortezomib specifically was piqued when these agents were shown to inhibit growth and cell proliferation potently in a standard National Cancer Institute (NCI) screen of 60 cell lines derived from multiple human tumors *(25)*. Additional studies in individual cell lines have subsequently confirmed the cytotoxicity of bortezomib in human breast carcinoma *(26)*, pancreatic cancer *(27)*, multiple myeloma cells *(1)*, and other cancers *(25,28)*. Importantly, unlike most anticancer agents, it has been shown that bortezomib can overcome multicellular drug resistance in vitro. Studies in several human ovarian and prostate carcinoma cell lines demonstrated that bortezomib showed equal or greater activity against spheroid cell cultures as it had against monolayer cultures *(9)*. Spheroid cultures mimic some of the features of solid tumors, and these results suggest that bortezomib may be effective against both solid tumors and hematologic malignancies.

3.1. Bortezomib Inhibits Tumor Growth in Murine Xenograft Models of Cancer

Despite reports of alternative PIs having antitumor activities in vivo *(5,29)*, bortezomib is the only such agent to have been studied in a wide range of murine xenograft models (Table 2). Bortezomib has been shown to inhibit potently the growth of tumors in mice bearing human squamous cell carcinoma *(28)*, prostate cancer xenografts *(25)*, and grafted murine mammary tumors (26). In fact, bortezomib induced the complete regression of prostate cancer xenografts in some animals *(25)*, and it prevented the development of tumors in human mantle cell lymphoma-xenografted mice *(30)*. As a single agent, bortezomib significantly inhibited the growth of xenografted human dexamethasone-resistant multiple myeloma tumors *(13)*. Tumor growth inhibition was observed after only 5 d of treatment, and complete tumor regression was seen in some mice. Furthermore, bortezomib was highly effective in preventing Lewis lung carcinoma metastases in mice *(26)*. Compared with control mice, animals receiving bortezomib treatment had fewer lung metastases and tended to have a lower percentage of large, vascularized metastases *(26)*.

3.2. Proteasome Inhibitors Enhance the Sensitivity of Cancer Cells to Traditional Anticancer Therapies

PIs appear to induce apoptosis via novel molecular mechanisms that can over-ride the prosurvival messages of Bcl-2 and the mutation of tumor suppressor genes such as *p53* *(31–33)*. Indeed, in the NCI human cancer screen, the cytotoxic "fingerprint" of bortezomib was found to be unique, with little similarity to 60,000 other standard or experimental anticancer drugs *(25)* (*see* Chap. 6). Therefore, the use of PIs (including bortezomib), combined with traditional chemotherapeutic agents, may prove particularly effective in inducing apoptosis in cancer cells refractory and resistant to standard cancer treatments.

Numerous studies have confirmed that proteasome inhibitors can enhance the sensitivity of tumor cells to chemotherapy (Table 1). These studies are described in detail in

Table 2
Animal Models Demonstrating the Antitumor Activities of Proteasome Inhibitors In Vivo

Model	Cells	Proteasome inhibitor	Combination drug
Athymic nude mice[a]	Human prostate cancer, PC-3	Bortezomib	None
Athymic nude mice[b]	Human MIA-PACa-2 pancreatic cancer	Bortezomib	Gemcitabine
Athymic nude mice[c]	Human LoVo colon cancer	Bortezomib	CPT-11 (SN-38)
Triple immune-deficient nude-XID mice[d]	Human RPMI 8226 myeloma cells with Matrigel basement membrane	Bortezomib	None
Athymic nude mice[e]	Human HT-29 ovarian cancer	Lactacystin	Etoposide
SCID mice[f]	Human Burkitt's lymphoma	Bortezomib	None
C57/B16 mice[g]	Murine TrampC1 prostate cancer	Bortezomib	Radiation (25 Gy)
SCID mice[h]	Human mantle cell lymphoma	Bortezomib	None
Athymic nude mice[i]	Human LoVo colon cancer	Bortezomib	Radiation (6 Gy)
Athymic nude mice[j]	Human pancreatic cancer, BxPc-3	Bortezomib	CPT-11
Balb/C SCID mice[k]	Squamous cell carcinoma: murine PAM-212, human UM-SCC-11B	Bortezomib	None
Lewis lung model; EMF-6 mouse model[l]	Murine lung cancer and human breast cancer	Bortezomib	Radiation, cyclophosphamide, cisplatin; 5-FU, paclitaxe[l], doxorubicin, cisplatin
Athymic nude mice[m]	Human LNCaP-Pro5 prostate cancer		Doxorubicin, etoposide, gemcitabine

CPT, campothecin; 5-FU, 5-fluorouracil; Z-LLF-CHO.
[a]Data from Adams et al. *(25).*
[b]Data from Bold et al. *(37).*
[c]Data from Cusack et al. *(38).*
[d]Data from LeBlanc et al. *(13).*
[e]Data from Ogiso et al. *(29).*
[f]Data from Orlowski et al. *(5).*
[g]Pervan et al. *(48).*
[h]Pham et al. *(30).*
[i]Russo et al. *(47).*
[j]Shah et al. *(27).*
[k]Sunwoo et al. *(28).*
[l]Teicher et al. *(26).*
[m]Williams et al. *(53).*

Chapter 6 and will be mentioned here in more general terms. Proteasome inhibition has been shown to enhance the cytotoxicity of many standard chemotherapies in cancer cells, including paclitaxel *(34,35)* and cisplatin *(36)*. In particular, bortezomib has shown activity in combination with dexamethasone *(1)*, gemcitabine *(37)*, melphalan *(2)*, campothecin (CPT)-11 *(27,38)*, doxorubicin *(39)*, etoposide *(39)*, and STI571 *(40)*. In addition, combination studies examining 5-fluorouracil (5-FU), CPT-11, paclitaxel, and docetaxel have been performed in human colon and pancreatic xenograft tumor models *(41)*; 5-FU, cyclophosphamide, paclitaxel, doxorubicin, and cisplatin have been tested in combination with bortezomib in a Lewis lung carcinoma tumor model in mice *(26)*. The combination of bortezomib with standard chemotherapies demonstrated improvement in mouse tumor regression and metastasis *(26,41)*, as well as increased tumor cell apoptosis and decreased tumor cell proliferation *(41)*. Notably, bortezomib also enhanced the effects of the experimental anticancer drugs tumor necrosis factor (TNF)-related apoptosis-inducing ligand (TRAIL) *(42,43)* and geldanamycin *(44)*.

Several studies have also examined the combination of bortezomib and radiation therapy in the treatment of human Hodgkin's lymphoma cells *(45)* and breast cancer cells *(46)* and found that proteasome inhibition sensitized these cells to ionizing radiation. A similar effect was observed in breast cancer cells treated by radioimmunotherapy *(46)*. Furthermore, bortezomib significantly enhanced the inhibitory effects of radiotherapy in mice bearing human colorectal or prostate tumors *(47,48)*, murine mammary tumors, and Lewis lung carcinomas *(26)*.

It has also been reported that proteasome inhibition may overcome the resistance of some cell types to conventional therapies; proteasome inhibitors have been shown to sensitize radiation-resistant murine lymphoma cells *(49)*, as well as etoposide-resistant colon cells and etoposide-sensitive ovarian cancer cells in vitro *(29)*. Similarly, bortezomib demonstrated activity against multiple myeloma *(1)* and CLL cells *(50,51)*, regardless of whether they were considered chemosensitive or chemoresistant. Bortezomib also sensitized resistant multiple myeloma cell lines, but not healthy bone marrow or peripheral blood mononuclear cells, to melphalan, doxorubicin, and mitoxantrone *(1,2,52)*.

In contrast, there are a few reports of proteasome inhibition blocking apoptosis induced by other tumoricidal agents, although this phenomenon appears to be dependent on cell type. Additionally, there have been reports of schedule-dependent antagonism between bortezomib and taxanes; taxane treatment prior to bortezomib treatment appears to promote the greatest extent of cytotoxicity and to stabilize proteins such as p27 in cancer cells *(39,53,54)*. When taxanes are given before bortezomib, less cytotoxicity is observed *(54)*. Such loss of synergism may occur because bortezomib induces cell cycle arrest *(25)*, and antitumor activities of taxanes occur in both phase-specific and nonspecific manners *(55)*. In vitro studies have shown that paclitaxel-induced apoptosis occurs by way of phosphorylation and subsequent proteasomal degradation of Bcl-2 in NIH-OVCAR-3 cells *(56)*. However, Bcl-2 overexpression does not block PI-induced apoptosis in prostate cells *(31,32)*, and therefore the abrogation of Bcl-2 elimination cannot explain the observed antagonism. The use of bortezomib and taxanes is further detailed in Chapter 12.

Remarkably few cell lines appear to resist proteasome inhibition itself *(57)*. There has been one report that multiple myeloma cells deliberately grown in the presence of bortezomib developed tolerance to the drug. Although the cells were less sensitive to bortezomib when grafted into mice, tumors established from adapted cell lines still responded to bortezomib treatment *(58)*. Therefore, in vitro bortezomib tolerance does not appear to be relevant to in vivo antitumor activity, because these cells also remained sensitive to alternative PIs such as proteasome-specific inhibitor (PSI), epoxomicin, and lactacystin. Studies on the behavior of these bortezomib-tolerant cells are ongoing *(58)* (*see* Chapter 13). The mechanisms by which proteasome inhibition overcomes cellular drug resistance are still unclear. In many cases, the ability of proteasome inhibitors to enhance the cytotoxicity of traditional tumoricidal agents has been associated with the inhibition of NF-κB activity *(27,34,38,39,46,47,50)*, but this is not always the case *(45,49)*. However, in a model of inducible chemoresistance, the inhibition of NF-κB with a "superrepressor," IkBa, enhanced tumor sensitivity to CPT-11 and TNF-α–resistant cells *(59)*, suggesting that the activation of NF-κB in response to chemotherapy is at least one potential mechanism of cancer cell chemoresistance. Thus, it is possible that the expression of antiapoptosis factors, which are mediated by NF-κB transcriptional activity such as c-IAP1, c-IAP2 *(18)*, and Bcl-2 *(60)*, are turned on as a part of the cell's survival response to stress *(61)*. Therefore, it is possible that proteasome inhibitors overcome chemoresistance at least partly through the inhibition of NF-κB transcriptional activity.

4. PROTEASOME INHIBITION INTERFERES WITH BONE MARROW INTERACTIONS

It has become clear that the resistance of some cancers to tumoricidal agents reflects not only the intrinsic resistance of the cancer cell itself, but also the protective interactions that may occur between the cancer cell and its environment. The bone marrow provides protection against apoptosis in multiple myeloma cells and also promotes tumor cell survival and cancer progression *(62)*. Furthermore, the bone marrow microenvironment appears to be involved in protecting cells and promoting cell adhesion-mediated multidrug resistance *(62)*. Damiano et al. *(63)* demonstrated that when myeloma cells were preadhered to fibronectin, they exhibited resistance to doxorubicin and melphalan compared with the same cells grown in suspension, suggesting that adherence of cancer cells may activate either growth-promoting signal transduction messages or antiapoptosis pathways.

In addition to the protective mechanisms that appear to be mediated by cancer cell adherence to the bone marrow microenvironment, myeloma cells probably benefit from the production of growth factors, such as IL-6, by bone marrow stromal cells *(64)*. IL-6 is particularly interesting, as its expression is thought to occur through both adhesion-induced TNF-α secretion *(65)* and NF-κB activation *(20)*. Importantly, bortezomib abrogated TNF-α–induced NF-κB activation, IL-6 secretion, the induction of intercellular adhesion molecule 1 (ICAM-1) and vascular cell adhesion molecule 1 (VCAM-1) expression, and myeloma cell adhesion to bone marrow stromal cells *(1,65,66)*.

Similarly, pretreatment of myeloma cells with lactacystin, MG-132, or bortezomib reversed adhesion-mediated drug resistance and sensitized cells to cytotoxic agents *(67)*. Bortezomib interfered with NF-κB–dependent gene expression and decreased the binding of multiple myeloma cells to bone marrow stromal cells by 50% *(1)*. Moreover, the proliferation of residual adherent multiple myeloma cells was inhibited by bortezomib

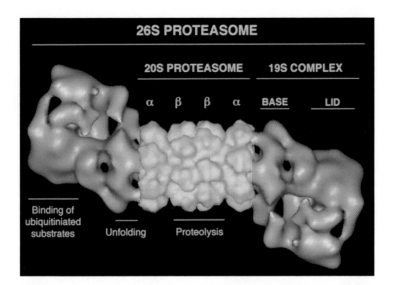

Color Plate 1, Fig. 3. 26S proteasome (*see* full caption and discussion in Ch. 2, p. 23.)

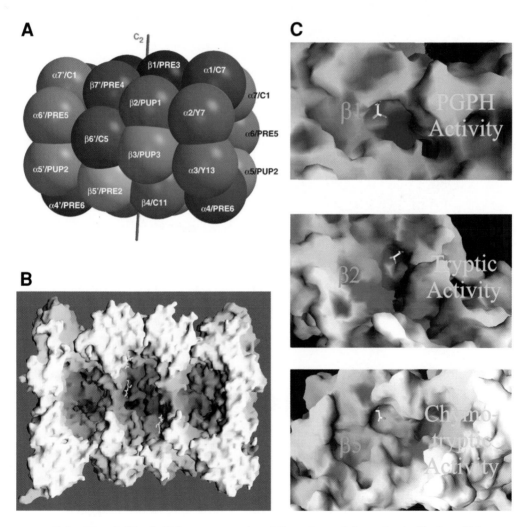

Color Plate 2, Fig. 1. 20S proteasome (*see* full caption and discussion in Ch. 3, p. 40.)

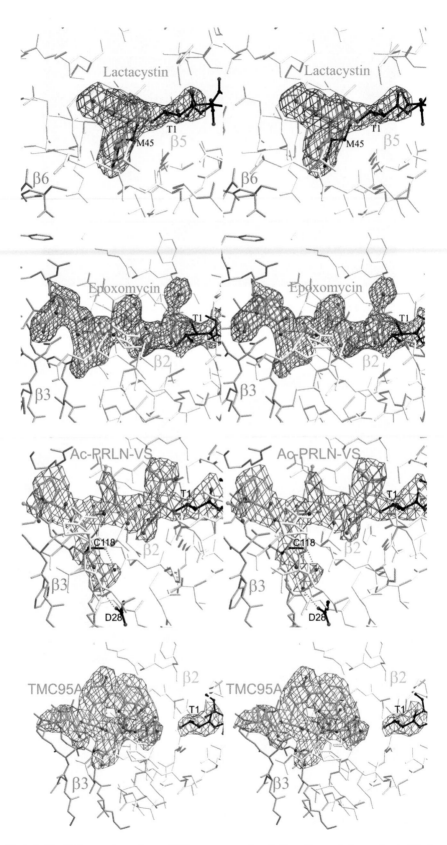

Color Plate 3, Fig. 2. Stereoview of yeast 20S proteasome (*see* full caption and discussion in Ch. 3, p. 42.)

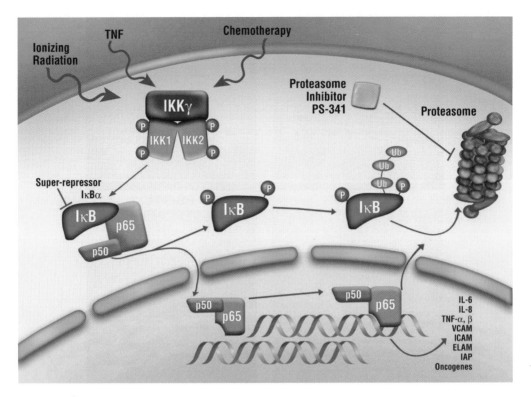

Color Plate 4, Fig. 1. Mechanism of NF-κB activation (*see* full caption and discussion in Ch. 11, p. 132.)

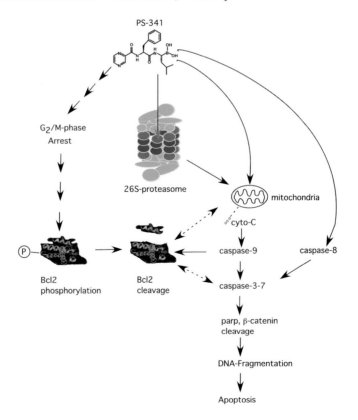

Color Plate 5, Fig. 10. Pleotropic activity of bortezomib (*see* full caption and discussion in Ch. 12, p. 157.)

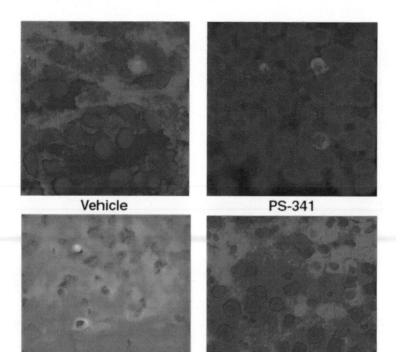

Color Plate 6, Fig. 1. Effect of bortezomib and Doxil® on MAPK activation in vitro (*see* full caption and discussion in Ch. 14, p. 174.)

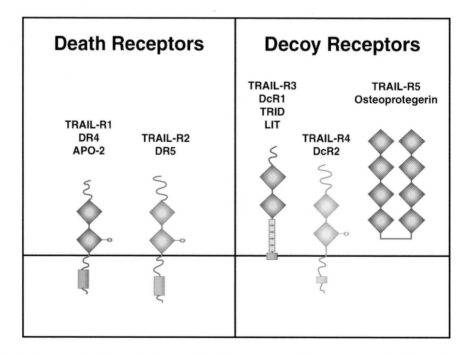

Color Plate 7, Fig. 1. Schematic of TRAIL death receptors and decoy receptors (*see* full caption and discussion in Ch. 15, p. 184.)

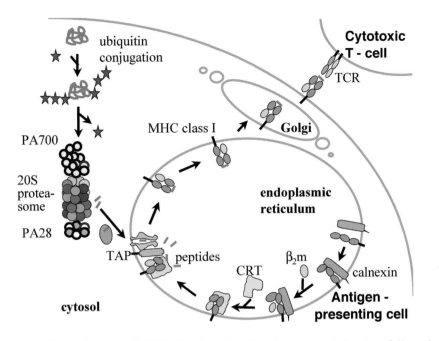

Color Plate 8, Fig. 2. Scheme of MHC class I restricted antigen presentation (*see* full caption and discussion in Ch. 17, p. 210.)

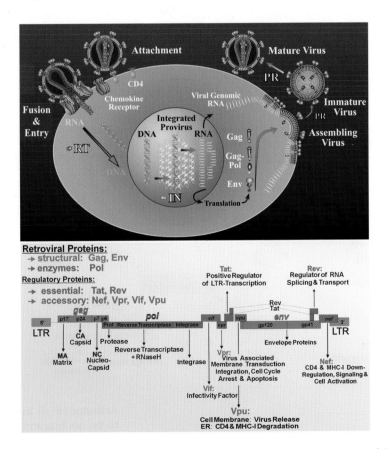

Color Plate 9, Fig. 1. HIV-1 replication cycle, genes, and functions of their products (*see* full caption and discussion in Ch. 18, p. 219.)

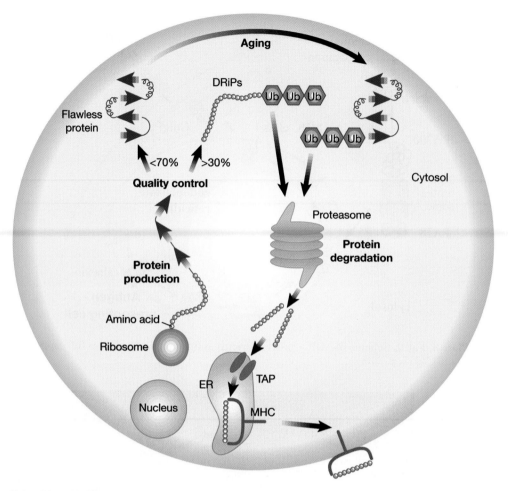

Color Plate 10, Fig. 5. Defective ribosomal product pathway (*see* full caption and discussion in Ch. 18, p. 227.)

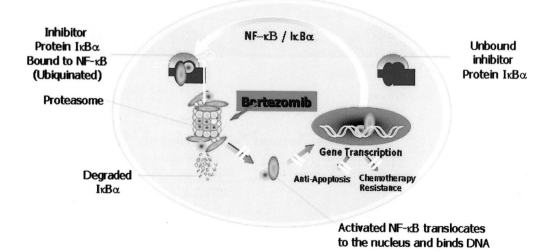

Color Plate 11, Fig. 2. Bortezomib and the ubiquitine-proteasome pathway (*see* full caption and discussion in Ch. 21, p. 290.)

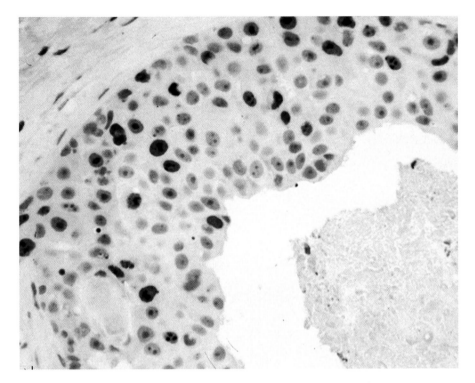

Color Plate 12, Fig. 3. Cell proliferation in breast cancer (*see* full caption and discussion in Ch. 21, p. 292.)

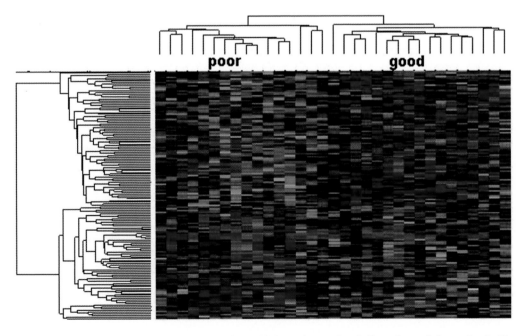

Color Plate 13, Fig. 5. Pharmacogenomics in multiple myleoma (*see* full caption and discussion in Ch. 21, p. 294.)

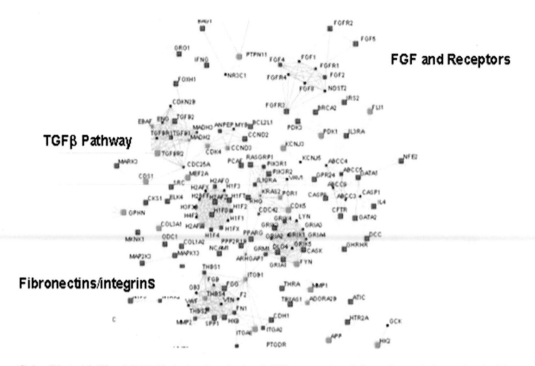

Color Plate 14, Fig. 6. PARIS-derived analysis of differences (*see* full caption and discussion in Ch. 21, p. 295.)

(1,66). Therefore, in addition to targeting cancer cells directly, studies in multiple myeloma cells suggest that PIs may overcome drug resistance in vivo by interfering with the protective interaction between cancer cells and the bone marrow *(1).*

5. PROTEASOME INHIBITORS AND ANGIOGENESIS

It is not known precisely how proteasome inhibition limits tumor growth in murine models of cancer. However, a number of studies suggest that, in addition to acting directly against tumor cells, proteasome inhibitors may have antiangiogenic properties.

Endothelial cell proliferation is required for the development of new blood vessels, and PIs have been shown to have greater activity against dividing endothelial cells than against quiescent cells *(7).* Importantly, PIs have also demonstrated direct inhibition of angiogenesis in the embryonic chick chorioallantoic membrane (CAM) angiogenesis model. Lactacystin treatment inhibited both the development of new vascular tissues and vascular endothelial tube formation in developing CAM tissues in a dose-dependent manner *(68).* Furthermore, proteasome inhibition prevented endothelial cells from producing plasminogen activator, a protease that plays an important role in the angiogenesis *(68).* In a later study, detailed histologic analysis revealed that PSI treatment resulted in massive apoptosis in the chick CAM. It was found that regions within the membrane were completely without blood flow, apparently because of apoptosis induction in endothelial cells *(7).*

Finally, a histologic analysis of blood vessel density in xenografted human squamous cell carcinoma tumors indicated that bortezomib had antiangiogenic activity in vivo *(28).* Sunwoo et al. *(28)* measured reductions in tumor blood vessel density, as well as NF-κB–dependent transcription and VEGF and growth-related protein α (Gro-α) production in tumor cells in vitro. Taken together, these data suggest that proteasome inhibition may inhibit angiogenesis through both the inhibition of growth factor production and the promotion of apoptosis in vascular endothelial cells.

6. NONCLINICAL DEVELOPMENT STUDIES OF BORTEZOMIB

Most of the nonclinical development studies were conducted by Millennium Pharmaceuticals, Inc., and the data are contained in unpublished company proprietary technical reports, except where indicated below.

6.1. Safety Pharmacology Studies

Safety pharmacology studies are designed to examine the potential for a test agent to induce undesirable pharmacologic effects on critical organ systems such as the cardiovascular (CV), nervous, and respiratory systems. CV safety pharmacology studies were conducted in cynomolgus monkeys with follow-up investigative studies conducted in vitro and in mice. In an initial study, telemetry-implanted, remotely monitored cynomolgus monkeys were administered bortezomib iv at 0.1 mg/kg and 32 d later at 0.3 mg/kg (1.2 and 3.6 mg/m^2). No bortezomib-related effects were detected on blood pressure, heart rate, or selected electrocardiographic (ECG) parameters. However at 0.3 mg/kg, the animals were euthanized moribund 12 h post dose. Since 0.3 mg/kg exceeded the maximum tolerated dose (MTD), a second study was performed in telemetered monkeys to examine a range of lower dosages. In this study, monkeys were administered bortezomib iv at doses of 0.10, 0.20, 0.25, and 0.30 mg/kg (1.2, 2.4, 3.0, and 3.6 mg/m², respectively). No bortezomib-related adverse clinical observations were observed at dosages ≤ 0.20 mg/kg. However, at dosages ≥ 0.25 mg/kg, the animals were euthanized moribund by 14 h post dose. No bortezomib-related effects were observed on ECG waveforms at any dosage. However, dosages ≥ 0.25 mg/kg (3.0 mg/m²) resulted in initial physiologically significant heart rate elevations, which preceded a profound hypotension and eventual bradycardia. The heart rate increase was considered a compensatory response to hypotension. The bortezomib-induced alterations in heart rate mirrored and may have been secondary to changes in body temperature.

To understand further the detailed kinetics and physiology of the CV effects of bortezomib in the monkey, a study was conducted in fully instrumented anesthetized cynomolgus monkeys. Animals were administered bortezomib iv at 0.03, 0.30, or 0.50 mg/kg (0.36, 3.60, and 6.00 mg/m², respectively). Heart rate, systemic arterial blood pressure, pulmonary arterial pressure, central venous pressure, left ventricular pressure, cardiac output, core body temperature, and ECG parameters were monitored for 6 h post dose. None of the animals died or exhibited significant adverse reactions during the period of monitoring at dosages at and above those previously shown to be acutely lethal within 14 h in conscious animals. There was no evidence of bortezomib-induced hypotension or heart rate effects. The lack of toxicologically significant findings correlating with those in the telemetry studies described above is best explained by the routine postoperative support provided to the animals, which included the maintenance of body temperature by a water-jacketed heating device and exposure to a heating lamp during the duration of the experiment.

To investigate further the possible mechanisms underlying the initial tachycardia, followed by progressive bradycardia and hypotension observed in telemetry studies, bortezomib was administered to BALB/c mice, and ECG tracings were recorded using a free-ranging remote ECG recording platform. Following a single iv injection of 0.1, 0.3, 1.0, 3.0, or 10.0 mg/kg (0.3, 0.9, 1.0, 9.0, and 30.0 mg/m², respectively), at 10 mg/kg there was initial tachycardia followed by a precipitous decrease in heart rate and a moribund state within 6–8 h. No noteworthy changes were seen at dosages ≤ 3.0 mg/kg. Increased parasympathetic vagal tone was not considered a contributing factor to the bradycardia since atropine treatment had no effect on bortezomib-induced bradycardia. There was a decrease in body temperature coincident with decreased heart rates. To confirm a direct association between body temperature and heart rate, additional animals were administered bortezomib intravenously, and body temperatures were maintained by ambient temperature control. During this period bradycardia was abrogated. Using an ex vivo perfused heart preparation, hearts from bortezomib-treated mice showed no difference in heart rate and force of contraction compared with untreated controls, indicating there was no direct effect of bortezomib on the heart *(69–71)*.

The possible role of bortezomib-induced soluble vasoactive factors as mediators of the terminal hypotension observed in monkeys was investigated. These experiments demonstrated that bortezomib promoted robust expression of the prostanoid vasoactive mediators prostaglandin (PG)E₂ and PGI₂ by human aortic endothelial cells. This was associated with induction of cyclooxygenase-2 (COX-2) mRNA and protein, an inducible mediator of vasodilation. Levels of the constitutive COX-1 mRNA and protein were not affected. These data on the CV effects of bortezomib indicate that acutely lethal intravenous dosages of bortezomib are associated with altered body temperature control that is correlated with parallel changes in heart rate, and ultimately terminal hypotension. These effects are abrogated by maintenance of body temperature and routine supportive care. Bortezomib induces the expression of COX-2 and associated prostanoids, and these soluble vasoactive mediators may play a role in the observed terminal hypotension. Lastly, bortezomib does not show direct effects on the heart or peripheral vascular systems.

Dedicated safety pharmacology studies were not conducted to assess the respiratory and central nervous systems. However, extensive evaluation of the nervous system was incorporated into 6-mo rat and 9-mo monkey toxicity studies including detailed clinical neurologic examinations in the 9-mo monkey study and extensive and specialized histopathology study of peripheral nerves, dorsal root ganglia, spinal cord, brain, and skeletal muscles, as well as immunohistochemistry for apoptotic cells in the dorsal root ganglion in both studies. These toxicology studies were also used for routine assessment of the respiratory system. No bortezomib-related effects have been observed on the central nervous system (CNS) or respiratory systems in these studies. Peripheral nerve axonal degeneration was observed in the 4-wk and 9-mo monkey toxicity studies, the 28-d gemcitabine and bortezomib combination toxicity study in the mouse, and an intraprostatic injection study in the dog.

6.2. Drug Metabolism and Pharmacokinetics (DMPK)

The objectives of the DMPK program were to measure exposure and pharmacodynamic effects of bortezomib, determine the pharmacokinetics in nonclinical species, determine the metabolic fate and transpecies differences in metabolism, characterize the distribution within the body, describe the rates, routes, and mechanism of elimination from the body, predict the potential for drug–drug interactions, and, lastly, examine the inter-relationships among dose, exposure, and effect (efficacy or toxicity). The information described below demonstrates that these objectives were accomplished.

6.3. Methods of Analyses

During the early nonclinical and clinical development of bortezomib, several liquid chromatography tandem mass spectroscopy (LC/MS/MS) assays were developed to determine plasma levels in toxicology and phase I clinical trials in cancer patients. The early rat and cynomolgus monkey plasma assays were fully validated to be compliant with the Food and Drug Administration Good Laboratory Practices (GLP) guidelines, but they did not have adequate sensitivity to characterize the pharmacokinetic (PK) properties of bortezomib in safety assessment studies. The human plasma assays used to support phase I studies in advanced cancer patients had sufficient sensitivity but were not formally validated.

The LC/MS/MS assays used to support definitive toxicology studies in rats, rabbits, and cynomolgus monkeys and phase II clinical trials in multiple myeloma patients were fully validated. The assays were sensitive, specific, and reproducible, with a quantifiable range of 0.5–30 ng/mL. [^{14}C]Bortezomib and its metabolites in various biologic matrices were quantified by radiochromatography, liquid scintillation spectrometry, and/or quantitative whole-body autoradiography (QWBA). Analysis of the radioactive samples conformed to GLP regulations.

The pharmacodynamic (PD) effects of bortezomib were determined using a novel ex vivo assay method that measured the chymotrypsin- and trypsin-like activities of the 20S proteasome from tissues or cells contained in whole blood *(70)*. Because bortezomib has activity only against the chymotrypsin-like catalytic site of the proteasome, measurement of both chymotrypsin- and trypsin-like activities allows for the normalization of activity as a ratio of these two activities. The analytical method was not validated. Analyses of PK data from nonclinical and clinical studies used noncompartmental methods contained in commercially available PK software.

6.4. Nonclinical Pharmacokinetics of Bortezomib

Single- and multiple-dose PK of bortezomib in rats and cynomolgus monkeys were determined as part of the toxicology studies. The doses used in the toxicology studies were in the same range as doses being evaluated in multiple myeloma patients. The sparse blood sampling design in the toxicology studies was adequate to determine systemic exposure of bortezomib but did not permit a detailed characterization of the PK properties of the compound.

After single-dose intravenous administration to rats and cynomolgus monkeys, plasma concentrations of bortezomib declined in a biphasic manner, with a rapid distribution phase followed by a longer terminal elimination phase. The elimination half-life in cynomolgus monkeys averaged 8–10 h following a single dose. The area under the plasma concentration-time curve (AUC) increased in a dose-dependent manner over the tested dosage range of 0.05 mg/kg (0.3 mg/m^2) to 0.20 mg/kg (1.2 mg/m^2) in rats and 0.05 mg/kg (0.6 mg/m^2) to 0.10 mg/kg (1.2 mg/m^2) in cynomolgus monkeys.

After multiple doses of bortezomib, there is a decrease in clearance that results in an increase in the terminal elimination half-life ($t_{1/2}$) and AUC in cynomolgus monkeys. Similar kinetics upon repeated dosing were observed in rats. An increase in half-life and AUC and a decrease in clearance were also observed in solid tumor patients. Table 3 summarizes the principal PK parameters in cynomolgus monkeys and cancer patients after single and multiple doses of 1.2 and 1.0 mg/m^2, respectively.

The PK of bortezomib was not a determinant in the dosing regimen used in multiple myeloma patients. In early clinical trials, the duration of 20S proteasome inhibition was used in guiding the dosing paradigm. In the later trials, the dose, frequency, and duration of intravenous administration were based on the clinical definition of MTD. However, the systemic exposure determined in the toxicology studies did serve as a basis to calculate traditional exposure multiples in animals vs humans.

6.5. Plasma Protein Binding and Blood Cell Partitioning

The extent of binding of bortezomib to rat, cynomolgus monkey, and human plasma proteins is similar across the three species. Over a bortezomib concentration range of 10–1000 ng/mL, which includes the clinically relevant concentrations observed in cancer patients, the in vitro binding averaged 84.9% in rat plasma, 72.4% in cynomolgus monkey plasma, and 82.9% in human plasma. The extent of binding was independent of the tested concentrations. Moderate binding of bortezomib to plasma proteins across species suggests that interspecies corrections for free fractions (non-protein-bound) are not necessary. Partition of [^{14}C]bortezomib between red blood cells (RBCs) and plasma in vitro using rat, cynomolgus monkey, and human blood was determined to be less than 1 in vitro in all three species.

Table 3
Pharmacokinetic Parameters of Bortezomib in Cynomolgus Monkeys and Solid Tumor
Patients After Single and Multiple Intravenous Doses

Species	Cynomolgus Monkeys		Solid Tumor Patients	
	Week 1	Week 5	Cycle 1, d 1	Cycle 1, d 8
Dose (mg/m^2)	1.2	1.2	1.0	1.0
No.	12	12	17	17
C_{max} (ng/mL)^a	80.6 ± 25.1	138 ± 51.4	157 ± 134	126 ± 87.6
$t_{1/2}$ (h)	7.78 ± 3.16	9.68 ± 2.59	5.45 ± 4.50	19.7 ± 11.6
AUC_{0-24} (ng/mL/h)	51.3 ± 10.6	111 ± 29.5	30.1 ± 15.3^b	54.0 ± 14.6
AUC (ng/mL/h)	61.3 ± 14.0	140 ± 45.2	36.8 ± 18.3	81.9 ± 25.7

^{a}Estimated.

^{b}Median time for last quantifiable measurement was approximately 6.5 h.

After intravenous administration of [^{14}C]bortezomib, total radioactivity (consisting of bortezomib and metabolites) was determined in rat and cynomolgus monkey. Total radioactivity in RBCs was several-fold higher than in plasma at all sampling time points. These results suggest that, in vivo, bortezomib metabolites may associate with the cellular components of blood, and these results are consistent with the extensive tissue distribution and slow elimination of bortezomib-related radioactivity.

6.6. Tissue Distribution

Tissue distribution of [^{14}C]bortezomib in rats and cynomolgus monkeys was evaluated by determining excised tissue content of total radioactivity and by QWBA. Both types of studies indicated rapid movement of radioactivity from the vascular compartment into all tissues with the exception of the CNS, testis, and various regions of the eye and optic nerve. Tissue/plasma concentration ratios of total radioactivity were greater than 1 in most tissues, in which there were measurable levels of radioactivity, at all time points evaluated. The extensive tissue penetration characteristics of bortezomib suggest that the compound should inhibit proteasome activity throughout the body, including cancer cells. Studies in a mouse model of efficacy indicated that the tumor/blood concentration ratio of [^{14}C]bortezomib at 1 h post dose was approximately 1. Many of the rat tissues had the highest total concentration of radioactivity at 1 h post dose, which is consistent with the observed rapid onset of 20S proteasome inhibition. The highest concentrations of total radioactivity were found in the organs of excretion and metabolism (i.e., kidneys and liver). Radioactivity was not detectable in the brain and spinal cord at any sampling time points.

Studies using genetically engineered cell lines have shown that bortezomib is unlikely to be a substrate for several drug efflux pumps that are often expressed in cancer, including P-glycoprotein (Pgp)-1, multidrug-resistance–associated protein (Mrp)3, and Mrp5. In addition, bortezomib was shown in Caco-2 cell culture to have similar flux values from the apical to basal and basal to apical directions, suggesting that bortezomib is not a substrate for Pgp.

6.7. Metabolism of Bortezomib

The metabolism of bortezomib in rats, cynomolgus monkeys, and cancer patients was extensively characterized in various biologic matrices and excreta. The metabolic profile in the three species is qualitatively quite similar. All the major in vitro and in vivo human metabolites are found in rats and/or cynomolgus monkeys. However, the available data preclude a conclusion on the quantitative similarities or differences among the three species.

Bortezomib is extensively metabolized by rats, cynomolgus monkeys, and humans, and little if any unchanged bortezomib was recovered in the excreta of rats and cynomolgus monkeys. More than 30 metabolites have been structurally confirmed with authentic standards or tentatively identified based on interpretation of mass spectra. In vitro and in vivo studies indicated that bortezomib is primarily oxidatively metabolized via cytochrome P450 and not via phase II pathways, e.g., glucuronidation and sulfation.

The major in vitro and in vivo bortezomib metabolic pathway is deboronation mediated by CYP3A4 and 2D6, forming M1 and M2. Deboronation accounted for greater than 90% of the total metabolism when bortezomib was incubated with human liver microsomes or major human recombinant expressed CYP isozymes. Hydroxylation of the deboronated metabolite was also observed. Glutathione and cysteinylglycine conjugates of deboronated bortezomib were identified when bortezomib was incubated with rat liver microsomes fortified with glutathione and rat glutathione-S-transferases.

All the deboronated metabolites formed in rat and human liver microsomal incubations were found in the plasma of rats, cynomolgus monkeys, and humans. The major metabolites found in rat, cynomolgus monkey, and human plasma were formed by deboronation of bortezomib, followed by hydroxylation of the corresponding acid. Rat bile contained many metabolites that are glutathione conjugates of deboronated bortezomib or hydroxylated deboronated bortezomib. Representative deboronated bortezomib metabolites formed in vitro and in vivo have been shown to be inactive as 20S proteasome inhibitors. In addition, cynomolgus monkey bile samples containing a mixture of bortezomib metabolites were also shown not to contain any inhibitory activity against 20S proteasome. The similarity in the in vitro and in vivo metabolic profile of bortezomib among rat, cynomolgus monkey, and cancer patients indicates that the rat and cynomolgus monkey, which have been used as the principal toxicology species, are appropriate species to assess the toxicity of bortezomib and its metabolites in cancer patients.

6.8. Inhibition and Induction of Metabolism

The assessment of potential drug-drug interactions was evaluated by the ability of bortezomib to inhibit and/or induce cytochrome P450 in vitro. Bortezomib was a poor inhibitor of recombinant human CYP P450 isozymes 1A2, 2C9, 2C19, 2D6, and 3A4, with median inhibitory concentration (IC_{50}) values of >18 μM (approx 7 µg/mL). These IC_{50} values are much higher than the observed bortezomib C_{max} of <0.5 μM in cancer patients at the efficacious doses. Additionally, bortezomib did not induce the activities of CYP3A4 and 1A2 in primary cultured human hepatocytes.Based on these results, it is unlikely that bortezomib will change the metabolic clearance of concomitant medications. However, the potential increase or decrease in bortezomib clearance by concomitant medications that are potent inducers or inhibitors of CYP3A4 or potent inhibitors of 2D6 has not been assessed.

6.9. Elimination

Four radioactive mass balance and excretion studies were conducted with [^{14}C]bortezomib in Sprague-Dawley rats and cynomolgus monkey. The first rat and cynomolgus monkey study used a ^{14}C-labeled bortezomib in which the nine carbons in the phenylalanine moiety were labeled with ^{14}C. Using this material, the recovery of total radioactivity was less than 50% in both species. The remainder of the administered radioactivity was found in the carcass after 72 and 144 h post dose in rats and cynomolgus monkeys, respectively. Owing to the low recovery of the administered radioactive dose, the studies were repeated using a ^{14}C-labeled bortezomib in which the carbonyl carbon was labeled with ^{14}C.

Using the carbonyl-labeled [^{14}C]bortezomib, biliary excretion was established to be the primary route of elimination of [^{14}C]bortezomib-derived radioactivity in rats. In bile duct-cannulated rats, 35.1% of the radioactivity was recovered in bile, 16.2% in urine, 7.75% in feces, and 1.20% in the expired air. Approximately 32% of the administered radioactivity was found in the tissues and carcass after 72 h. In total, more than 95% of the administered dose was accounted for.

Urinary and biliary excretions were established to be the primary routes of elimination of [^{14}C]bortezomib-derived radioactivity in cynomolgus monkeys. Within the first 24 h, 30–40% of the total recovered radioactivity was excreted via urine or feces. The remaining 60–70% of the recovered radioactivity was eliminated slowly during the next 120 h. Overall, approx 25 and 15% of the administered radioactivity was recovered in urine and feces, respectively at 144 h post dose; the cage washes accounted for 15% of the radioactivity. Selected tissues (gastrointestinal [GI] tract, heart, kidneys, liver, lungs, and pancreas) and the carcass still contained 12 and 19%, respectively, of the administered radioactivity at 144 h post dose. A total 65–80% of the administered radioactivity was accounted for in 144 h.

The slow elimination and incomplete recovery of the administered radioactivity in rats and cynomolgus monkeys are probably due to the extensive tissue distribution and retention of bortezomib and/or metabolites and slow release of the radioactive material from the tissues.

Oxidative deboronation of bortezomib is the primary mechanism for inactivation and subsequent elimination. Elimination of [^{14}C]bortezomib-derived radioactivity via both urinary and biliary routes in rats and cynomolgus monkeys suggests that bortezomib may be administered safely to cancer patients with compromised renal function.

6.10. Pharmacokinetic and Pharmacodynamic Relationships

In the initial absence of sensitive bioanalytical methods for measuring plasma concentrations of bortezomib, the ex vivo proteasome chymotruptic/tryptic (ChT/T) ratio assay was employed as a PD marker of bortezomib presence in the systemic circulation and tissues. Inhibition of 20S proteasome activity in the tissues was correlated with the inhibition levels observed in the cellular component of circulating whole blood. Because of this relationship, the whole blood 20S proteasome activity was believed to be an appropriate indirect measure of pharmacologic activity in the tissues.

In the long-term toxicity studies in rats and cynomolgus monkeys, the mean exposure to bortezomib and inhibition of proteasome activity at 30 min increased with doses of 0.05–0.15 mg/kg (0.3–0.9 mg/m^2) and 0.05–0.1 mg/kg (0.6–1.2 mg/m^2), respectively. Similarly, studies in phase I advanced cancer patients indicated a dose-related increase in mean inhibition of 20S proteasome activity across the explored dose range of 1.3–2 mg/m^2 with maximal inhibition of activity observed within 60 min. The time-course of recovery from 20S proteasome inhibition in rats, cynomolgus monkeys, and cancer patients after a single dose of 1.2, 1.2, and 1.6 mg/m^2, respectively, is shown in Fig. 1.

In the cynomolgus monkey, the PK/PD relationship can be described by a simple maximum effect (E_{max}) model with a plasma EC$_{50}$ of 3.91 ng/mL. There is a steep increase in the inhibition of 20S proteasome activity between bortezomib plasma levels of 1 and 5 ng/mL. However, at concentrations >5 ng/mL, proteasome inhibition appears to reach a plateau of approx 70–80% (Fig. 2). Observations in initial rat and cynomolgus monkey toxicity studies resulted in the presumption that a complete or nearly complete recovery of 20S proteasome activity between doses was a critical determinant in the dosing schedule. Subsequent nonclinical studies and clinical experience have shown that complete recovery of 20S proteasome activity is not an absolute determinant of the safety and efficacy of the compound. Complete recovery of proteasome activity to pretreatment levels does not occur clinically at 72 h. However, the twice-weekly dosing schedule has been well tolerated over several cycles in patients.

In the cynomolgus monkey, the PK/PD relationship can be described by a simple maximum effect (E_{max}) model with a plasma EC$_{50}$ of 3.91 ng/mL. There is a steep increase in the inhibition of 20S proteasome activity between bortezomib plasma levels of 1 and 5 ng/mL. However, at concentrations >5 ng/mL, proteasome inhibition appears to reach a plateau of approx 70–80% (Fig. 2).

In cancer patients, the PK/PD relationship is similarly described by a simple E_{max} model with a plasma EC$_{50}$ of 1.48 ng/mL, a steep portion of the concentration-response curve up to 2 ng/mL followed by a plateau at approximately 70–80% inhibition, at which point even doubling or tripling of the concentration results in marginal increase in 20S proteasome inhibition (Fig. 3). Therefore, the relationship between 20S proteasome activity assay and plasma concentration has a narrow dynamic range but is useful to define concentrations of bortezomib in the pharmacologically active concentration range.

7. TOXICOLOGY

The objectives of the nonclinical toxicity program were to establish the pharmacologic safety in critical organ systems, establish the potential of bortezomib for genotoxic effects, determine the potential developmental toxicity, identify the target organs of toxicity, assess reversibility to toxicity, determine relationships of toxicity to exposure and PD, examine the potential for important toxicologic drug interactions, understand the mechanism of potential important toxicities, and establish the potential occupational hazards associated with exposure to bortezomib. These objectives were fully accomplished through the series of studies outlined below.

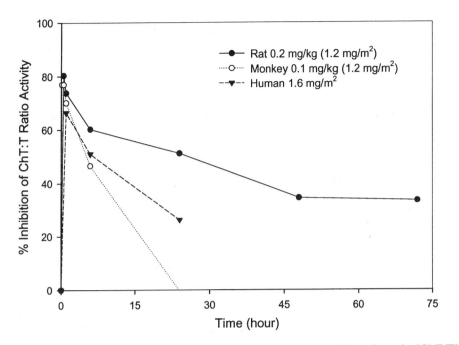

Fig. 1. Percent inhibition of 20S proteasome activity (chymotryptic/tryptic ratio [ChT/T]) in whole blood from rats, monkeys, and humans following a single intravenous dose of bortezomib.

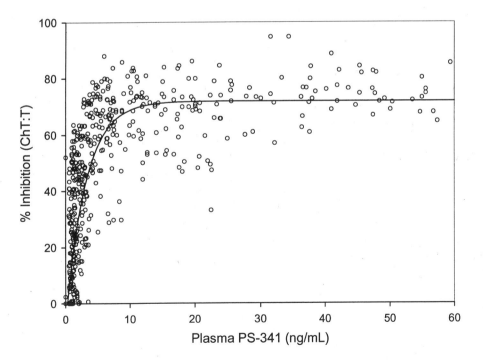

Fig. 2. Relationship of plasma concentrations of bortezomib (PS-341) and inhibition of 20S proteasome activity (chymotryptic/tryptic ratio [ChT/T]) in cynomolgus monkeys (E_{max} model; clinical study RPT-00039).

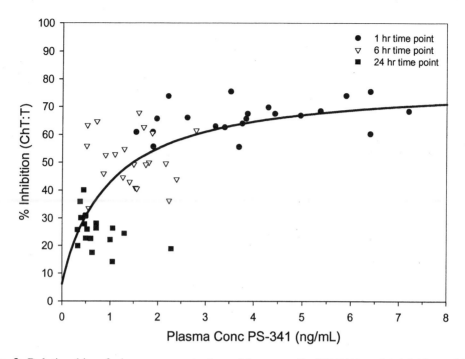

Fig. 3. Relationship of plasma concentration of bortezomib (PS-341) and inhibition of 20S proteasome activity (chymotryptic/tryptic ratio [ChT/T]) in advanced cancer patients (E_{max} model; clinical study DM98-194).

7.1. Single-Dose Toxicity Studies

Intravenous and intraperitoneal routes of administration were initially compared in pilot single-dose bortezomib toxicity studies in female BALB/c mice. These studies were designed to determine which route of administration would be better tolerated as observed by mortality and body weight effects and, therefore, would be appropriate for further tolerability and efficacy studies in mice. The tolerability of intravenous and intraperitoneal administration was comparable, and the intravenous route was selected as the preferred route of administration and the intended route for human clinical studies.

The toxicity of bortezomib administered intravenously as a single dose was assessed in mice, rats, female beagle dogs, and cynomolgus monkeys. The MTDs of bortezomib administered as an iv bolus dose to mice, rats, female dogs, and monkeys were determined to be 1.0 mg/kg (3.0 mg/ m²), 0.10 mg/kg (0.6 mg/m²), 0.18 mg/kg (3.6 mg/m²), and 0.10 mg/kg (1.2 mg/m²), respectively. These dosages in the mouse, rat, dog, and monkey are 2.3-, 0.46-, 2.8-, and 0.92-fold the proposed clinical dosage of 1.3 mg/m², respectively. In general, a specific cause of death was not determined in these studies. Common clinical signs included fecal changes (liquid, reduced, or absent feces), loss of appetite, emesis, hypoactivity, and reduced body weight. Based on the single-dose toxicity profile, the comparative MTDs, and the observed pharmacologic responsiveness, the rat and monkey were considered the most sensitive and most appropriate species for the definitive toxicology studies. Additionally, evaluation of the in vitro metabolic profiles in rat and monkey revealed comparable metabolism of bortezomib compared with human.

To determine whether bortezomib would be better tolerated by lengthening the time of dose administration, the single-dose toxicity of bortezomib was assessed following a 24-h intravenous infusion in monkeys and compared with the results of the intravenous bolus study described above. The overall profile of toxicity and the MTD in this study (0.1 mg/kg or 1.2 mg/m^2) were equivalent to those observed in the intravenous bolus study. Owing to the lack of difference in the MTD, bolus intravenous administration was used for all additional toxicology studies and in clinical trials.

7.2. Repeat-Dose Toxicity Studies

7.2.1. Pilot Rodent Repeat-Dose Studies

A series of exploratory/pilot toxicity studies were conducted to determine the MTD using daily and various intermittent dosing regimens for bortezomib in rodents. Daily ip administration studies were conducted in male C57BL/6 mice for 10–14 d at dosages ranging from 0.03 to 10.00 mg/kg/d (0.09 to 30.00 mg/m^2/d). On the basis of mortality and body weight effects, the once-daily ip administration MTD in the C57BL/6 mouse was 0.30 mg/kg/d (0.90 mg/m^2). Daily iv dosing studies using dosages of 0.01–0.30 mg/ kg/d (0.06–1.80 mg/m^2/d) were conducted in female Lewis rats for 7 d. On the basis of mortality and body weight effects, the once-daily iv administration MTD in the Lewis rat was 0.05 mg/kg/d (0.30 mg/m^2/d). Additional exploratory intravenous tolerability studies were conducted utilizing various intermittent dosing regimens in rats to investigate the effect of regimen on tolerability. Bortezomib was administered iv to female Lewis rats at dosages ranging from 0.01 to 0.30 mg/kg/dose (0.06–1.80 mg/m^2/dose) every other day for 14 d. In these studies, on the basis of mortality and body weight effects the every-other-day iv administration MTD in the Lewis rat was 0.10 mg/kg/dose (0.60 mg/ m^2/dose). Twice-weekly iv administration of bortezomib in male Sprague-Dawley rats for 14 d at dosages ranging from 0.01 to 0.35 mg/kg/dose (0.06 to 2.10 mg/m^2/dose) resulted in an MTD of 0.20 mg/kg/dose (1.80 mg/m^2/dose). One additional study investigated the iv administration of bortezomib to female Lewis rats once-weekly for 8 wk at dosages of 0.03, 0.10, and 0.30 mg/kg/dose (0.18, 0.60, and 1.80 mg/m^2/dose). On the basis of mortality and body weight effects, the once-weekly iv apparent MTD was 0.10 mg/kg/dose (0.60 mg/m^2/dose) in the Lewis rat. In general, these exploratory studies suggested that bortezomib is better tolerated over a sustained dosing regimen with intermittent administration. Results from these studies, together with the observed duration of PD and in vivo pharmacology studies in xenograft models, suggested that twice-weekly administration of bortezomib at the MTD was the optimal dosing strategy for further development.

7.2.2. Two-Week Twice-Weekly Intravenous Toxicity Study in Rats

A GLP-compliant 2-wk, twice-weekly iv toxicity study with bortezomib was performed in Sprague-Dawley rats at 0, 0.10, 0.20, and 0.25 mg/kg (0, 0.6, 1.2, and 1.5 mg/ m^2) with subgroups allowed a 2-wk recovery period. The objectives of this study were to determine the MTD, the target organs of toxicity, and the reversibility of toxicity.

No mortality or adverse clinical signs were observed. The principal bortezomib-related microscopic changes at $\geq$ 0.10 mg/kg were renal tubular changes of minimal to mild karyomegaly (enlarged nuclei), tubular dilation, tubular regeneration, mineralization, and/or lymphocytic infiltration. These changes were partially reversed after 2 wk of recovery. Mild edema and/or chronic inflammation in the colon were observed at 0.25 mg/kg in males only, with reversal following 2 wk of recovery. No toxicokinetic (TK) evaluations were performed. A dose-dependent inhibition of proteasome activity was observed with recovery of activity noted between dose administrations.

Based on microscopic kidney changes at all dosages, a no observable adverse effect level (NOAEL) was not established, and based on the lack of life-threatening toxicity at any dosage, the MTD was 0.25 mg/kg (1.5 mg/m^2). At the MTD 1 h post dose on d 1, the 20S proteasome was inhibited 87 and 73% in males and females, respectively, relative to concurrent controls. The MTD dosage was comparable (1.15 times) to the proposed clinical dosage of 1.3 mg/m^2 administered twice weekly.

7.2.3. Two-Week Once-Daily Intravenous Range-Finding Toxicity Study in Cynomolgus Monkeys

A non-GLP-compliant range-finding 2-wk, once-daily, intravenous toxicity study in cynomolgus monkeys with a 24-d recovery period was conducted to define initially the toxicity profile and an MTD for future studies. Bortezomib was administered once daily iv at 0, 0.045, 0.067, and 0.100 mg/kg/d (0, 0.54, 0.80, and 1.20 mg/m^2/d) for up to 2 wk. However, owing to severe toxicity, with mortality at all dosages, neither a NOAEL nor an MTD were established for daily intravenous administration of bortezomib to monkeys. Because of the poor tolerability of this regimen and the then emerging knowledge of the duration of PD effects, no further studies using daily intravenous dosing were conducted.

7.2.4. Four-Week Twice-Weekly Intravenous Toxicity Study in Cynomolgus Monkeys

A GLP-compliant 4-wk, twice-weekly, intravenous toxicity study in cynomolgus monkeys with a 2-wk recovery period was conducted to establish the MTD, the target organs of toxicity, and recovery from toxicity. Bortezomib was administered twice weekly iv at 0, 0.045, 0.067, and 0.100 mg/kg (0, 0.54, 0.80, and 1.20 mg/m^2). A subgroup of animals was allowed a 2-wk recovery period. Bortezomib-related mortality was observed in one male at 0.100 mg/kg on d 26. A definitive cause of death was not determined. Bortezomib-related clinical signs included increased incidence of red skin on limbs and GI toxicity (emesis and liquid, mucoid, nonformed, absent, or few feces) at 0.100 mg/kg. Body weight loss was observed at 0.100 mg/kg and in one male at 0.067 mg/kg. Decreased food consumption was more frequent at 0.100 mg/kg. These signs were reversible following the 2-wk recovery period.

Bortezomib-related hematologic findings included decreased lymphocyte counts and increased monocyte counts at dosages $\geq$ 0.067 mg/kg. Other changes at 0.100 mg/kg included mildly lower erythrocytic parameters in males, mild to moderate decreased total protein, and moderately higher fibrinogen. Except for the decreased lymphocyte counts in one recovery male, these findings were fully reversed at the end of the 2-wk recovery period. Bortezomib-related increases in absolute and relative (to body weight) liver weight were seen in males at 0.100 mg/kg. Decreased ovarian weights were noted in females at 0.100 mg/kg/dose.

Bortezomib-related microscopic changes were seen in the kidneys, spleen, thymus, and sciatic nerve. Mild tubular nephrosis characterized by degeneration of tubular epithelium was observed in the kidneys at 0.100 mg/kg. This finding was associated with subacute inflammation and slight glomerular changes in some affected animals. Slight lymphocytic depletion in various lymphoid tissues was observed in a few animals at 0.100 mg/kg. Minimal to slight axonal degeneration of the sciatic nerve was observed in 2 of 10 animals at 0.100 mg/kg. All pathology findings except axonal degeneration were fully reversible following recovery.

PD analyses on d 1 showed dosage-related decreased 20S proteasome specific activity at all dosage levels 1 h post dose. No gender differences were noted. Recovery was generally observed within 72 h. Comparable reductions in 20S proteasome activities were observed 1 h post dose on d 22 of study. Toxicokinetics were not assessed. Based on the observation of decreased lymphocyte counts at 0.067 mg/kg (0.80 mg/m^2), the NOAEL was 0.045 mg/kg (0.54 mg/m^2), and owing to the mortality at 0.100 mg/kg (0.80 mg/m^2), the MTD was 0.067 mg/kg (0.80 mg/m^2). The mean 20S proteasome-specific activities were inhibited 54 and 73% on d 1 at the NOAEL and MTD, respectively. The MTD is 0.62 times the clinical dosage of 1.3 mg/m^2, twice weekly.

7.2.5. Six-Month (Nine-Cycle) Intravenous Toxicity Study in Sprague-Dawley Rats With A Three-Month Interim Sacrifice

The objective of this GLP-compliant study was to investigate the potential toxicity of bortezomib when administered to Sprague-Dawley rats by intravenous injection over five or nine 3-wk cycles (i.e., twice-weekly administrations for 2 wk followed by a 1-wk rest period), and recovery from toxicity following an 8-wk recovery period. Bortezomib was administered iv at 0.05, 0.1, and 0.20 mg/kg (0.3, 0.6, and 1.2 mg/m^2) with a concurrent vehicle control group. On d 28/29, the high dosage was decreased from 0.20 to 0.15 mg/kg (1.2 to 0.9 mg/m^2) due to toxicity. Animals from each group were assigned to three subsets of 10 animals/sex/subset. One subset was sacrificed after five 3-wk cycles (14 wk), and the second and third subsets were sacrificed after nine 3-wk cycles (26 wk) and at the end of an 8-wk recovery period, respectively. Traditional toxicologic parameters, as well as extensive neuropathologic evaluation, TK, and proteasome activity were assessed. Bortezomib-related mortality was observed in several male (4 of 30) and female (7 of 30) animals at 0.20/0.15 mg/kg, with several deaths occurring before the dosage reduction and few thereafter. Bortezomib-related microscopic changes observed in the GI, hematopoietic, and lymphoid systems were considered to be contributing factors to the debilitated state and early death of these animals.

Dosage-related clinical observations were noted at all dosages and were primarily referable to GI toxicity. Reduced body weights or weight gains were seen at ≥0.10 mg/ kg, and reduced food consumption was seen at 0.20/0.15 mg/kg. Bortezomib-related clinical signs, body weight, and food consumption effects were reversible during the recovery period. The principal clinical pathology effects were dosage-related decreases in platelets at all dosages, with maximal decreases of approx 50% at 0.20/0.15 mg/kg, variable increases in neutrophils and/or fibrinogen at all dosages, and minimal decreases in red cell mass at $0.1. These changes were fully or largely reversible. The pathogenesis of the decreased platelet counts is not known, and the white blood cell and fibrinogen changes correlate with inflammatory lesions described histologically. Clinical chemistry changes included dosage-related increases in serum glucose at all dosages, with increases up to 73% at 0.20/0.15 mg/kg, slight to moderate decreased cholesterol in males at all dosages, and decreased total protein at 0.20/0.15 mg/kg. Only slight increases in serum glucose in males remained at the end of recovery. A cause for increased serum glucose was not established. The changes in serum cholesterol most likely relate to the increased liver weights and resultant changes in lipid metabolism, and the decreased serum proteins probably reflect GI losses resulting from the lesions described histologically. Bortezomib-related changes in organ weights included dosage-related increased liver weights at all dosages, increased kidney weights at ≥ 0.10 mg/kg, and decreased thymus and epididymal weights at 0.20/0.15 mg/kg. These changes were correlated with microscopic changes in these organs.

Widespread bortezomib-related microscopic changes were seen in preterminal and scheduled euthanasia animals. At wk 26, the predominant changes observed at all dosages included hepatocellular hypertrophy, vacuolation and pigment accumulation, cecal mucosal hyperplasia, salivary gland hypertrophy of the mucous cells, and single-cell necrosis of ovarian corpora luteal cells in females. At dosages ≥ 0.10 mg/kg, bone marrow hypocellularity and/or necrosis, renal tubular dilation, minimal to marked atrophy and/or single cell necrosis in the thymus and secondary lymphoid organs, subacute inflammation in the nasolacrimal ducts, GI tract mucosal hyperplasia and/or single cell necrosis of the lamina propria, acinar cell necrosis of the lacrimal gland, and single cell necrosis of the red pulp and lymphoid cells in the spleen were observed. Additionally, renal changes including tubular cell hypertrophy, as well as renal interstitial inflammation and proteinaceous material in tubules and glomeruli, were observed in females at dosages ≥ 0.10 mg/kg, and subacute inflammation in fat was observed in males at dosages ≥ 0.10 mg/kg. Changes observed only at 0.20/0.15 mg/kg included subacute to chronic vascular inflammation in various tissues and testicular degeneration with epididymal hypospermia and anterior uveitis in a few males.

Animals sacrificed at 14 wk had comparable lesions in the liver, GI tract, lymphoid organs, salivary glands, and lacrimal glands, but several additional changes in target organs were seen at wk 26, as described above. Preterminal animals generally had more severe changes in the target organs outlined above but also showed additional changes associated with a moribund state. After 8 wk of recovery, microscopic changes persisted in several tissues including lymphoid tissues, liver, kidney, bone marrow, and the nasolacrimal duct, but these tissues showed evidence of recovery compared with the wk 26 sacrifice. TK analyses revealed dose-dependent increases in mean AUC_{0-24} and C_{max} values at wk 1, 14, and 26. No gender differences were observed. Additionally, increases in mean AUC_{0-24} and C_{max} values were observed from wk 1 to 14. The AUC_{0-24} and C_{max} values at wk 14 were similar to those observed at Week 26. PD analysis at wk 1, 14, and 26 revealed general dose-dependent decreases in 20S proteasome activity. The mean 20S proteasome activities at 1 h post dose for wk 1 were 49, 42, and 23% of the control values for males and 44, 31, and 24% of control values for females at 0.05, 0.10, and 0.20/0.15 mg/kg, respectively. Partial recovery of proteasome activity was observed by 72 h post dose. At wk 26, the mean 20S proteasome activities at 1 h post dose were 25, 19, and 17% of control values for males and 28, 16, and 18% of control values for females at 0.05, 0.10 and 0.20/0.15 mg/kg, respectively. Recovery to predose levels was noted at 72 h post dose. The PD results from wk 14 were similar to the wk 26 results.

Based on changes in clinical pathology and histologic changes observed at all dosages, a NOAEL was not determined in this study. The most important target organs were considered to be the GI tract and the hematopoietic and lymphoid tissues. At the lowest dosage of 0.05 mg/kg (0.3 mg/m^2), there were numerous minor changes, but this was considered a minimal effect dosage and resulted in mean AUC_{0-24} and C_{max} values of 84.7 h · ng/mL and 4.7 ng/mL at wk 26. The mean peak inhibition of 20S proteasome activity was 73% at this dosage at wk 26. The MTD based on mortality at 0.20/0.15 mg/kg (1.2/0.9 mg/m^2) was 0.10 mg/kg (0.6 mg/m^2). This dosage was associated with mean AUC_{0-24} and C_{max} values of 134 h · ng/mL and 10.9 ng/mL and mean peak inhibition of 20S proteasome activity of 82% at wk 26. Eight weeks of recovery was insufficient for full recovery of bortezomib-related changes; however there were indications of reversibility of most of the changes seen during the treatment period.

7.2.6. NINE-MONTH (13-CYCLE) INTRAVENOUS TOXICITY STUDY IN CYNOMOLGUS MONKEYS

The objective of this GLP-compliant study was to investigate the potential toxicity of bortezomib when administered to cynomolgus monkeys by intravenous injection over 13 3-wk cycles (i.e., twice-weekly administrations for 2 wk followed by a 1-wk rest period) and to assess recovery from toxicity following an 8-wk recovery period. Bortezomib was administered iv at 0.050, 0.075, and 0.100 mg/kg (0.6, 0.9, and 1.2 mg/m^2, respectively), with a concurrent vehicle control group. Three animals/sex were scheduled for sacrifice at the end of the treatment period, and an additional three animals/sex from the control and 0.100-mg/kg groups were scheduled for an 8-wk recovery period. However, owing to mortality observed over the course of the study, only two females at 0.100 mg/kg were retained for recovery, and, owing to hematologic changes, one female at 0.050 mg/kg was added to the recovery subset. Traditional parameters of toxicity, as well as intensive neurologic, neuropathologic, TK, and proteasome activity, were assessed.

Bortezomib-related mortality was observed at dosages ≥ 0.075 mg/kg. One of six males and two of six females at 0.100 mg/kg were euthanized on each of d 50, 172, and 197, which corresponded to the 3rd, 9th, and 10th cycles of administration, respectively. At 0.075 mg/kg, one of three females was euthanized on d 179, which corresponded to the ninth cycle of dosing. In the preterminal animal at 0.100 mg/kg euthanized on d 50 (third cycle), the predominant findings were GI intolerance and dehydration; these findings was correlated with histologic changes of diffuse GI mucosal hyperplasia, which was considered the major cause of the deteriorating condition and the reason for euthanasia of this animal. In contrast, in the three preterminal animals euthanized between d 172 and 197 (ninth and tenth cycles), there were marked decreases in red cell mass (75–92%), with evidence of a regenerative response, marked decreases in platelet count (82–93%), and leukopenia in two of the these three animals. These hematologic changes were associated with bone marrow suppression histopathologically. Severe anemia and thrombocytopenia were considered major contributors to the deteriorating condition and euthanasia of these three animals.

Bortezomib-related clinical signs observed throughout the treatment period included soft feces, diarrhea, emesis, and/or decreased activity; these signs were dosage-dependent and were seen in all animals at ≥ 0.075 mg/kg. Salivation and prostration were seen in one of five surviving males at 0.100 mg/kg. There were no bortezomib-related clinical observations during the recovery period. Administration of up to 13 cycles of bortezomib was associated with dosage-dependent mildly to moderately lower mean erythrocyte, leukocyte (neutrophil and lymphocyte), and platelet parameter values. The onset of the hematologic changes occurred between d 72 (fourth cycle) and d 170 (ninth cycle) and appeared to be nonprogressive once observed. The bortezomib-related changes tended to be more pronounced at higher dosages ($\geq$ 0.075 mg/kg, with the exception of lower erythrocyte values in one female at 0.050 mg/kg). These hematologic changes are consistent with bone marrow suppression, but with hematologic, bone marrow smear, and histologic evidence of regenerative hematopoiesis maintained throughout the study. Additionally, there was a tendency for bortezomib-treated animals to have slightly higher mean fibrinogen values at time points $\geq$ d 170 (ninth cycle), suggesting an ongoing inflammatory process. This change was more pronounced in selected individuals. There were no consistent bortezomib-related effects on serum chemistry parameters values. Following an 8-wk recovery period, there was evidence of recovery of the hematology parameters. However, one female at 0.050 mg/kg and one male at 0.100 mg/kg had decreased red cell parameters and platelet counts compared with pretreatment values, but with an increase in reticulocyte percentage, decreased myeloid/erythroid (M/E) ratio due to an increase in erythroid component, and bone marrow hypercellularity noted histologically, indicating continued hematopoietic recovery.

Peripheral blood immunophenotyping after 12 complete dosing cycles showed that bortezomib at $\geq$ 0.050 mg/kg induced decreases in total lymphocyte numbers, primarily through reductions in numbers of CD2$^+$, CD4$^+$, and CD8$^+$ T-cells and, to a lesser extent, CD16$^+$ natural killer (NK) cells and CD20$^+$ B-cells. Treatments during the 13th dosing cycle resulted in additional transient (<24 h), potentially stress-related decreases in numbers of total lymphocytes and most cell types in all groups, including controls. At 0.100 mg/kg, a 26- or 55-d recovery after the 13th dosing cycle generally resulted in the return of CD8$^+$ T, CD16$^+$ NK, and CD20$^+$ B-cell numbers to values comparable to those of controls. However, incomplete recovery of CD2$^+$ and CD4$^+$ T cells and, thus, total lymphocyte numbers. These observations were consistent with the general bone marrow suppressive effects of bortezomib.

At completion of the main phase, bortezomib-related organ weight changes were dosage-dependent increases in relative and absolute liver and kidney weights in both males ($\geq$0.050 mg/kg) and females ($\geq$0.050 and $\geq$0.075 mg/kg for liver and kidney weights, respectively). These organ weight increases were reversible in the 8-wk recovery period. Bortezomib-related macroscopic changes at the main scheduled euthanasia occurred in the kidneys as dark areas/foci (2/3, 2/3, and 1/2 males at 0.05, 0.075 and 0.100 mg/kg, respectively, and 1/2 females at 0.100 mg/kg) and pale foci (1/3 males at 0.075 mg/kg). These changes were reversible following 8-wk of recovery.

At the completion of the main phase, bortezomib-related microscopic findings were observed in the bone marrow (hematopoietic hypocellularity) or lymphoid organs/tissues (lymphoid atrophy and/or single cell necrosis) of males and/or females given $\geq$0.050 mg/kg; in the peripheral nervous system (sensory peripheral neuropathy) and kidney (tubular degeneration/hypertrophy and/or glomerulopathy) of males and/or females administered $\geq$0.075 mg/kg; and in the intestinal tract (GI mucosal hyperplasia) and liver/gallbladder (sinusoidal leukocytosis or biliary hyperplasia and inflammation) of males administered $\geq$0.075 mg/kg. After 8-wk of recovery, the bone marrow, mandibular lymph nodes, and spleen demonstrated a reversible hyperplastic response, whereas the kidney, thymus, and peripheral nervous system showed minimal to slight residual lesions, indicating incomplete reversibility.

Because prior observations of peripheral neuropathy in the monkey, mouse, and dog, as well as in clinical trials resulted in a desire to evaluate the entire nervous system thoroughly, this study included repeated clinical neurologic examinations and extensive neuropathology evaluation. Specifically, neuropathology included traditional paraffin-embedded hematoxlin and eosin (H&E)-stained histopathology evaluation of the brain (all major regions), peripheral nerves (five peripheral nerves), spinal cord (three levels), spinal nerve roots including dorsal root ganglia (dorsal and ventral at three levels of the spinal cord), and skeletal muscle (for evidence of denervation changes). Additionally, plastic-embedded thin sections stained with toluidine blue for each peripheral nerve, spinal nerve root, and dorsal root ganglia were evaluated. Lastly, immunohistochemistry for detection of apoptotic cells was performed on dorsal root ganglia. These evaluations definitively diagnosed minimal to moderate peripheral sensory neuropathy in 1 of 6 animals at 0.075 mg/kg and 8 of 12 animals at 0.100 mg/kg. Peripheral neuropathy was observed in preterminal (0.100 mg/kg only), main sacrifice (0.075 and 0.100 mg/kg), and recovery sacrifice (0.100 mg/kg) animals. The affected recovery animals had fewer peripheral nerves with lesions, suggesting partial recovery following 8 wk of recovery. There were no bortezomib-related degenerative changes (or apoptosis) in the neurons of the dorsal root ganglia, which are the cell bodies for the peripheral sensory nerves, further supporting the predicted reversibility of these lesions. There were no primary bortezomib-related changes in the CNS, and no evidence of a motor component to the peripheral neuropathy.

TK analyses revealed dosage-dependent increases in mean AUC_{0-24} and C_{max} values at wk 1, 5, 37, and 38. Increases in mean AUC_{0-24} and C_{max} values were observed from wk 1 to wk 5, but with comparable AUC_{0-24} and C_{max} values at wk 5, 37, and 38. In general, dosage-dependent decreases in mean 20S proteasome activity were observed at wk 1, 5, 37, and 38, compared with predose levels. The 20S proteasome activities observed at 10 min post dose on wk 1 were 129, 37, 22, and 19% of d 1 predose values at 0, 0.050, 0.075, and 0.100 mg/kg, respectively. Similar findings were observed at wk 5, 37, and 38.

In conclusion, based on changes observed at all dosages in clinical pathology, immunology, gross pathology and histopathology, organ weights, and bone marrow evaluation, a NOAEL was not determined for the administration of bortezomib by intravenous injection to the cynomolgus monkey over 13 cycles of twice-weekly administration for 2 wk followed by a 1-wk rest period. The MTD, based on mortality at ≥0.075 mg/kg primarily attributable to either GI or hematologic toxicity, was 0.050 mg/kg. This dosage was associated with mean AUC_{0-24} and C_{max} values of 83.1 h · ng/mL and 48.2 ng/mL and peak inhibition of 20S proteasome ChT/T ratio proteasome activity of 75% at wk 38. Complete or partial recovery was observed after an 8-wk recovery period for most of the bortezomib-related effects, with the exception of minimal to slight histopathologic changes seen in the kidney, thymus, and peripheral nervous system.

7.3. Reproductive Toxicology Studies

The potential developmental toxicity (Segment 2) of bortezomib was evaluated in the Sprague-Dawley rat and New Zealand white rabbit. These studies were conducted with daily intravenous administration rather than the twice-weekly clinical regimen to ensure continuous bortezomib exposure to the dam and developing fetus during the period of organogenesis. No evaluation of effects on fertility or peri- and postnatal development (Segments 1 and 3, respectively) were conducted. However, the potential effects of bortezomib on primary and secondary sex organs were assessed during microscopic evaluation in the 6-mo rat study and the 9-mo monkey study. In the 6-mo rat toxicity study, testicular seminiferous tubule degeneration was observed in males at the highest dosage (0.20/0.15 mg/kg), and ovarian luteal cell necrosis was observed in females at all dosages (≥0.05 mg/kg). Therefore, although fertility studies have not been performed, it is considered possible that bortezomib could affect fertility.

7.3.1. DEVELOPMENTAL TOXICITY STUDIES IN THE RAT

In a range-finding developmental toxicity study, time-mated Sprague-Dawley rats were administered bortezomib once daily iv at 0, 0.05, 0.10, 0.15, and 0.20 mg/kg (0, 0.3, 0.6, 0.9, and 1.2 mg/m^2, respectively). Because of to the mortality observed at 0.10 mg/kg (0.6 mg/m^2) and the lack of maternal or fetal toxicity at 0.05 mg/kg (0.3 mg/m^2), the dosage of 0.075 mg/kg (0.45 mg/m^2) was selected as the high dosage for the definitive study.

In the definitive developmental toxicity study, bortezomib was administered once daily iv to time-mated Sprague-Dawley rats at dosages of 0, 0.025, 0.050, and 0.075 mg/kg (0, 0.15, 0.30, and 0.45 mg/m^2, respectively) from gestation d 6 to 17, inclusive. Maternal body weights and food consumption were decreased at 0.075 mg/kg (0.83 mg/m^2) between d 6 and 9. One female at this dosage had persistent weight losses up to gestation d 15. This female had fetuses with the minor skeletal anomaly of reduced numbers of caudal vertebrae, which that was considered secondary to maternal toxicity and generalized growth retardation since the fetal weights for this litter were low. Based on these results, there was no evidence of selective effects on embryo-fetal development at dosages up to 0.075 mg/kg (0.45 mg/m^2). The NOAEL for maternal and fetal effects was 0.050 mg/kg/d (0.3 mg/m^2/d), and this daily intravenous dosage is approximately 0.23 times the proposed twice-weekly intravenous clinical dosage of 1.3 mg/m^2.

7.3.2. DEVELOPMENTAL TOXICITY STUDIES IN THE RABBIT

Range-finding, once-daily intravenous, toxicity studies were conducted first in nonpregnant female New Zealand white rabbits and then in presumed pregnant New Zealand white rabbits. Because of the test article-related mortality, clinical signs, body weight and food consumption decreases, clinical pathology changes, and macroscopic changes in nonpregnant female rabbits at dosages ≥0.075 mg/kg (0.83 mg/m^2), the dosages selected for the range-finding iv developmental toxicity study in presumed pregnant rabbits were 0, 0.010, 0.025, 0.040, and 0.050 mg/kg/d (0, 0.11, 0.28, 0.44, and 0.55 mg/m^2/d, respectively) from gestation d 7 to 19, inclusive. No maternal toxicity was observed. One doe at 0.050 mg/kg had an abortion. There was no clear evidence of embryo lethality or fetotoxicity. Based on these findings and those of the nonpregnant rabbit range-finding study, the dosage of 0.050 mg/kg/d (0.55 mg/m^2/d) was selected as the high dosage for the definitive developmental toxicity study in rabbits.

In the definitive developmental toxicity study in rabbits, bortezomib was administered once daily iv to presumed pregnant rabbits at dosages of 0, 0.010, 0.025, and 0.050 mg/kg (0, 0.11, 0.28, 0.55 mg/m^2, respectively) from gestation d 7 to 19, inclusive. Bortezomib-related maternal mortality, abortion, clinical signs, and decreased body weight gain and food consumption were observed at 0.050 mg/kg (0.55 mg/m^2). Embryo lethality was evidenced at 0.050 mg/kg by increased numbers of resorptions and a decreased live litter size and lower fetal weights indicating mild fetotoxicity. The incidence of litters and fetuses with major malformations was unaffected by treatment. There was no clear teratologically significant effect on the incidences of minor external, visceral, and skeletal anomalies or percentage of fetuses with rib and sternebral variants compared with controls. The NOAEL for maternal toxicity and embryo-fetal development was 0.025 mg/kg/d (0.28 mg/m^2/d), which is 0.21 times the proposed twice-weekly iv clinical dosage of 1.3 mg/m^2. Based on the results of the rat and rabbit teratology studies, bortezomib did not cause developmental toxicity in the rat or rabbit at the highest maternally tolerated dosages.

7.4. Combination Tolerability Studies of Bortezomib With Other Chemotherapeutics

Pilot/exploratory tolerability studies in mice were conducted with bortezomib in combination with carboplatin, cyclophosphamide, doxorubicin, irinotecan, gemcitabine, taxol, and 5-FU. These studies generally assessed body weight and mortality as tolerability endpoints. In general, when dosages of the individual agents were in toxic ranges, additive toxicity was observed when cytoxic agents were combined with bortezomib.

In a GLP-compliant combination toxicity study with bortezomib and gemcitabine, bortezomib was administered iv either alone or in combination with gemcitabine at 0, 0.3, 0.6, 1.0, and 2.0 mg/kg bortezomib (0, 0.9, 1.8, 3.0, and 6.0 mg/m^2) to female BALB/c mice. Bortezomib was administered using the clinical dosing regimen of twice-weekly for two consecutive weeks followed by a week of rest and then twice-weekly for two additional consecutive weeks. Gemcitabine was administered iv once-weekly throughout the study either alone or in combination with bortezomib at 0, 265, and 333 mg/kg/dose (0, 795, and 1000 mg/m^2). Bortezomib-related microscopic lesions included vacuolar changes in the hepatocytes at dosages $\geq$1.0 mg/kg, minimal to moderate axonal degeneration of the sciatic nerve at dosages $\geq$1.0 mg/kg, and skin lesions at the injection sites at all doses. These lesions were not affected by concomitant gemcitabine administration. Bortezomib elicited a dosage-dependent inhibition of 20S proteasome-specific activity (40–65%) 1 h post-dose, which was not affected by coadministration of gemcitabine. The target organ-related toxicities of gemcitabine and bortezomib each appeared to be independent of coadministration. The toxicity of coadministered gemcitabine and bortezomib was additive but not synergistic. These studies indicate that additive toxicity is generally seen when cytotoxic anticancer agents are combined with bortezomib. Therefore, caution is warranted when cytotoxic agents are used in combination with bortezomib.

7.5. Tissue Irritation Study in the Rabbit

A GLP-compliant local tissue irritation study was conducted in male New Zealand white rabbits with the proposed commercial formulation of bortezomib to assess the potential for erythema, edema, and microscopic changes following administration of a single injection either via the intended route of administration (intravenous) or an accidental route of administration. Perivascular (PV), intravenous, subcutaneous and intramuscular (im) routes were examined. Animals were administered 0.1 mg/kg (1.1 mg/m^2) bortezomib at the clinical concentration of 1.0 mg/mL by pv, iv, sc, or im routes. Based on the results of this study, bortezomib was considered a slight tissue irritant when administered at the clinical concentration of 1 mg/mL by iv, pv, and im routes. No tissue reaction was seen after subcutaneous administration. Consistent with these results, the mannitol ester formulation of bortezomib has been well tolerated at the injection site in clinical trials.

7.6. Genotoxicity Studies

GLP-compliant assays were conducted to determine the mutagenicity/clastogenicity of bortezomib in both in vitro and in vivo systems. In the first bacterial reverse mutation assay conducted, bortezomib was plated at concentrations up to 1000 µg/plate and was determined to be negative for mutagenicity. A subsequent bacterial reverse mutation assay was conducted to conform fully to recent ICH guidelines for inclusion of an *Escherichia coli* tester strain. Dosage levels of up to 5000 µg/plate were used. Bortezomib was nonmutagenic in this second bacterial reverse mutation assay. Low recovery of bortezomib in the formulation analyses was observed in the two preliminary and one of the two confirmatory phases of this study. The study was considered adequate since either dosage-limiting toxicity was observed for each tester strain or each tester strain was tested up to the ICH concentration limit in at least one phase of this study with the stated exceptions (TA98 in the absence of S9 and TA1535 in the absence and presence of S9). Bortezomib was determined to be positive for induction of structural aberrations when evaluated at concentrations of 3.125, 12.5, and 100 µg/mL in the in vitro chromosomal aberration test in Chinese hamster ovary cells. However, it was negative for the formation of micronucleated polychromatic erythrocytes in the in vivo mammalian erythrocyte micronucleus test in mice following a single iv dose up to 1 mg/kg (3 mg/m^2; the MTD). The positive response in the in vitro chromosomal aberrations assay is believed to be due to the interruption of the cell cycle and related to the pharmacologic action of proteasome inhibition. The Sponsor has observed consistently positive clastogenicity results with proteasome inhibitors from divergent chemical series (unpublished observations). This general effect of proteasome inhibitors may be caused by cell cycle arrest resulting from the inhibition of proteasome-dependent degradation of cyclins. The absence of micronuclei in the in vivo study is probably a consequence of much lower bortezomib concentrations achievable in vivo due tolerability limitations.

7.7. Immunotoxicity

The immuntoxicologic potential of bortezomib was assessed in two non-GLP studies in mice using twice-weekly intraperitoneal administration for 28 d. In the first study, female BALB/c mice were administered bortezomib twice-weekly ip at 0, 0.3, and 0.6 mg/kg (0, 0.9, and 1.8 mg/m^2). Immunotoxicity was assessed by examining hematology and lymphocyte subset analysis from whole blood, lymph nodes, spleen, and thymus. No toxicologically relevant changes to body weight, hematology, and lymphocyte subset analyses from the blood, lymph nodes, spleen, or thymus were observed. The NOAEL for immunotoxicologic effects with bortezomib was 0.6 mg/kg (1.8 mg/m^2).

The second study was conducted in female SJL/J mice to assess the potential immunomodulatory effects of twice-weekly intraperitoneal administration of bortezomib for 28 d on an active immunization model of autoimmune disease, experimental allergic encephalomyelitis (EAE).

Groups of female SJL/J mice were administered bortezomib twice-weekly ip at 0, 0.5 or 2.0 mg/kg (0, 1.5, and 6.0 mg/m^2) and were immunized with proteolipid peptide, the EAE precipitating antigen, on d 1. Because of considerable clinical toxicity and mortality at 2.0

mg/kg, this dosage level was terminated early, and that group was unavailable for analysis of immunomodulatory effects. There were no bortezomib-related effects at 0.5 mg/kg on body weight, lymphocyte subsets as determined by flow cytometry analysis from whole blood, lymph nodes, spleen, and thymus, hematologic parameters, or the ability of T-cells to respond to a mitogen, specific antigens, or anti-CD3. The NOAEL for immunomodulatory effects with bortezomib was the highest tolerated dosage of 0.5 mg/kg (1.5 mg/m^2). Based on the results of these two immunotoxicity studies in mice up to MTDs, bortezomib was shown not to have adverse immunotoxic or immunomodulatory effects.

7.8. Toxicology Evaluation and Conclusions

The objectives of the nonclinical toxicity program were to establish the pharmacologic safety levels for critical organ systems, establish the potential of bortezomib for genotoxic effects, determine the potential developmental toxicity, identify the target organs of toxicity, assess reversibility to toxicity, determine relationships of toxicity to exposure and PD, examine the potential for important toxicologic drug interactions, and understand the mechanism of potential important toxicities with bortezomib. These objectives have been fully accomplished through the series of studies outlined. The program has conformed to the available worldwide regulatory guidance and contemporary practices for the development of anticancer agents.

7.8.1. TARGET ORGANS OF TOXICITY

Acute lethality has been demonstrated in several species following single intravenous dose administration of bortezomib. The single-dose MTDs of bortezomib administered as an iv bolus dose to mice, rats, female dogs, and monkeys were determined to be 1.0 mg/kg (3.0 mg/m^2), 0.10 mg/kg (0.6 mg/m^2), 0.18 mg/kg (3.6 mg/m^2), and 0.10 mg/kg (1.2 mg/m^2), respectively. Although a definitive cause of acute lethality has not been demonstrated in these studies, results from the cynomolgus monkey cardiovascular safety studies suggest that cardiovascular collapse due to secondary events is the penultimate cause of death. Mechanism-based intervention studies suggest that routine supportive care can abrogate many of the events preceding lethality. Acute toxicity has been most thoroughly studied in the cynomolgus monkey, in which the observed MTD is 1.2 mg/m^2 and the observed minimum lethal dose is 3.0 mg/m^2. Therefore, within a species, there is not a large margin between the MTD and a potentially lethal dose, and this characteristic warrants caution with the appropriate control of administered dosage.

In repeated-dose toxicity studies, the target organs of toxicity have been thoroughly characterized. In rat toxicity studies, the principal target organ systems are dosage-related hyperplastic mucosal changes throughout the GI tract, decreased platelet counts sometimes associated with bone marrow hypocellularity, lymphoid tissue atrophy due to apoptosis of lymphocytes, and increased liver weight with hepatocellular hypertrophy and/or vacuolization. All findings were determined to be partly or completely reversible within 8 wk.

The most important target organ is considered to be proliferative mucosal changes in the GI tract, and these changes are the likely cause of death or moribund sacrifice for unscheduled death of animals in repeated-dose toxicity studies in the rat. These changes may be secondary to low-grade apoptosis and regenerative hyperplasia in this tissue. The pathogenesis of dosage-related decreased platelet counts is not fully known, but it is sometimes associated with visible bone marrow hypocellularity and may be myelosuppressive in origin. The monkey toxicity studies provide a better model to evaluate fully the hematologic effects of bortezomib. Hematopoietic effects are generally not severe and are reversible at and below the MTD. Atrophy of lymphoid tissues through apoptosis of lymphocytes may be a direct proapoptotic pharmacologic effect of bortezomib but may be in part secondary to systemic stress since other target organs of toxicity are seen at all affected dosage levels. In vivo cytochrome P450 enzyme induction studies have not been conducted to determine the likely role of P450 induction as the cause of liver weight increases and hepatocellular hypertrophy. The identification of the GI tract and lymph nodes as target organs correlated with their identification as areas of high concentration of bortezomib-derived radioactivity in QWBA study in rats.

In cynomolgus monkey repeated-dose toxicity studies, effects on the principal target organs were sporadic and sometimes included severe anemia and thrombocytopenia associated with bone marrow suppression, GI intolerance characterized by emesis and diarrhea and associated with GI mucosal hyperplasia, decreased circulating lymphocyte counts and lymphoid tissue atrophy/single cell necrosis, renal tubular degeneration/hypertrophy and/or glomerulopathy, and peripheral neuropathy characterized by axonal degeneration of peripheral sensory nerves.

Partial or full reversal was observed following recovery of up to 8 wk with minimal residual sensory neuropathy, kidney changes, and lymphoid atrophy. Sporadic anemia and thrombocytopenia has been seen at all dosages studied and was the cause of moribund sacrifice for three of four animals in the 9-mo study. The pathogenesis of this change appears to be hematopoietic bone marrow suppression affecting all cell lineages. This toxicity showed a dosage response in incidence and severity but tended to affect some animals within any given dosage group to a greater extent than others. This toxicity was readily monitorable hematologically and showed bone marrow recovery following discontinuation of dosing.

GI intolerance was the most consistent dosage-related toxicity and the likely cause of moribund sacrifice for one early death animal without severe anemia and/or thrombocytopenia from the 38-wk study. The histologic correlate for GI intolerance, as in the rat, is GI mucosal hyperplasia and these changes may be secondary to low-grade apoptosis and regenerative hyperplasia, in this tissue. Decreased circulating lymphocytes and lymphoid tissue atrophy may be a direct effect of bortezomib and may be related to bone marrow and secondary lymphoid organ suppression but is also likely to be partially secondary to systemic stress since other toxicities are seen at all affected dosage levels. Minimal to moderate renal tubular degeneration and hypertrophy and membranous glomerulopathy were observed predominantly in the 38-wk study. These lesions were not associated with evidence of impaired renal function and appeared to be at least partially reversible after an 8-wk recovery period. The mechanism of this bortezomib-related change is not known.

Minimal to moderate peripheral nerve degeneration was observed in both the 4- and 38-wk cynomolgus monkey toxicity studies. This same lesion has also been observed in mice and in dogs (after intraprostatic injection of bortezomib). The lesion was confined to axons associated with the peripheral nervous system, affected only anatomic pathways carrying sensory nerves, and was not associated with degeneration of the nerve cell bodies of the sensory nerve axons. Although full reversibility has not been demonstrated, following an 8-wk recovery period, animals showed partial recovery, and the lack of cell death in the dorsal root ganglia also suggests that eventual recovery would be expected. No primary bortezomib-related lesions were observed in the CNS. The mechanism of bortezomib-induced peripheral neuropathy is not known.

When one considers the most commonly reported adverse events associated with administration of bortezomib in clinical trials, there is good overlap with what is seen in animals, suggesting that the species selected, especially the monkey, have good general predictive power for the human toxicity associated with bortezomib. For example, the most commonly reported adverse events in the pivotal clinical trials (including nausea, vomiting, anorexia, diarrhea, fatigue, pyrexia, thrombocytopenia, and peripheral neuropathy) were either observed or inferred (i.e., nausea) in animal studies. Importantly, all the principal nonclinical toxicities observed show a dosage-response relationship, appear to be readily monitorable, and have been shown to be fully or partially reversible during the recovery periods assessed, as has been the experience in clinical trials.

7.8.2. SAFETY MARGINS

Safety margins for bortezomib have been examined on the basis of dosage (mg/m^2), exposure (AUC), and, to a limited extent, PD (20S proteasome activity). Because of the limited amount of PK/TK data from both nonclinical and clinical studies and the inherent variability of the PD assay, analysis of safety margins using dosage is preferred. For a cytotoxic oncology product, safety margins are most appropriately expressed by comparing the MTD (mg/m2) from comparable studies across species.

The MTD following nine cycles (6 mo) of administration of bortezomib in the rat was 0.10 mg/kg or 0.6 mg/m^2. In the monkey the MTD following 13 cycles (9 mo) was 0.05 mg/kg or 0.6 mg/m^2. The proposed clinical dose in multiple myeloma patients is 1.3 mg/m^2. Thus, the safety margin expressed on the basis of dosage is less than 1 when comparing MTDs from comparable nonclinical studies with the clinical studies. This is not an unusual finding with cytoxic anticancer agents. The ultimate objectives of the nonclinical toxicity studies with products of this type are as follows; to determine a safe starting dose for clinical trials; to characterize the target organs of toxicity and their reversibility in order to predict potential toxicity in humans; to relate nonclinical findings to the experience in humans; and to define mechanisms of important toxicities when appropriate. These objectives have been accomplished. Notably, bortezomib is comparatively well tolerated as a chemotherapeutic agent in humans. Considering these factors and the intended use of bortezomib as a chemotherapeutic agent, the lack of a nonclinical/clinical safety margin is acceptable.

In the definitive toxicity studies, both TK and PD assessments were conducted. In the 6-mo iv toxicity study in rats, the mean AUC_{0-24} and C_{max} at the MTD of 0.10 mg/kg (0.6 mg/m^2) at wk 26 were 134 h·ng/mL and 10.9 ng/mL, respectively, with a mean 20S proteasome (ChT/T) inhibition of 83%. In the 9-mo iv toxicity study in the monkey, the MTD was the lowest dosage studied, 0.05 mg/kg (0.6 mg/m^2) and resulted in mean AUC_{0-24} and C_{max} values of 83.1 h·ng/mL and 48.2 ng/mL at wk 38. The mean peak of 20S proteasome (ChT/T) inhibition was 75% at wk 38 for this dosage. These compare with the best available PK data from cancer patients administered 1.0 mg/m^2: the AUC_{0-24} and C_{max} were 54.0 h·ng/mL and 126 ng/mL (Table 3), respectively, and the mean proteasome inhibition was 60–70%. Therefore, on the basis of AUC, the safety margins are 2.5- and 1.5-fold greater at the MTDs in the rat and monkey, respectively, compared with the human clinical AUC. However, on the basis of C_{max}, the comparable safety margins are less than 1. As described previously, the relationship between plasma concentration and proteasome inhibition is characterized by an E_{max} model in which a plateau of effect is achieved at greater than approx 80% inhibition. The proteasome inhibition data from toxicity studies and clinical trials indicate that the MTD is generally associated with dosages that produce approx 70–80% inhibition.

7.9. Nonclinical Studies Have Provided a Rationale for the Proposed Clinical Dosing Regimen

The pivotal in vivo pharmacology studies with bortezomib were murine xenograft studies. Most cancer chemotherapeutics are administered with dosing strategies that employ an MTD and a regimen that is defined either empirically or on the basis of maximizing overall dose intensity. Because bortezomib works through a novel molecular mechanism, a variety of dose regimens were explored to determine whether a traditional MTD approach was optimal. In a number of in vivo murine tumor models, it has been repeatedly demonstrated that the higher the dosage administered, the greater the antitumor effect until the MTD is surpassed and bortezomib-related toxicity compromises the host's health. These observations justify an MTD dosage strategy in the use of bortezomib.

The PD action of bortezomib is well established and can be measured through an ex vivo assay (20S proteasome activity). Proteasome inhibition is sustained for a duration beyond the time point when bortezomib can reliably be measured in the systemic circulation. Therefore, proteasome inhibition was used as a PD endpoint to guide dosing intervals. In nonclinical and clinical studies, the duration of proteasome inhibition has been shown to have a $t_{1/2}$ of approx 24 h and generally shows return to baseline activity by 72–96 h. Thus, a twice-weekly dosing regimen allows return of proteasome activity toward baseline between administration of individual doses. This theoretical advantage of allowing cells to recover some proteasome function for normal cellular housekeeping functions between doses is supported by the toxicity data described below.

To investigate the effect of the dosing regimen on bortezomib tolerability, pilot studies were conducted comparing daily, every-other-day, twice-weekly (at least 72 h apart) and once-weekly intravenous administration of bortezomib. In these pilot studies in rats, twice-weekly dosing allowed for the administration of the highest MTD of bortezomib compared with daily or every-other-day dosing over a 7–14-d period. In the 2-wk GLP toxicity study in the Sprague-Dawley rat using the twice-weekly dosing regimen, the MTD was 1.5 mg/m². In the developmental toxicity range-finding study in pregnant female Sprague-Dawley rats with daily iv dose administration for 12 d, the MTD was determined to be 0.3 mg/m². Thus, the MTD in the Sprague-Dawley rat is fivefold greater with the twice-weekly regimen compared with daily administration in a comparable duration study. These observations indicate that greater overall dose intensity (both dosage level and total dosage delivered over time) can be accomplished with the twice-weekly regimen compared with daily dose administration.

Results from these toxicity studies, in combination with the observed PD of bortezomib, and the results of the pharmacology xenograft studies support the twice-weekly administration of bortezomib as an appropriate dosing strategy for human use. During the clinical development of bortezomib, it was further determined that a cyclical regimen of twice weekly for 2 wk followed by 1 wk of rest allowed better overall tolerance than the continuous twice-weekly regimen through multiple cycles of administration.

8. CONCLUSIONS

Preclinical studies indicate that proteasome inhibition has both in vitro and in vivo activity against a wide range of cancers. The ability of proteasome inhibitors to reduce or eliminate tumor growth in cell culture and animal tumor models appears to occur through multiple mechanisms, including (1) induction of cell cycle arrest and apoptosis, (2) inhibition of cell proliferation, (3) abrogation of angiogenesis, and (4) interference with tumor cell interactions with the bone marrow microenvironment. Studies of the proteasome inhibitor bortezomib in animal models have indicated that the drug was present and active in almost all tissues studied and that toxic effects were managable, dose-dependent, and reversible.

REFERENCES

1. Hideshima T, Richardson P, Chauhan D, et al. The proteasome inhibitor PS-341 inhibits growth, induces apoptosis, and overcomes drug resistance in human multiple myeloma cells. *Cancer Res* 2001;61:3071–3076.
2. Berenson JR, Ma HM, Vescio R. The role of nuclear factor-κB in the biology and treatment of multiple myeloma. *Semin Oncol* 2001;28:626–633.
3. Masdehors P, Omura S, Merle-Beral H, et al. Increased sensitivity of CLL-derived lymphocytes to apoptotic death activation by the proteasome-specific inhibitor lactacystin. *Br J Haematol* 1999;105:752–757.
4. Delic J, Masdehors P, Omura S, et al. The proteasome inhibitor lactacystin induces apoptosis and sensitizes chemo- and radioresistant human chronic lymphocytic leukaemia lymphocytes to TNF-alpha-initiated apoptosis. *Br J Cancer* 1998;77:1103–1107.
5. Orlowski RZ, Eswara JR, Lafond-Walker A, Grever MR, Orlowski M, Dang CV. Tumor growth inhibition induced in a murine model of human Burkitt's lymphoma by a proteasome inhibitor. *Cancer Res* 1998;58:4342–4348.
6. MacLaren AP, Chapman RS, Wyllie AH, Watson CJ. p53-dependent apoptosis induced by proteasome inhibition in mammary epithelial cells. *Cell Death Differ* 2001;8:210–218.
7. Drexler HC, Risau W, Konerding MA. Inhibition of proteasome function induces programmed cell death in proliferating endothelial cells. *FASEB J* 2000;14:65–77.
8. Kisselev AF, Goldberg AL. Proteasome inhibitors: from research tools to drug candidates. *Chem Biol* 2001;8:739–758.
9. Frankel A, Man S, Elliott P, Adams J, Kerbel RS. Lack of multicellular drug resistance observed in human ovarian and prostate carcinoma treated with the proteasome inhibitor PS-341. *Clin Cancer Res* 2000;6:3719–3728.
10. Almond JB, Snowden RT, Hunter A, Dinsdale D, Cain K, Cohen GM. Proteasome inhibitor-induced apoptosis of B-chronic lymphocytic leukaemia cells involves cytochrome c release and caspase activation, accompanied by formation of an approximately 700 kDa Apaf-1 containing apoptosome complex. *Leukemia* 2001;15:1388–1397.
11. Kumatori A, Tanaka K, Inamura N, et al. Abnormally high expression of proteasomes in human leukemic cells. *Proc Natl Acad Sci USA* 1990;87:7071–7075.
12. Palermo A, Mulligan G, D'Cruz C, et al. Coordinate regulation of proteasome genes in cancer. In: *Proceedings of the 2001 AACR-NCI-EORTC International Conference on Molecular Targets and Cancer Therapeutics*, 2001:7.
13. LeBlanc R, Catley LP, Hideshima T, et al. Proteasome inhibitor PS-341 inhibits human myeloma cell growth in vivo and prolongs survival in a murine model. *Cancer Res* 2002;62:4996–5000.
14. Grimm LM, Goldberg AL, Poirier GG, Schwartz LM, Osborne BA. Proteasomes play an essential role in thymocyte apoptosis. *EMBO J* 1996;15:3835–3844.
15. Sadoul R, Fernandez PA, Quiquerez AL et al. Involvement of the proteasome in the programmed cell death of NGF-deprived sympathetic neurons. *EMBO J* 1996;15:3845–3852.
16. Theuer J, Dechend R, Muller DN et al. Angiotensin II induced inflammation in the kidney and in the heart of double transgenic rats. *BMC Cardiovasc Disord* 2002;2:3.
17. Chen C, Edelstein LC, Gelinas C. The Rel/NF-κB family directly activates expression of the apoptosis inhibitor Bcl-x$_L$. *Mol Cell Biol* 2000;20:2687–2695.

18. Wang CY, Mayo MW, Korneluk RG, Goeddel DV, Baldwin AS Jr. NF-κB antiapoptosis: induction of TRAF1 and TRAF2 and c-IAP1 and c-IAP2 to suppress caspase-8 activation. *Science* 1998;281:1680–1683.

19. Bancroft CC, Chen Z, Dong G, et al. Coexpression of proangiogenic factors IL-8 and VEGF by human head and neck squamous cell carcinoma involves coactivation by MEK-MAPK and IKK-NF-kappaB signal pathways. *Clin Cancer Res* 2001;7:435–442.

20. Chauhan D, Uchiyama H, Akbarali Y, et al. Multiple myeloma cell adhesion-induced interleukin-6 expression in bone marrow stromal cells involves activation of NF-κB. *Blood* 1996;87:1104–1112.

21. Naujokat C, Sezer O, Zinke H, Leclere A, Hauptmann S, Possinger K. Proteasome inhibitors induced caspase-dependent apoptosis and accumulation of p21[WAF1/Cip1] in human immature leukemic cells. *Eur J Haematol* 2000;65:221–236.

22. Wagenknecht B, Hermisson M, Groscurth P, Liston P, Krammer PH, Weller M. Proteasome inhibitor-induced apoptosis of glioma cells involves the processing of multiple caspases and cytochrome c release. *J Neurochem* 2000;75:2288–2297.

23. Fan XM, Wong BC, Wang WP, et al. Inhibition of proteasome function induced apoptosis in gastric cancer. *Int J Cancer* 2001;93:481–488.

24. Adams J, Behnke M, Chen S, et al. Potent and selective inhibitors of the proteasome: dipeptidyl boronic acids. *Bioorg Med Chem Lett* 1998;8:333–338.

25. Adams J, Palombella VJ, Sausville EA, et al. Proteasome inhibitors: a novel class of potent and effective antitumor agents. *Cancer Res* 1999;59:2615–2622.

26. Teicher BA, Ara G, Herbst R, Palombella VJ, Adams J. The proteasome inhibitor PS-341 in cancer therapy. *Clin Cancer Res* 1999;5:2638–2645.

27. Shah SA, Potter MW, McDade TP, et al. 26S proteasome inhibition induces apoptosis and limits growth of human pancreatic cancer. *J Cell Biochem* 2001;82:110–122.

28. Sunwoo JB, Chen Z, Dong G, et al. Novel proteasome inhibitor PS-341 inhibits activation of nuclear factor-κB, cell survival, tumor growth, and angiogenesis in squamous cell carcinoma. *Clin Cancer Res* 2001;7:1419–1428.

29. Ogiso Y, Tomida A, Lei S, Omura S, Tsuruo T. Proteasome inhibition circumvents solid tumor resistance to topoisomerase II-directed drugs. *Cancer Res* 2000;60:2429–2434.

30. Pham L, Tamayo A, Lo P, Yoshimura L, Ford RJ. Antitumor activity of the proteasome inhibitor PS-341 in mantle cell lymphoma B cells. *Blood* 2001;98:465a.

31. Feinman R, Gangurde P, Miller S et al. Proteasome inhibitor PS-341 inhibits constitutive NF-κB activation and bypasses the anti-apoptotic bcl-2 signal in human multiple myeloma cells. *Blood* 2001;98:640a.

32. Herrmann JL, Briones F, Jr, Brisbay S, Logothetis CJ, McDonnell TJ. Prostate carcinoma cell death resulting from inhibition of proteasome activity is independent of functional Bcl-2 and p53. *Oncogene* 1998;17:2889–2899.

33. An WG, Hwang SG, Trepel JB, Blagosklonny MV. Protease inhibitor-induced apoptosis: accumulation of wt p53, p21WAF1/CIP1, and induction of apoptosis are independent markers of proteasome inhibition. *Leukemia* 2000;14:1276–1283.

34. Oyaizu H, Adachi Y, Okumura T et al. Proteasome inhibitor 1 enhances paclitaxel-induced apoptosis in human lung adenocarcinoma cell line. *Oncol Rep* 2001;8:825–829.

35. Soligo D, Servida F, Delia D et al. The apoptogenic response of human myeloid leukaemia cell lines and of normal and malignant haematopoietic progenitor cells to the proteasome inhibitor PSI. *Br J Haematol* 2001;113:126–135.

36. Li QQ, Yunmbam MK, Zhong X et al. Lactacystin enhances cisplatin sensitivity in resistant human ovarian cancer cell lines via inhibition of DNA repair and ERCC-1 expression. *Cell Mol Biol* (Noisy-le-grand) 2001;47 Online Pub:OL61–OL72.

37. Bold RJ, Virudachalam S, McConkey DJ. Chemosensitization of pancreatic cancer by inhibition of the 26S proteasome. *J Surg Res* 2001;100:11–17.

38. Cusack JC Jr, Liu R, Houston M et al. Enhanced chemosensitivity to CPT-11 with proteasome inhibitor PS-341: implications for systemic nuclear factor-kappaB inhibition. *Cancer Res* 2001;61:3535–3540.

39. Williams S, Logothetis CJ, Papandreou C, McConkey DJ. Preclinical evaluation of PS-341-based combination chemotherapy in prostate cancer. In: *Proceedings of the American Association for Cancer Research*, 2001:7.

40. Gatto SR, Scappini B, Verstovsek S et al. In vitro effects of PS-341 alone and in combination with STI571 in BCR-ABL positive cell lines both sensitive and resistant to STI571. *Blood* 2001;98:101a.

41. Pink M, Pien CS, Worland P, Adams J, Kauffman MG. PS-341 enhances chemotherapeutic effect in human xenograft models. In: *Proceedings of the American Association for Cancer Research*, 2002;43:158.

42. Mitsiades CS, Treon SP, Mitsiades N, et al. TRAIL/Apo2L ligand selectively induces apoptosis and overcomes drug resistance in multiple myeloma: therapeutic applications. *Blood* 2001;98:795–804.

43. Sayers TJ, Brooks A, Seki N, Murphy WJ, Elliott P. The proteasome inhibitor PS-341 sensitizes tumor cells to TRAIL-mediated apoptosis. In: *Proceedings of the 2001 AACR-NCI-EORTC International Conference on Molecular Targets and Cancer Therapeutics*, 2001;7.

44. Mimnaugh EG, Neckers L. Biologic rationale for the combination of an Hsp90 antagonist with a proteasome inhibitor. In: *Proceedings of the 2001 AACR-NCI-EORTC International Conference on Molecular Targets and Cancer Therapeutics*, 2001:7.

45. Pajonk F, Pajonk K, McBride WH. Apoptosis and radiosensitization of Hodgkin cells by proteasome inhibition. *Int J Radiat Oncol Biol Phys* 2000;47:1025–1032.

46. Ng B, Kramer E, Devitt ML et al. Proteasome inhibitor, PS-341, enhances in vitro radiosensitivity of human breast cancer cells treated with radiotherapy or radioimmunotherapy. In: *Proceedings of the 2001 AACR-NCI-EORTC International Conference on Molecular Targets and Cancer Therapeutics*, 2001:7.

47. Russo SM, Tepper JE, Baldwin AS et al. Enhancement of radiosensitivity by proteasome inhibition: implications for a role of NF-κB. *Int J Radiat Oncol Biol Phys* 2001;50:183–193.

48. Pervan M, Pajonk F, Sun JR, Withers HR, McBride WH. Molecular pathways that modify tumor radiation response. *Am J Clin Oncol* 2001;24:481–485.

49. Kurland JF, Meyn RE. Protease inhibitors restore radiation-induced apoptosis to Bcl-2- expressing lymphoma cells. *Int J Cancer* 2001;96:327–333.

50. Chandra J, Niemer I, Gilbreath J et al. Proteasome inhibitors induce apoptosis in glucocorticoid-resistant chronic lymphocytic leukemic lymphocytes. *Blood* 1998;92:4220–4229.

51. McConkey DJ, Pahler JC, Szanto S, Faderl S, Keating M. Efficacy and mechanisms of proteasome inhibitor-induced apoptosis in chronic lymphocytic leukemia. In: *Proceedings of the 2001 AACR-NCI-EORTC International Conference on Molecular Targets and Cancer Therapeutics*, 2001:7.

52. Ma MH, Parker KM, Manyak S et al. Proteasome inhibitor PS-341 markedly enhances sensitivity of multiple myeloma cells to chemotherapeutic agents and overcomes chemoresistance through inhibition of the NF-kappaB pathway. *Blood* 2001;98:437a.

53. Williams SA, Papandreou C, McConkey D. Preclinical effects of proteasome inhibitor PS-341 in combination chemotherapy for prostate cancer. In: *Proceedings of the American Society of Clinical Oncology-37th Annual Meeting*, 2001;20:169b.

54. Gumerlock PH, Moisan LP, Lau AH, Mack PC, Lara PN, Gandara DR. Docetaxel followed by PS-341 results in phosphorylation and stabilization of p27 and increases response in non-small cell lung carcinoma (NSCLC). *Clin Cancer Res* 2001;7:157.

55. Pienta KJ. Preclinical mechanisms of action of docetaxel and docetaxel combinations in prostate cancer. *Semin Oncol* 2001;28:3–7.

56. Chadebech P, Brichese L, Baldin V, Vidal S, Valette A. Phosphorylation and proteasome-dependent degradation of Bcl-2 in mitotic-arrested cells after microtubule damage. *Biochem Biophys Res Commun* 1999;262:823–827.

57. Adams J. Development of the proteasome inhibitor PS-341. *Oncologist* 2002;7:9–16.

58. Steiner P, Neumeier H, Lightcap ES, et al. Generation of PS-341-adapted human multiple myeloma cells as experimental tools for analysis of proteasome function in cancer. *Blood* 2001;98:310a.

59. Wang CY, Cusack JC Jr, Liu R, Baldwin AS Jr. Control of inducible chemoresistance: enhanced anti-tumor therapy through increased apoptosis by inhibition of NF-κB. *Nat Med* 1999;5:412–417.

60. Wang CY, Guttridge DC, Mayo MW, Baldwin AS, Jr. NF-κB induces expression of the Bcl-2 homologue A1/Bfl-1 to preferentially suppress chemotherapy-induced apoptosis. *Mol Cell Biol* 1999;19:5923–5929.

61. Cusack JC, Liu R, Baldwin AS. NF-kappa B and chemoresistance: potentiation of cancer drugs via inhibition of NF-kappa B. *Drug Resist Updat* 1999;2:271–273.

62. Shain KH, Landowski TH, Dalton WS. The tumor microenvironment as a determinant of cancer cell survival: a possible mechanism for de novo drug resistance. *Curr Opin Oncol* 2000;12:557–563.

63. Damiano JS, Cress AE, Hazlehurst LA, Shtil AA, Dalton WS. Cell adhesion mediated drug resistance (CAM-DR): role of integrins and resistance to apoptosis in human myeloma cell lines. *Blood* 1999;93:1658–1667.

64. Uchiyama H, Barut BA, Mohrbacher AF, Chauhan D, Anderson KC. Adhesion of human myeloma-derived cell lines to bone marrow stromal cells stimulates interleukin-6 secretion. *Blood* 1993;82:3712–3720.

65. Hideshima T, Chauhan D, Schlossman R, Richardson P, Anderson KC. The role of tumor necrosis factor alpha in the pathophysiology of human multiple myeloma: therapeutic applications. *Oncogene* 2001;20:4519–4527.

66. Hideshima T, Chauhan D, Podar K, Schlossman RL, Richardson P, Anderson KC. Novel therapies targeting the myeloma cell and its bone marrow microenvironment. *Semin Oncol* 2001;28:607–612.

67. Landowski TH, Dalton WS. Myeloma cell adhesion to fibronectin activates NF-κB and induces the expression of genes contributing to cell adhesion-mediated drug resistance. *Blood* 2001;98:377a.

68. Oikawa T, Sasaki T, Nakamura M et al. The proteasome is involved in angiogenesis. *Biochem Biophys Res Commun* 1998;246:243–248.

69. Rottman J, Csizmadia V, Ozkaynak E, Kadambi V, Ganley K, Cardoza K. Investigative cardiovascular study of the proteasome inhibitor PS-341 in the mouse. Presented at the 42nd Annual Meeting of the Society of Toxicology, March 9–13, 2003, Salt Lake City, UT.

70. Lightcap ES, McCormack TA, Pien CS, Chau V, Adams J, Elliott PJ. Proteasome inhibition measurements: clinical application. *Clin Chem* 2000;46:673–683.

71. Csizmadia V, Rottman J, Bouchard P, Raczynski A, Juedes M, White P. The proteasome inhibitor PS-341 induces COX-2 in murine and human endothelial cells. Presented at the 42nd Annual Meeting of the Society of Toxicology, March 9–13, 2003, Salt Lake City, UT.

72. Bargou RC, Leng C, Krappmann D, et al. High-level nuclear NF-κB and Oct-2 is a common feature of cultured Hodgkin/Reed-Sternberg cells. *Blood* 1996;87:4340–4347.

73. Davis RE, Brown KD, Siebenlist U, Staudt LM. Constitutive nuclear factor κB activity is required for survival of activated B cell-like diffuse large B cell lymphoma cells. *J Exp Med* 2001;194:1861–1874.

74. Rath PC, Aggarwal BB. Antiproliferative effects of IFN-α correlate with the downregulation of nuclear factor-κB in human Burkitt lymphoma Daudi cells. *J Interferon Cytokine Res* 2001;21:523–528.

75. Wolchok JD, Goodman AR, Vilcek J. Activation of NF-κB may be necessary but is not sufficient for induction of H-2 antigens by TNF in J558L murine myeloma cells. *J Leukoc Biol* 1994;55:7–12.

76. Borset M, Hjorth-Hansen H, Johnsen AC, et al. Apoptosis, proliferation and NF-κB activation induced by agonistic Fas antibodies in the human myeloma cell line OH-2: amplification of Fas-mediated apoptosis by tumor necrosis factor. *Eur J Haematol* 1999;63:345–353.

77. Feinman R, Koury J, Thames M, Barlogie B, Epstein J, Siegel DS. Role of NF-κB in the rescue of multiple myeloma cells from glucocorticoid-induced apoptosis by bcl-2. *Blood* 1999;93:3044–3052.

78. Mori N, Fujimori M, Ikeda S, et al. Constitutive activation of NF-κB in primary adult T-cell leukemia cells. *Blood* 1999;93:2360–2368.

79. Kordes U, Krappmann D, Heissmeyer V, Ludwig WD, Scheidereit C. Transcription factor NF-κB is constitutively activated in acute lymphoblastic leukemia cells. *Leukemia* 2000;14:399–402.

80. Furman RR, Asgary Z, Mascarenhas JO, Liou HC, Schattner EJ. Modulation of NF-κB activity and apoptosis in chronic lymphocytic leukemia B cells. *J Immunol* 2000;164:2200–2206.

81. Munzert G, Kreitmeier S, Bergmann L. Normal structure of NFκB2, C-REL and BCL-3 gene loci in lymphoproliferative and myeloproliferative disorders. *Leuk Lymphoma* 2000;38:395–400.

82. Guzman ML, Neering SJ, Upchurch D, et al. Nuclear factor-κB is constitutively activated in primitive human acute myelogenous leukemia cells. *Blood* 2001;98:2301–2307.

83. Lindholm PF, Bub J, Kaul S, Shidham VB, Kajdacsy-Balla A. The role of constitutive NF-κB activity in PC-3 human prostate cancer cell invasive behavior. *Clin Exp Metastasis* 2001;18:471–479.

84. Gasparian AV, Yao YJ, Kowalczyk D, et al. The role of IKK in constitutive activation of NF-κB transcription factor in prostate carcinoma cells. *J Cell Sci* 2002;115:141–151.

85. Nakshatri H, Bhat-Nakshatri P, Martin DA, Goulet RJ Jr, Sledge GW Jr. Constitutive activation of NF-κB during progression of breast cancer to hormone-independent growth. *Mol Cell Biol* 1997;17:3629–3639.

86. Sovak MA, Bellas RE, Kim DW, et al. Aberrant nuclear factor-κB/Rel expression and the pathogenesis of breast cancer. *J Clin Invest* 1997;100:2952–2960.

87. Palayoor ST, Youmell MY, Calderwood SK, Coleman CN, Price BD. Constitutive activation of IκB kinase α and NF-κB in prostate cancer cells is inhibited by ibuprofen. *Oncogene* 1999;18:7389–7394.

88. Bours V, Dejardin E, Goujon-Letawe F, Merville MP, Castronovo V. The NF-κB transcription factor and cancer: high expression of NF-κB- and IκB-related proteins in tumor cell lines. *Biochem Pharmacol* 1994;47:145–149.

89. Reuning U, Wilhelm O, Nishiguchi T, et al. Inhibition of NF-κB-Rel A expression by antisense oligodeoxynucleotides suppresses synthesis of urokinase-type plasminogen activator (uPA) but not its inhibitor PAI-1. *Nucleic Acids Res* 1995;23:3887–3893.

90. Grundker C, Schulz K, Gunthert AR, Emons G. Luteinizing hormone-releasing hormone induces nuclear factor κB-activation and inhibits apoptosis in ovarian cancer cells. *J Clin Endocrinol Metab* 2000;85:3815–3820.

91. Lind DS, Hochwald SN, Malaty J, et al. Nuclear factor-κ B is upregulated in colorectal cancer. *Surgery* 2001;130:363–369.

92. Wang W, Abbruzzese JL, Evans DB, Larry L, Cleary KR, Chiao PJ. The nuclear factor-κB RelA transcription factor is constitutively activated in human pancreatic adenocarcinoma cells. *Clin Cancer Res* 1999;5:119–127.

93. Arlt A, Vorndamm J, Muerkoster S, et al. Autocrine production of interleukin 1β confers constitutive nuclear factor kB activity and chemoresistance in pancreatic carcinoma cell lines. *Cancer Res* 2002;62:910–916.

94. Mukhopadhyay T, Roth JA, Maxwell SA. Altered expression of the p50 subunit of the NF-κB transcription factor complex in non-small cell lung carcinoma. *Oncogene* 1995;11:999–1003.

20 Phase I Trials

Bortezomib Alone and in Combination With Standard Chemotherapies

Dixie-Lee W. Esseltine and David P. Schenkein

Contents

ABSTRACT

The Phase I development of the proteasome inhibitor, bortezomib (formerly known as PS-341), in patients with advanced cancer began in 1998. Since that time clinical trials have studied both single agent bortezomib and bortezomib in combination with other chemotherapy agents. The side effect profile that has emerged from dose escalation trials suggests manageable toxicities. Gastrointestinal side effects such as diarrhea and nausea were dose-related and peripheral sensory neuropathy was dose-limiting in some patients with solid tumors. Indications of efficacy in multiple myeloma (including a durable complete remission), non-Hodgkin's lymphoma, and selected solid tumors were also reported. The recommended dose and schedule for Phase II development was 1.3 mg/m^2/dose given twice weekly for 2 wk with 10 d rest.

Key Words

PS-341, Phase 1 trials, bortezomib.

1. INTRODUCTION

Bortezomib, a modified dipeptidyl boronic acid derived from leucine and phenylalanine, is a novel chemical entity that potently, specifically, and reversibly inhibits the proteolytic activity of the proteasome. Because numerous proteins involved in cell cycle control and apoptosis have been shown to be regulated by proteasome degradation, proteasome inhibition was of interest for its potential application to the treatment of

From: *Cancer Drug Discovery and Development: Proteasome Inhibitors in Cancer Therapy*
Edited by: J. Adams © Humana Press Inc., Totowa, NJ

cancer. Importantly, numerous published studies have reported that cancer cells are more sensitive to the proapoptotic effects of proteasome inhibition than nontransformed normal cells (1–8). In the in vitro cytotoxicity screen conducted by the National Cancer Institute (NCI) in 60 cell lines, bortezomib demonstrated potent cytotoxicity, with a distinct cytotoxicity pattern compared with a historical file of approx 60,000 compounds studied in this screen (9). Additionally, bortezomib affected tumor growth in a wide variety of solid tumor xenograft models, both as a single agent and in combination with chemotherapy and radiation. In the single-agent preclinical studies, the efficacy of bortezomib was dose-dependent, and the agent was most effective when administered at or near the maximum tolerated dose (MTD). Once-weekly and twice-weekly schedules of administration were tolerated in nonhuman primates (10). As measured by an in vitro assay (11), intermittent proteasome inhibition was better tolerated across species, and greater toxicity was observed at higher levels of proteasome inhibition as measured with the 20S assay (12).

Because bortezomib has advanced to phase III trials and has been studied in hundreds of patients both as a single agent and in combination with other drugs, it is appropriate to review the phase I studies that initiated the human development of this compound. Several combination trials are being supported by Millennium Pharmaceuticals (Cambridge, MA) (see Table 3), and more than 20 phase I and phase II studies are ongoing at NCI-Cancer Treatment Evaluation Program (NCI-CTEP) cancer centers throughout North America. Information on NCI-CTEP–sponsored bortezomib trials is available on the NCI's web site (http://www.cancer.gov/search/clinical_trials).

The human clinical development of bortezomib began in 1998 when the first patient was dosed with bortezomib in a phase I dose-escalation cancer trial at the M.D. Anderson Cancer Center (MDACC; Houston, TX) (13). Based on the MTD in nonhuman primates of 0.8 mg/m^2, the initial dose was 0.13 mg/m^2 (i.e., one-sixth of the MTD observed in monkeys). Subsequently, two other phase I dose-escalation trials were initiated at Memorial Sloan-Kettering Cancer Center (MSKCC; New York, NY) and at the Lineberger Comprehensive Cancer Center/University of North Carolina (LCC/UNC; Chapel Hill, NC). Table 1 shows that these three phase I dose-escalation studies examined three schedules of drug administration in patients with advanced hematologic or solid tumors. One schedule required the drug to be administered intravenously once weekly for 4 wk (the least dose intensive), another twice weekly for 2 wk (moderate intensity), and another twice weekly for 4 wk (the most intensive). Each treatment period was followed by a period of rest (10–17 d). The primary objectives of these studies were to establish the bortezomib-related dose-limiting toxicities (DLTs) and the MTD of bortezomib in the patient population studied. The secondary objectives were to define further the pharmacodynamics (PD), the pharmacokinetics (PK), and the antitumor activity of bortezomib.

Achieving the pharmacodynamic objectives required an assay to show that bortezomib effectively inhibited its target, the chymotryptic-like peptidase activity of the proteasome (11). Nonclinical studies had demonstrated that proteasome inhibition measured after

Table 1
Millennium-Sponsored Single-Agent Phase I Bortezomib Trials

Testing center (study no.)	Treatment schedule	Cycle length (d)	DLT (mg/m^2)	MTD (mg/m^2)
MDACC (98-194)	1×/wk × 4 wk	35	2.0 and 1.8	1.6
MSKCC (98-104)	2×/wk × 2 wk	21	1.56	1.3
UNC/MSKCC (9834 and 0031)	2×/wk × 4 wk	42	1.38, 1.2	1.04

DLT, dose-limiting toxicity; MDACC; M.D. Anderson Cancer Center; MSKCC, Memorial Sloan-Kettering Cancer Center; MTD, maximum tolerated dose; UNC; University of North Carolina.

dosing was both dose-dependent and reversible across species *(14)*. This assay, therefore, was critical to the early clinical development of bortezomib.

2. PHASE I SINGLE-AGENT TRIAL RESULTS

2.1. Phase I Study in Advanced Solid Tumors: Primarily Patients With Androgen-Independent Prostate Cancer

The phase I dose-escalation study conducted at the MDACC enrolled 53 patients with advanced solid tumors, 48 of whom had a diagnosis of androgen-independent prostrate cancer (AIPC) *(15)*. Bortezomib was administered once weekly for 4 wk, followed by 14 d of rest after the fourth dose (Table 1). Dose escalation proceeded from 0.13 mg/m^2/dose to 2.0 mg/m^2/dose. Patients received a mean of 10 doses (range, 1–57 doses). The total number of completed cycles was 128, and 29 of 53 patients (55%) completed at least two treatment cycles.

Preliminary data from this trial in patients with AIPC have been presented *(12–14,16,17)*. Papandreou et al. *(12)* reported that the extent of bortezomib-induced proteasome inhibition achieved in the whole blood of 45 patients was dose-dependent and that no grade 3 toxicities were reported in the 37 patients whose proteasome inhibition did not exceed 65%. In contrast, some patients who attained proteasome inhibition greater than 70% (n = 33) experienced grade 3 hypotension (n = 1), diarrhea (n = 2), and fatigue (n = 1), and patients who progressed on to cycle 2 were more likely to suffer greater intensities of toxicities *(12)*. Additionally, the serum level of interleukin-6 (sIL-6) was measured in 41 AIPC patients with metastatic bone disease *(17)*, and it was shown that patients who achieved over 70% proteasome inhibition experienced decreases in sIL-6 levels that correlated with the dose of bortezomib received. Similarly, a dose-dependent decline in prostate-specific antigen (PSA) slope was observed, and patients reported decreases in B symptoms *(17)*. Evidence of antitumor activity was seen in two prostate cancer patients; both experienced a partial response (PR), as evidenced by a reduction in the size of retroperitoneal lymph nodes. One patient also had a 50% reduction in PSA. These patients were treated at doses of 0.4 and 1.6 mg/m^2/dose, respectively. DLTs occurred at doses of 1.8 and 2.0 mg/m^2 and included diarrhea, syncope, and orthostatic hypotension. The MTD for this schedule of administration was determined to be 1.6 mg/m^2/dose.

Nix et al. *(14,18)* have reported the preliminary PK results from this study based on samples from 24 of the 26 patients treated at doses of 1.45–2.0 mg/m^2. The PK profile fits a two-compartment model, with a rapid initial (α) distribution half-life (30 min), followed by a more sustained terminal (β) elimination half-life (8.7–14.8 h). No clear dose relationship was observed in the values of C_{max} over this limited dose range, but a trend of increased exposure (AUC$_{INF}$) to bortezomib was observed. After dose administration, the distribution of bortezomib in the systemic circulation was rapid and extensive. Estimates of the mean volume of distribution exhibited a wide range, from 721 to 1270 L, and steady-state volumes of distribution ranged from 416 to 979 L. Figure 1 displays, by dose group, the mean plasma bortezomib profiles among patients treated with a single dose of 1.45, 1.6, 1.8, and 2.0 mg/m^2.

Blood samples were taken and assessed for proteasome inhibition in the 20S proteasome assay in 45 patients at all dose levels. The maximum percentage inhibition of 20S proteasome activity was observed within 1 h after dosing. This was a dose-dependent increase in the mean percentage inhibition of 20S proteasome activity consistent with a sigmoid model of maximum obtainable effect (E_{max}). At 1 h after the first bortezomib dose on d 1, cycle 1, the E_{max} model showed a relatively steep dose-response curve up to 1.3 mg/m^2, followed by a tendency to plateau at higher doses, with a calculated median effective dose (ED)$_{50}$ of 0.89 mg/m^2 and an E_{max} of 92%. The time-course of inhibition of 20S proteasome activity showed a progressive and substantial return toward predose levels from a postdose peak at 1 h through the next 7 d, although a few patients experienced a complete return to pretreatment baseline in 20S proteasome activity before the subsequent dose.

The relationship between plasma bortezomib concentrations and the extent of proteasome inhibition was evaluated in 21 patients for whom combined PK/PD data points were available. Such a concentration-effect relationship was well characterized by a simple E_{max} model with a steep slope up to plasma concentrations of 3 ng/mL, followed by a plateau. The median effective concentration (EC)$_{50}$ plasma concentration relationship with 20S proteasome inhibition was calculated to be 1.48 ng/mL.

2.2. Phase I Study in Advanced Solid Tumors

Aghajanian and colleagues at MSKCC *(19)* conducted a phase I trial of bortezomib in patients with a variety of advanced solid tumors. Investigators administered iv doses of bortezomib ranging from 0.13 to 1.56 mg/m^2 given twice weekly for 2 wk, followed by 10 d of rest (Table 1). A total of 89 cycles of treatment were administered in 43 heavily pretreated patients. At this dosing schedule, the MTD was found to be 1.3 mg/m^2, with dose-limiting diarrhea and sensory neuropathy occurring in some patients at the 1.56-mg/m^2 dose level. Grade 3 diarrhea was seen in 2 of 12 patients treated at the highest dose, but each of these patients responded to loperamide treatment. Additionally, 2 of 12 patients treated with 1.56 mg/m^2 bortezomib experienced a painful grade 3 peripheral sensory neuropathy, as did 1 patient at the 1.3-mg/m^2 dose level. No hematologic DLTs were noted. Other side effects were fatigue, fever, anorexia, nausea, vomiting, rash, pruritus, and headache. One patient with non-small cell lung cancer (bronchioloalveolar type) experienced a partial response to therapy *(19)*. This patient had received prior

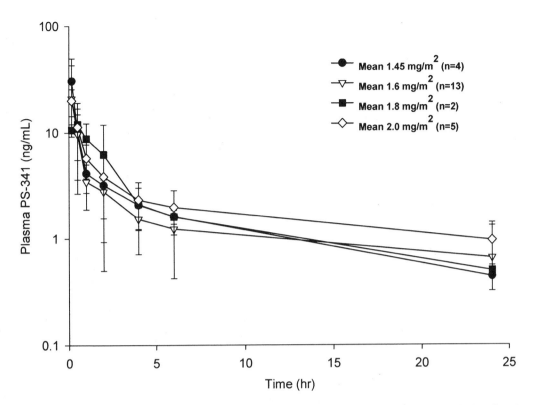

Fig. 1. Mean single-dose plasma bortezomib (PS-341) profiles. (Reprinted with permission from Nix D, et al. Clinical development of a proteasome inhibitor, PS-341, for the treatment of cancer. In: *Proceedings of the American Society of Clinical Oncology-37th Annual Meeting*, 2001;20:86a.)

therapy with at least five regimens that included neurotoxic agents. Symptomatic improvement was noted after one cycle. Although therapy was stopped because of neuropathy, the response lasted approximately 3 mo. Three other patients (with nasopharyngeal carcinoma, metastatic melanoma, and renal cell carcinoma) had stable disease for 2.5–5 mo.

The level of proteasome inhibition at 1 h was dose-related. The 20S proteasome assay showed that six patients in the 1.56-mg/m^2 dose cohort had an absolute percentage inhibition of over 80% at one time point at least (data on file, Millennium Pharmaceuticals). The mean percentage inhibition at 1 h was over 60% in patients treated at doses between 1.0 and 1.5 mg/m^2 bortezomib. No patient had value greater than 80% in those dose cohorts.

2.3. Phase I Study in Advanced Hematologic Malignancies

Patients with advanced hematologic malignancies were eligible for a phase I bortezomib trial conducted at two centers, the LCC/UNC and MSKCC. Patients in this study received intravenous doses of drug twice a week for 4 wk followed by 14 d of rest *(20)*. In total, 27 patients received 293 doses of drug, and 24 complete cycles were administered. The MTD was determined to be 1.04 mg/m^2 with this dosing regimen. DLTs observed at doses greater than 1.04 mg/m^2 were hyponatremia, hypokalemia, fatigue, and malaise. Although not defined as dose-limiting by protocol, grade 3 thrombocytopenia did lead to doses being held or modified in this study. Continued therapy also revealed one case of postural hypotension, one systemic hypersensitivity reaction, and a grade 4 elevation in liver enzymes in a patient with hepatitis C and excess acetaminophen ingestion.

In nine evaluable, heavily pretreated patients with plasma cell dyscrasias who completed one cycle, there was one complete response, and eight patients experienced variable reductions in paraprotein levels and/or bone marrow plasmacytosis [20]. One patient with mantle cell lymphoma and another with follicular cell lymphoma had reductions in nodal tumors (Table 2) documented as partial responses, both of which were durable [20].

The 20S proteasome inhibition was determined to be time- and dose-dependent, with an incomplete return to normal of proteasome inhibition prior to the next dose without obvious clinical consequences.

3. PRELIMINARY PHASE I COMBINATION TREATMENT TRIAL RESULTS

Phase I combination studies were initiated based on bortezomib's ability to enhance the effects of standard chemotherapies in solid tumor xenograft models—in particular, its activity in combination with gemcitabine in a pancreatic cancer model [21], with CPT-11 in colon and pancreatic cancer models [22,23], and with docetaxel in an ovarian cancer model [24]. Subsequently, an investigator-sponsored trial, developed by Orlowski and Dees [25] based on their work at UNC at Chapel Hill with anthracyclines in combination with bortezomib, explored the use of bortezomib with a pegylated liposomal doxorubicin (Doxil) [26]. Zangari and colleagues [27] have also investigated the combination of bortezomib and thalidomide in resistant myeloma in a phase I dose-escalation study.

Preliminary results from these phase I combination trials were reported at the 2002 annual meetings of the American Society of Clinical Oncology and the American Society of Hematology [26–29]. Limited follow-up data are available. In the bortezomib/ gemcitabine combination trial [28,30], bortezomib was given twice weekly, on d 1, 4, 8, and 11, and gemcitabine was given once weekly, on d 1 and 8, to a total of 31 patients (Table 3). The MTD in previously treated patients was determined to be 1.0 mg/m^2 bortezomib and 1000 mg/m^2 gemcitabine. There was no evidence of additive toxicity in patients receiving the combination. DLTs were observed in two patients within the expanded cohort of patients receiving 1.0 mg/m^2 bortezomib and 1000 mg/m^2 gemcitabine and included grade 3 thrombocytopenia and grade 3 leukopenia [30]. Four of four patients receiving 1.3 mg/m^2 bortezomib and 800 mg/m^2 gemcitabine experienced DLTs, which included transient neutropenia (grade 4), small bowel obstruction (grade 3), nausea and vomiting (grade 3), and two episodes of transient thrombocytopenia (grade 3). Two of four chemotherapy-naïve patients also experienced DLTs, with one myocardial infarction and one grade 3 transaminitis. A PR was documented (by response evaluation criteria in solid tumors [RECIST] criteria) in one of five patients with relapsed metastatic non-small cell lung cancer [30]. PD and PK results are pending.

Preliminary findings of a clinical trial of bortezomib in combination with irinotecan in a similar 21-d cycle were also recently reported [29,31]. Bortezomib was given on d 1, 4, 8, and 11, and a 90-min irinotecan infusion was given on d 1 and 8, to a total of 51 patients. The MTD of this study has been determined to be 1.3 mg/m^2 bortezomib and 125 mg/m^2 irinotecan [31], with two of five patients having DLTs at the 1.5/125-mg/m^2 dose

Table 2

Reported Antitumor Activity from Single-Agent Bortezomib Phase I Trials

Malignancy	No./cell type treated (ITT)[a]	Evaluation criteria	Treatment schedule
Non-small cell lung cancer (bronchioloalveolar type)[b]	1/8	Radiograph (CT)	2×/wk × 2; 1.56 mg/m^2
Mantle cell lymphoma[c]	1/3	Radiograph (CT)	2×/wk × 4; 1.38 mg/m^2
Follicular cell lymphoma[c]	1/1	Radiograph (CT)	2×/wk × 4; 1.38 mg/m^2
Multiple myeloma[c]	9/11	Quantitative immunoglobulins (immunofixation) Bone marrow	2×/wk × 4; 1.04 mg/m^2 and 1.2 mg/m^2
Waldenstrom's macroglobulinemia[c]	1/1	IgM Bone marrow	2×/wk × 4; 1.2 mg/m^2
Androgen-independent prostate cancer (AIPC)[d]	3/48	Radiograph (CT) with or without PSA	1×/wk × 4; 0.4 and 1.6 mg/m^2

CT, computed tomography; PSA, prostate-specific antigens.
[a]ITT, intent to treat population. The denominator reflects all patients dosed.
[b]Data from Aghajanian et al. *(19)*.
[c]Data from Orlowski et al. *(20)*.
[d]Data from Papandreou et al. *(12)*.

level (one with grade 3 nausea and vomiting and one with grade 3 rash and diarrhea). There was no evidence of additive toxicities with this combination therapy at the doses examined, and the regimen was well tolerated; the most common complaints were fatigue, diarrhea, and nausea. Antitumor activity was reported in two patients: one with gastroesophageal junction adenocarcinoma and one with ovarian cancer *(31)*. The PK profiles of both bortezomib and irinotecan were assessed in the 125-mg/m^2 irinotecan dosing cohorts on d 1 of cycle 1 and d 8 of cycle 2 *(32)* and were not observed to be altered when the two agents were given in combination.

The data from the phase I combination trial of bortezomib and pegylated liposomal doxorubicin in 19 patients with advanced hematologic malignancies were recently reported *(26)*. Twice-weekly bortezomib (d 1, 4, 8, and 11) was given with a single dose of liposomal doxorubicin (30 mg/m^2 on d 4) in a 21-d cycle (Table 3). At the first dose level tested (0.90 mg/m^2 bortezomib), DLTs of grade 3 diarrhea, hypotension, syncope, and confusion were experienced by one patient with underlying Crohn's disease. Non-DLT grade 3 toxicities, which included low blood counts, fatigue, and palmar plantar erythrodysesthesia, were seen in other patients at higher doses. Of the 14 patients with multiple myeloma, 10 were evaluable for response. The investigators reported three patients with complete remission, four with PRs, one with minor response, one with

Table 3
Millennium Pharmaceuticals-Sponsored Phase I Bortezomib Combination

Major tumor type (study no.)	Cycle length (d)	Bortezomib Treatment Doses (mg/m^2)	Treatment days in cycle	Adjunct treatment		Established MTD bortezomib adjunct (mg/m^2)
				Dose range (mg/m^2)	Treatment days in cycle	
Solid tumors (027)[a]	21	1.0/1.3	1, 4, 8, 11	Gemcitabine 500–1000	1, 8	1.0/1000
Solid tumors (028)[b]	21	1.0/1.3	1, 4, 8, 11	Irinotecan 50–125	1, 8	1.3/125
AIPC (033)[c]	21	1.0/1.3/1.8	2, 9	Docetaxel 25–40	1, 8	Not yet established
Lung and other solid tumors (034)[d]	21	1.0/1.3	1, 4, 8, 11	Docetaxel 60–75 1	1	Not yet established
Anthracycline-resistant breast cancer (035)[e]	21	1.0/1.3/1.5	1, 4, 8, 11	Docetaxel 60–100	1	Not yet established
Hematologic malignancies (001)[f]	21	0.90/ 1.05/ 1.20/ 1.30	1, 4, 8, 11	Liposomal doxorubicin 30	4	Not yet established

AIPC, androgen-independent prostate cancer; MTD, maximum tolerated dose.
[a]Data from Appleman et al. *(30)*.
[b]Data from Ryan et al. *(31)*.
[c]Data from Roth et al. (33).
[d]Data on file, Millennium Pharmaceuticals.
[e]Data from Albanell et al. *(35)*.
[f]Data from Orlowski et al. *(26)*.

stable disease, and one with progressive disease. The MTD of the combination has not yet been determined, and accrual to the trial continues.

Of interest also is the report by Zangari et al. *(27)* concerning the combination of bortezomib and thalidomide. Bortezomib was added to the second cycle of a dose-escalation study with thalidomide in patients resistant to post-transplant salvage therapy. The authors observed activity (as assessed by reductions in M-protein), particularly in those with chromosome 13 abnormalities. It was also encouraging that the preliminary data did not suggest additive neurotoxicity. Further study will allow a determination of the exact contribution of bortezomib to the efficacy of thalidomide.

Additional combination studies are in progress investigating bortezomib and docetaxel for the treatment of advanced solid tumors in patients with prostate, lung, and breast cancers (Table 3). Preliminary results suggest that these combinations are quite tolerable, although no study has reached the MTD. All have reported that some patients have completed eight or more cycles of combination therapy.

The phase I/II study in patients with advanced AIPC and progressive disease *(33)* has reached an expanded cohort at doses of 1.3 mg/m^2 bortezomib and 40 mg/m^2 docetaxel.

The schedule of drug administration is unique and is based on preclinical evidence *(34)*: docetaxel is given on d 1 and 8 with dexamethasone premedication, and bortezomib is given on d 2 and 9 in a 21-d cycle. The MTD has not been reached. Of the 12 patients enrolled in the initial cohorts, 2 patients each had grade 3 diarrhea and hyperglycemia, and 1 patient had grade 3 hyponatremia, hematuria, and a pathologic fracture; there were no grade 4 toxicities. Four patients had a PSA response ($\geq$ 50% decline from baseline).

The phase I study in patients with advanced breast cancer who had received prior therapy with anthracyclines *(35)* employs a 21-d cycle in which bortezomib is administered by intravenous bolus on d 1, 4, 8, and 11, and docetaxel is given 1 h before bortezomib on d 1. The MTD has not been reached, and the study has reached a dose level of 1.0 mg/m^2 bortezomib and 100 mg/m^2 docetaxel. Adverse events resulted in discontinuation in two patients with grade 3 neuropathy. One patient had peripheral sensory neuropathy and the other a radiation-recall mononeuropathy. Investigators have reported tumor shrinkage in six of the nine evaluable patients who had measurable disease (RECIST criteria).

A third docetaxel combination trial is under way in patients with advanced solid tumors, primarily those with non-small cell lung cancer. Bortezomib is given on d 1, 4, 8, and 11, and docetaxel is given on d 1 before bortezomib. The MTD has not been reached, and the study has reached a dose level of 1.0 mg/m^2 bortezomib and 75 mg/m^2 docetaxel (data on file, Millennium Pharmaceuticals).

Chapter 23 reviews additional information on the phase II development of bortezomib in multiple myeloma, in which there was also the opportunity to study dexamethasone in combination with bortezomib.

4. DISCUSSION

There was a sound rationale for the development of bortezomib as an antineoplastic agent. The PD assay monitoring proteasome activity in blood cells was used extensively in nonclinical development with multiple species and provided a guide to dose and schedule selection for the phase I program. Although observations in the initial rat and cynomolgus monkey toxicity studies suggested that a complete or nearly complete recovery of 20S proteasome activity between doses was a critical determinant in the dosing schedule, subsequent nonclinical studies as well as clinical experience have shown that complete recovery of 20S proteasome activity is not an absolute determinant of the safety and efficacy of the compound. Recovery of proteasome activity to pretreatment levels is not complete at 72 h, but the degree of recovery at that time point nevertheless appears sufficient, since the twice-weekly dosing schedule has been well tolerated over several cycles in many patients. Therefore, 72 h has been the recommended minimal interval between doses.

The relationship between the 20S proteasome activity assay and plasma bortezomib concentrations is useful to define concentrations of bortezomib in the pharmacologically active concentration range. In addition, using a sensitive assay, PK studies have established that the drug had a mean terminal elimination half-life of approx 8.7–14.8 h, with a rapid α-distribution half-life *(14)*.

Based on the phase I studies conducted under the Millennium Pharmaceuticals, Investigational New Drug application assessing three schedules of single-agent bortezomib administration (Table 1), the twice-weekly for 2 wk regimen was selected for phase II clinical trials. At the 1.3-mg/m^2 dose and the 21-d schedule, bortezomib produced on average over 60% proteasome inhibition in the blood *(14)*. Furthermore, this twice-weekly dosing regimen can be integrated into the treatment schemes of other standard chemotherapies (Table 3).

DLTs for the preferred 21-d schedule of administration in patients with advanced solid tumors were peripheral sensory neuropathy and diarrhea. The side-effect profile in the 123 patients treated in the phase I studies with the single agent bortezomib was very similar to that observed in sensitive animal species. The adverse events were generally managable. There was a dose relationship with most of the gastrointestinal adverse events, although these could be managed with appropriate support medications. Thrombocytopenia was rarely more severe than grade 3 and was not associated with significant bleeding. Its occurrence was least common in the solid tumor patients and most common in the patients with advanced hematologic malignancies and compromised bone marrows. Of note was the rarity of significant renal, hepatic, and cardiac toxicity. The occurrence of neutropenia and febrile neutropenia, in particular, was uncommon.

Peripheral sensory neuropathy was described in the single-agent trials and was dose-limiting in a few cases *(19,20)*. Risk factors have not been established definitively for this side effect, but its occurrence was described more often in patients with prior exposure to neurotoxic agents. Peripheral neuropathy was experienced in 5 of 43 (12%) patients with advanced solid tumors who were dosed with bortezomib twice weekly for 2 wk, including 3 patients in the 1.56-mg/m^2 group and 1 patient each in the 1.08- and 1.30-mg/m^2 dose groups *(19)*. It also occurred in 5 of 27 (19%) patients with hematologic malignancies who received bortezomib twice weekly for 4 wk. It was not common in the weekly administration schedule in mainly prostate cancer patients, occurring in 2 of 53 patients (4%). Additional investigations were incorporated into the phase II program trials to characterize this side effect further (*see* Chap. 23).

Preliminary results to date from combination studies do not indicate any unexpected or additive toxicities when bortezomib is used in combination with gemcitabine *(28,30)*, irinotecan *(29,31)*, liposomal doxorubicin *(26)*, or docetaxel *(33,35)*.

Although the single-agent phase I studies were not designed to assess anticancer activity, preliminary evidence of biologic activity was reported in patients with non-small cell lung cancer, AIPC, multiple myeloma, and non-Hodgkin's lymphoma (Table 2). Further experience with combination therapy is needed to assess the impact of combination vs single-agent therapy in effecting responses in solid tumors.

The occurrence of antitumor activity verifies that proteasome inhibition is a useful target for the treatment of both hematologic and solid tumors. The observation of activity in multiple myeloma was pursued in phase II studies of bortezomib in patients with refractory and relapsed myeloma. Subsequently, an international, multicenter, randomized phase III study comparing bortezomib with high-dose dexamethasone in relapsed myeloma patients was initiated in 2002.

Bortezomib is a first-in-class compound and has many potential clinical applications. Although the mechanisms of cytotoxicity mediated by bortezomib continue to be evaluated at a cellular level, its safety and efficacy for the treatment of cancer—both as a single agent and in combination with standard chemotherapies, biologic agents, and radiation therapy—will continue to be explored.

REFERENCES

1. Orlowski RZ, Eswara JR, Lafond-Walker A, Grever MR, Orlowski M, Dang CV. Tumor growth inhibition induced in a murine model of human Burkitt's lymphoma by a proteasome inhibitor. *Cancer Res* 1998;58:4342–4348.
2. Delic J, Masdehors P, Omura S, et al. The proteasome inhibitor lactacystin induces apoptosis and sensitizes chemo- and radioresistant human chronic lymphocytic leukaemia lymphocytes to TNF-alpha-initiated apoptosis. *Br J Cancer* 1998;77:1103–1107.
3. Kudo Y, Takata T, Ogawa I, et al. p27Kip1 accumulation by inhibition of proteasome function induces apoptosis in oral squamous cell carcinoma cells. *Clin Cancer Res* 2000;6:916–923.
4. Masdehors P, Merle-Beral H, Maloum K, Omura S, Magdelenat H, Delic J. Deregulation of the ubiquitin system and p53 proteolysis modify the apoptotic response in B-CLL lymphocytes. *Blood* 2000;96:269–274.
5. Hideshima T, Chauhan D, Schlossman R, Richardson P, Anderson KC. The role of tumor necrosis factor alpha in the pathophysiology of human multiple myeloma: therapeutic applications. *Oncogene* 2001;20:4519–4527.
6. Hideshima T, Richardson P, Chauhan D, et al. The proteasome inhibitor PS-341 inhibits growth, induces apoptosis, and overcomes drug resistance in human multiple myeloma cells. *Cancer Res* 2001;61:3071–3076.
7. Ma MH, Parker KM, Manyak S, et al. Proteasome inhibitor PS-341 markedly enhances sensitivity of multiple myeloma cells to chemotherapeutic agents and overcomes chemoresistance through inhibition of the NF-kappaB pathway. *Blood* 2001;98:437a.
8. Soengas MS, Capodieci P, Polsky D, et al. Inactivation of the apoptosis effector Apaf-1 in malignant melanoma. *Nature* 2001;409:207–211.
9. Adams J, Palombella VJ, Sausville EA, et al. Proteasome inhibitors: a novel class of potent and effective antitumor agents. *Cancer Res* 1999;59:2615–2622.
10. Investigator Brochure. Millennium Pharmaceuticals, Inc. Cambridge, MA; 2003.
11. Lightcap ES, McCormack TA, Pien CS, Chau V, Adams J, Elliott PJ. Proteasome inhibition measurements: clinical application. *Clin Chem* 2000;46:673–683.
12. Papandreou C, Daliani D, Millikan RE, et al. Phase I study of intravenous (I.V.) proteasome inhibitor PS-341 in patients (Pts) with advanced malignancies. In: *Proceedings of the American Society of Clinical Oncology-37th Annual Meeting*, 2001;20:86a.
13. Papandreou CN, Pagliaro L, Millikan R, et al. Phase I study of PS-341, a novel proteasome inhibitor, in patients with advanced malignancies. In: *Proceedings of the 1999 AACR-NCI-EORTC International Conference on Molecular Targets and Cancer Therapeutics*, 1999:5.
14. Nix DJ, Pien C, LaButti J, Maden T, Adams J, Elliott P. Clinical pharmacology of the proteasome inhibitor PS-341. In: *Proceedings of the 2001 AACR-NCI-EORTC International Conference on Molecular Targets and Cancer Therapeutics*, 2001:7.
15. Papandreou CN, Daliani DD, Yang H, et al. Phase I trial of the proteasome inhibitor bortezomib in patients with advanced solid tumors with observations in androgen-independent prostate cancer. *J Clin Oncol* 2003; in press.
16. Papandreou CN, Pagliaro L, Millikan R, et al. Phase I study of PS-341, a novel proteasome inhibitor, in patients with advanced malignancies. In: *Proceedings of the American Society of Clinical Oncology-36th Annual Meeting*, 2000;19:190a.
17. Logothetis CJ, Yang H, Daliani D, et al. Dose-dependent inhibition of 20S proteasome results in serum IL-6 and PSA decline in patients (pts) with androgen-independent prostate cancer (AI PCa) treated with the proteasome inhibitor PS-341. In: *Proceedings of the American Society of Clinical Oncology-37th Annual Meeting*, 2001;20:186a.
18. Nix D, Pien C, Maden T, et al. Clinical development of a proteasome inhibitor, PS-341, for the treatment of cancer. In: *Proceedings of the American Society of Clinical Oncology-37th Annual Meeting*, 2001;20:86a.
19. Aghajanian C, Soignet S, Dizon DS, et al. A phase I trial of the novel proteasome inhibitor PS341 in advanced solid tumor malignancies. *Clin Cancer Res* 2002;8:2505–2511.
20. Orlowski RZ, Stinchcombe TE, Mitchell BS, et al. Phase I trial of the proteasome inhibitor PS-341 in patients with refractory hematologic malignancies. *J Clin Oncol* 2002;20:4420–4427.

21. Bold RJ, Virudachalam S, McConkey DJ. Chemosensitization of pancreatic cancer by inhibition of the 26S proteasome. *J Surg Res* 2001;100:11–17.

22. Cusack JC Jr, Liu R, Houston M, et al. Enhanced chemosensitivity to CPT-11 with proteasome inhibitor PS-341: implications for systemic nuclear factor-kappaB inhibition. *Cancer Res* 2001;61:3535–3540.

23. Shah MA, Schwartz GK. Cell cycle-mediated drug resistance: an emerging concept in cancer therapy. *Clin Cancer Res* 2001;7:2168–2181.

24. Pink M, Pien CS, Worland P, Adams J, Kauffman MG. PS-341 enhances chemotherapeutic effect in human xenograft models. In: *Proceedings of the American Association for Cancer Research*, 2002;43:158.

25. Orlowski RZ, Dees EC. The role of the ubiquitination-proteasome pathway in breast cancer: applying drugs that affect the ubiquitin-proteasome pathway to the therapy of breast cancer. *Breast Cancer Res* 2003;5:1–7.

26. Orlowski RZ, Hall M, Voorhees P, et al. Phase I study of the proteasome inhibitor bortezomib (PS-341, Velcade™) in combination with pegylated liposomal doxorubicin (Doxil®) in patients with refractory hematologic malignancies. *Blood* 2002;100:105a.

27. Zangari M, Barlogie B, Prather J, et al. Marked activity also in Del 13 multiple myeloma (MM) of PS-341 (PS) and subsequent thalidomide (THAL) in a setting of resistance to post-autotransplant salvage therapies. *Blood* 2002;100:105a.

28. Ryan DP, Eder JP, Winklemann J, et al. Pharmacokinetic and pharmacodynamic phase I study of PS-341 and gemcitabine in patients with advanced solid tumors. In: *Proceedings of the American Society of Clinical Oncology-38th Annual Meeting*, 2002;21:95a.

29. Clark JW, Ryan D, Dees C, et al. Phase I dose-escalation study of the proteasome inhibitor, PS-341, plus irinotecan in patients with advanced solid tumors. In: *Proceedings of the American Society of Clinical Oncology-38th Annual Meeting*, 2002;21:93a.

30. Appleman LJ, Ryan DP, Clark JW, et al. Phase I dose escalation study of bortezomib and gemcitabine safety and tolerability in patients with advanced solid tumors. In: *Proceedings of the American Society of Clinical Oncology-39th Annual Meeting*, 2003;22:209.

31. Ryan DP, O'Neil B, Lima CR, et al. Phase I dose-escalation study of the proteasome inhibitor, bortezomib, plus irinotecan in patients with advanced solid tumors. In: *Proceedings of the American Society of Clinical Oncology-39th Annual Meeting*, 2003;22:228.

32. Supko JG, Eder JP, Lynch TJ, et al. Pharmacokinetics of irinotecan and the proteasome inhibitor bortezomib in adult patients with solid tumor malignancies. In: *Proceedings of the American Society of Clinical Oncology-39th Annual Meeting*, 2003;22:136.

33. Roth B, Dreicer R, Berg W, et al. Phase I/II trial of bortezomib plus docetaxel in patients with advanced androgen-independent prostate cancer. In: *Proceedings of the American Society of Clinical Oncology-39th Annual Meeting*, 2003;22:424.

34. Gumerlock PH, Kawaguchi T, Moisan LP, et al. Mechanisms of enhanced cytotoxicity from docetaxel → PS-341 in combination in non-small cell lung carcinoma (NSCLC). In: *Proceedings of the American Society of Clinical Oncology-38th Annual Meeting*, 2002;21:304a.

35. Albanell J, Baselga J, Guix M, et al. Phase I study of bortezomib in combination with docetaxel in anthracycline-pretreated advanced breast cancer. In: *Proceedings of the American Society of Clinical Oncology-39th Annual Meeting*, 2003;22:16.

21 Clinical Molecular Diagnostics for Proteasome Inhibitors in Cancer Therapy

Jeffrey S. Ross, Gerald P. Linette,
Geoffrey S. Ginsburg, William Trepicchio,
Oscar Kashala, Rebecca Mosher, Jeffrey Brown,
George Mulligan, Jim Deeds, and James Stec

CONTENTS

ABSTRACT

The field of molecular diagnostics is in a state of rapid evolution featuring continuous technology developments and new clinical opportunities for drug selection, predicting efficacy and toxicity, and monitoring disease outcome. The introduction of new anticancer agents targeting the proteasome has created opportunities for the development of companion diagnostics to guide drug use and patient selection. In this chapter the field of molecular diagnostics is reviewed relevant to cancer, and a series of established prognostic factors known to predict the clinical course of multiple myeloma is presented. Biomarkers impacted by the proteasome pathway that may become clinically useful predictors of therapy related outcome are also included. The chapter concludes with a consideration of the emerging field of pharmacogenomics and its potential use for the prediction of drug response for patients treated with proteasome inhibitors.

From: *Cancer Drug Discovery and Development: Proteasome Inhibitors in Cancer Therapy*
Edited by: J. Adams © Humana Press Inc., Totowa, NJ

KEY WORDS

Proteasome, proteasome inhibitors, NF-κB, myeloma, bortezomib, pharmacogenomics

1. INTRODUCTION

The field of molecular diagnostics is in a state of rapid evolution featuring continuous technology developments and new clinical opportunities for drug selection, predicting efficacy and toxicity, and monitoring disease outcome *(1–3)*. The approvals of Herceptin® (trastuzumab) for the treatment of HER-2/*neu* over-expressing breast cancer and Gleevec® for the treatment of chronic myelogenous leukemia featuring a *bcr/abl* translocation and gastrointestinal stromal tumors with selective c-*kit* oncogene-activating mutations have brought to the diagnostic laboratory an expanding role for the testing of patients to determine their eligibility to receive these new therapies *(4,5)*. As seen in Table 1, the current molecular diagnostics industry consists of a market greater than $3 billion that is currently growing at approx 25% per year. It is widely believed that in the next 5–10 yr, the clinical application of molecular diagnostics will further revolutionize the drug discovery and development process, customize the selection, dosing, route of administration of existing and new therapeutic agents, and truly personalize medical care *(6,7)*. As proteasome inhibitors are introduced into clinical trials and move through the approval process, a wide array of techniques and procedures have and will be performed on patients to customize their dosing and combination therapy strategies in order to maximize the beneficial effects of these novel anticancer therapeutics

Emerging genomic and proteomic technologies are now resulting in the molecular subclassification of disease as the basis for diagnosis, prognosis, and therapeutic selection. Expanded knowledge of the molecular basis of cancer has shown that significant differences in gene expression patterns can guide therapy for a variety of solid tumors and hematologic malignancies *(8,9)*. Genetic variants in the drug target itself, disease pathway genes, or drug-metabolizing enzymes may all be used as predictors of drug efficacy or toxicity.

2. MOLECULAR DIAGNOSTIC PROGRAMS IN ONCOLOGY

2.1. Pharmacogenetics

More than one million genetic markers known as single-nucleotide polymorphisms (SNPs) have recently become available for genotyping and phenotyping studies *(9,10)*. The use of a variety of techniques for cloning and sequencing, as well as an evolving number of informatics approaches leading to the successful mining of high-quality sequence variations, has uncovered numerous loci that appear to have significant potential to generate clinically useful data for patient management. The application of genotyping strategies to predict anticancer drug efficacy has recently emerged in a variety of clinical settings *(11,12)*. For example, in colorectal cancer, pretreatment genotyping on peripheral blood samples is currently being used to select therapy based on the prediction of resistance associated with certain genetic polymorphisms *(13)*. SNP discovery and genotyping in cancer management has featured the evaluation of variations in drug metabolism associated with genomic variations in drug-metabolizing enzymes such as the cytochrome system *(14)*. Other detoxification pathways associated with SNP-based

Table 1
Estimated World-wide Molecular Diagnostics Markets[a]

By diagnostic technique	2000	2005	2010
DNA probes	240	400	850
PCR-based	1,450	2,200	4,350
FISH	600	850	2,350
Arrays	400	1,300	3,300
Others	450	750	1,150
Total	3,140	5,500	12,000
By Clinical Setting			
Infections	2,080	2,920	5,100
Cancer	337	900	1,900
Genetic tests	320	792	2,007
Food supply testing	110	198	400
Others	293	690	1,593
Total	3,140	5,500	12,000

FISH, fluorescence *in situ* hybridization; PCR, polymerase chain reaction.
[a]In millions of US dollars. Modified from Jain KK. *Molecular Diagnostics: Technologies, Markets, Companies*. Jain PharmaBiotech Publications, Basel, 2002.

variations in drug metabolism have been described *(15)*, but, in comparison with the cytochrome gene system, these markers have not yet achieved significant clinical utility.

2.2. Pharmacogenomics

Pharmacogenomics can best be defined as the application of whole genome technologies (e.g., gene and protein expression data) for prediction of the sensitivity or resistance of an individual's disease to a single drug or a group of drugs *(16,17)*. cDNA microarrays were introduced in the mid-1990s *(18)* and have achieved widespread use for the expression profiling of human clinical samples and in drug and biomarker target discovery. This technique has generated a wealth of new information in the fields of leukemia/lymphoma, solid tumor classification, drug and biomarker target discovery, and pharmacogenomic drug efficacy testing *(19,20)*. Using cDNA microarrays, several groups have now reported on their success in discovering gene expression that can be linked to resistance and responsiveness to standard of care chemotherapy *(21–23)*. The current status of research concerning the discovery of pharmacogenomic markers predictive of the response to proteasome inhibition will be discussed in more detail below.

2.3. Pharmacodynamics

In addition to the pharmacogenetic and pharmacogenomic tests, a series of bioassays, gene expression profiles, and tissue-based biomarkers has recently emerged to guide the dose, timing, and route of administration for novel therapeutics. These tests are used to speed the preclinical and early phase clinical development of drugs by enhancing the achievement of the ideal therapeutic dose while avoiding dose-related toxicity. Recent examples of these novel assays include the blood-based bioassay (Fig. 1) of the proteasome designed to guide the use of the proteasome inhibitor bortezomib (Velcade™; formerly known as PS-341) for the treatment of multiple myeloma and solid tumors (24–26) and the immunohistochemical determination of the epidermal growth factor receptor (EGFR) target and cell proliferation markers on skin biopsies of patients receiving the anti-EGFR small molecule tyrosine kinase inhibitor Iressa® (27). In Fig. 1, the graph shows 20S proteasome inhibition data taken 1.0 h after dosing in blood samples collected from over 130 cancer patients treated with bortezomib in multiple phase I clinical trials. The data points were compiled regardless of age, sex, race, dosing regimen, or cancer type and showed a dose relationship between 20S proteasome inhibition and the dose of bortezomib. In the phase I clinical trials, doses of bortezomib in the 1.1–1.3 mg/m^2 range produced an average 30% of expected 20S proteasome activity (70% inhibition). In these phase I clinical trials, at this dosage, with interval administrations timed to allow proteasome recovery, managable toxicity biologic activity was observed in patients with a variety of hematopoietic and solid tumors.

2.4. Toxicogenomics

Toxicogenomics is the study of gene expression patterns using high-throughput microarrays, automated reverse transcriptase (RT)-polymerase chain reaction (PCR), nuclear magnetic resonance (NMR), and proteomic strategies designed to detect up- and downregulation of genes associated with drug toxicity risk (28–31). Toxicogenomic markers for adverse side effects may influence selection and optimization of lead compounds prior to human studies. The limitations and uncertainties of gene expression profiling associated with data mining constraints on mechanistic and predictive toxicology have recently been emphasized, and the clinical value of toxicogenomics is currently mostly unrealized (31).

3. TECHNIQUES AND PATHWAYS IN MOLECULAR DIAGNOSTICS OF PROTEASOME INHIBITORS IN ONCOLOGY

A wide variety of techniques are currently in clinical development and clinical use for the detection of predisposition, screening, diagnosis, prognosis, and prediction of response to therapy for cancer patients (32). In Table 2, the methods and procedures used to discover clinically relevant biomarkers and prognostic and predictive tests in cancer are summarized. For the emerging proteasome inhibitors, molecular diagnostics investigations have focused on the use of biomarkers known to predict disease outcome for a specific tumor type that, based mostly on preclinical evidence, are also impacted by altering proteasome activity. As seen in Fig. 2, current opinion has it that inhibition of the proteasome by bortezomib may alter the following major pathways that can influence cancer outcome: nuclear signaling and chemoresistance via nuclear factor-κB (NF-κB), antiapoptosis and chemoresistance via bcl2, angiogenesis via vascular endothelial growth factor (VEGF), and cell proliferation via regulation of the G$_1$/S and G$_2$/M transitions by cyclins, cyclin regulators, oncogenes, and tumor suppressor genes. Ubiquitination and proteasome degradation of inhibitor κB (IκB) releases NF-κB into the cytoplasm; it can then move into the nucleus and induce transcription of cytokine and chemokine signaling,

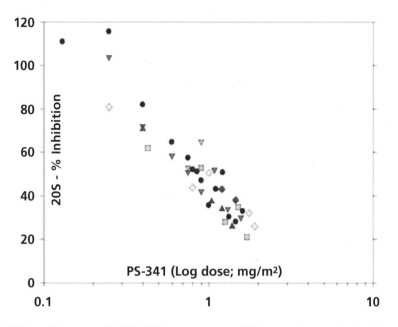

Fig. 1. Effect of bortezomib (PS-341) treatment on 20S proteasome activity in humans.

cell proliferation, angiogenesis, and resistance to apoptosis. The proteasome inhibitor bortezomib (Millennium Pharmaceuticals), a boron-containing dipeptide, blocks IκB degradation in a dose-dependent manner, thereby blocking NF-κB activity and decreasing its downstream signaling effects on pathways including apoptosis, angiogenesis, and cell proliferation.

3.1. The NF-κB Pathway

A pivotal regulatory protein degraded by the proteasome is the transcription factor NF-κB *(33)*. This factor binds to multiple DNA sequences, initiating the transcription of gene products including various cytokines (e.g., interleukin-1 [IL-1], IL-6, IL-8, tumor necrosis factor [TNF]), angiogenesis factors (e.g., VEGF), cell adhesion molecules (e.g., intercellular adhesion molecule 1 [ICAM-1] and vascular cell adhesion molecule 1 [VCAM-1]), enzymes (e.g., cyclo-oxygenase 2 [COX-2], nitric oxide synthase [NOS]), and antiapoptotic factors (e.g., bcl-2 and survivin). In a variety of tumors, the use of chemotherapy and/or radiation has been accompanied by an increased expression of NF-κB, rendering these neoplasms less sensitive to subsequent therapy *(34,35)*. Activation of NF-κB and cytoprotective genes in cancer may result from signal-induced phosphorylation and proteasome-dependent degradation of IκB, the inhibitor of NF-κB function *(36)*. Chromosomal rearrangement of genes coding for the viral oncoprotein Rel and NF-κB has been noted in many human hematopoietic and solid tumors *(34)*. Studies of NF-κB in cancer have emphasized the interplay between NF-κB signaling and the relative expression of antiapoptotic proteins such as *bcl2* and proapoptotic proteins such as *bax* *(36,37)*. Multiple myeloma has been known for some time to signal via the NF-κB pathway *(38–40)*. Exposure of myeloma cells to chemotherapy leads to an increase in IκB phosphorylation and reduces the levels of this inhibitor of NF-κB function. Chemo-

Table 2
Summary of Molecular Diagnostic Techniques in Oncology

Target	Method	Testing samples	Current clinical examples	Future status
DNA	Routine cytogenetics	Blood Bone marrow Fresh tissues	Classification Leukemia Lymphoma Sarcomas	Limited by low sensitivity and resolution
	ISH, FISH FISH and CISH and CISH	Blood Bone marrow Fresh Tissues Paraffin blocks	*Bcr/abl* translocation in CML HER-2/*neu* amplification N-*myc* amplification Sarcoma translocations HPV genotyping in gynecologic cytology	Selected growth Limited by low resolution
	CGH CGH Arrays	Blood Bone marrow Fresh Tissue	Detection of chromosomal and single gene gains and losses in tumor tissues vs normal tissues for research	Predominantly for research use only Continued development Major bioinformatics challenges
	SNPs	Blood	Uncommon familial cancer predisposition Prediction of metabolism and toxicity of anticancer drugs	Continued discovery of new applications Limited by low throughput
	PCR sequencing	Blood Bone marrow Fresh tissues	Common familial cancer predisposition *BRCA1* and 2 and others Tumor suppressor gene mutations *p53* and others Oncogene-activating mutations *ckit* in GIST Gene rearrangements in lymphoma Minimal residual disease after BMT High-risk HPV detection	
	Southern blot	Blood Bone marrow Fresh tissues	Gene rearrangements in lymphoma N-*myc* gene amplification in neuroblastoma	Little further utility owing to dilutional effects and lack of automation

	Technique	Clinical application	Sample type	Growth potential
RNA	Microsatellite instability	Colorectal cancer predisposition; Resection margin status; Urothelial carcinoma metastasis	Fresh tissues; Urine	Growth potential for selected clinical situations
	Transcriptional profiling	Pharmacogenomic discovery	Blood; Bone marrow; Fresh tissues	Substantial growth
	Northern blot		Fresh tissues	
	RT-PCR	Minimal residual disease after BMT; Micrometastasis detection in sentinel lymph nodes; Oncogene activation; CpG island hypermethylation to detect prostate cancer; TS/DPD levels to predict 5-FU response	Blood; Bone marrow; Fresh tissues (?Paraffin blocks)	Substantial growth
	ISH, FISH, and CISH	Melastatin detection for melanoma prognosis	Blood (after cell capture assays); Bone marrow; Fresh tissues	Limited growth
Protein	Western blot	Serology-immunology tests; Infectious agents	Blood	Limited
	2D PAGE	Discovery of novel proteins and peptides	Blood; Bone marrow; Fresh tissues	Research only
	MALDI-TOF	Protein and peptide identification and sequencing; SNP detection	Blood; Bone marrow; Body fluids	Requires automation to increase throughput

(continued on next page)

289

Table 2
Summary of Molecular Diagnostic Techniques in Oncology (*Continued*)

Target	Method	Testing samples	Current clinical examples	Future status
	SELDI	Blood	Detection of early-stage ovarian and prostate cancer	Technique undergoing validation Tremendous potential for early cancer detection and therapy monitoring
	IHC	Bone marrow Fresh tissues	Immunophenotyping of lymphoma Solid tumor classification ER/PR status in breast cancer HER-2/*neu* status in breast cancer	Enormous potential if technique can be standardized and reproducibility improved
BioAssays	PCR-based	Fresh tissues Urine	Telomerase TRAP assay	Limited
	Ligand-receptor assays	Fresh tissues	Hormone receptor (ER/PR) Others	Limited
	Truncated protein assays	Blood Bone marrow	Familial polyposis (APC) detection	Limited
General Enabling Techniques				

Technique	Sample	Application	Status/Potential
Laser capture Microdissection	Fresh tissues	Biomarker discovery	Research only
Tissue microarrays	Paraffin blocks Fresh tissues Paraffin blocks	Biomarker discovery	Research only
Quantitative digital image analysis	Tissue sections	Biomarker Validation Quantification of ISH and IHC	Prognostic and predictive marker assessment
Microcapillary electrophoresis	Blood Body fluids Tissue-derived fluids	High-throughput sequencing Microsatellite instability High-throughput proteomics	Substantial potential
Immunomagnetic cell capture assays	Blood Bone Marrow Body fluids	Detection of cancer in blood Parmacogenomic testing Pharmacogenomic testing	Unknown potential

APC, antigen-presenting cell; BMT, bone marrow transplant; CGH, comparative genome hybridization; CISH, competitive in situ hybridization; CML, chronic myeloid leukemia; FISH, fluorescence in situ hybridization; 5-FU, 5-fluorouracil; GIST, gastrointestinal stromal tumor; HPV, human papillomavirus; IHC, immunohistochemistry; ISH, in situ hybridization, MALDI-TOF, matrix-assisted laser desorption/ionization-time of flight; PCR, polymerase chain reaction; PR, progesterone recepto; RT, reverse transcriptase; SELDI, surface-enhanced laser desorption ionization; SNP, single-nucleotide polymorphism; TRAP, telomeric repeat amplification protocol; TS/DPD, thymidylate synthase/dihydropyrimidine dehydrogenase; 2D PAGE, two-dimensional polyacrylamide gel electrophoresis.

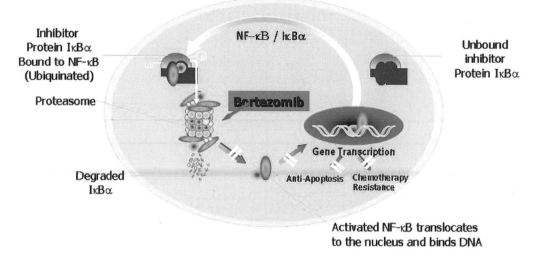

Fig. 2. Bortezomib and the ubiquitin-proteasome pathway. IκBα, inhibitor κBα; NF-κB, nuclear factor-κB.

resistant myeloma cell lines have increased NF-κB activity compared with sensitive lines *(41)*. Preclinical studies using IκB kinase inhibitors to block NF-κB expression selectively however, indicate that the antitumor impact of proteasome inhibition in myeloma includes effects on other pathways *(42)*. To date, no publications have correlated NF-κB expression at either the mRNA or the protein level before proteasome inhibitor treatment with response to the proteasome inhibitors. However, it is conceivable that in the future, diagnostic procedures (e.g., immunohistochemistry) designed to quantify NF-κB expression will be used for the selection of proteasome inhibitors in both multiple myeloma and solid tumor chemotherapy strategies.

3.2. Apoptosis and the bcl2 Pathway

Studies of NF-κB in cancer have emphasized the interplay between NF-κB signaling and the relative expression of antiapoptotic proteins such as bcl2 and proapoptotic proteins such as bax *(35,36)*. The resistance to apoptosis seen in chemotherapy-treated cancer cell lines transfected with extra copies of the *bcl-2* gene was overcome when the cells were exposed to bortezomib *(43,44)*. A number of studies have linked overexpression of bcl-2 with resistance to conventional chemotherapy and adverse outcome in a variety of hematopoietic and solid tumors (see below) *(45,46)*. To date, bcl-2 and bax measurements on clinical samples have not been used to select patients prospectively for proteasome inhibitor-based therapy.

3.3. Angiogenesis and the VEGF Pathway

Many factors associated with tumor angiogenesis including cell adhesion molecules, cytokines, and growth factors such as VEGF are regulated through the proteasome *(47–*

Table 3
Common Cancer Biomarkers Associated With Cell Proliferation Believed
to Be Regulated by Proteasome Degradation

Category	Protein involved	Protein function
Cyclins and regulators	Cyclins A, B, D, E CDK inhibitors	Regulates cell cycle
Tumor suppressors	p53	Transcription factor
Oncogenes	c-fos/c-jun; c-myc; N-myc	Transcription factors
Inhibitory proteins	IκB	Inhibits NF-κB
	p130	Inhibits E2F-1
Enzymes	cdc25 phosphatase	CDK1/cyclin B phosphatase
	Tyrosine amino transferase	Tyrosine metabolism
Others	Ki -67	PCN degradation

CDK, cyclin-dependent kinase; IκB, inhibitor κB; NF-κB, nuclear factor-κB, PCN.

50). In preclinical studies, the proteasome inhibitor lactacystin significantly reduced tumor angiogenesis *(50).* Bortezomib has been shown to limit angiogenesis, reduce VEGF expression, and lower the frequency and number of metastases in several experimental cancer systems *(43,44).* Thus, proteasome inhibitors may have potential as antiangiogenesis agents impacting both primary tumor growth and the development of cancer metastasis. However, to date, no clinical studies attempting to correlate levels of VEGF expression or tumor microvessel density with response to proteasome inhibition have been published.

3.4. Cell Proliferation and the G_1/S and G_2/M Transitions

Numerous cell cycle-related regulatory proteins are degraded by the proteasome, including cyclins, tumor suppressor genes, oncogenes, inhibitory proteins that control the activity of other regulatory proteins, and enzymes *(51–53)* (Table 3). The correctly synchronized production and degradation of these proteins is critical to their function and to the orderly progression of cells through the cell cycle. A number of cell cycle-dependent biomarkers have been studied as prognostic factors in cancer patients (see below). In general, the most prevalent clinical method of determining cell proliferation in cancer is MIB-1 immunohistochemistry (IHC) *(54).* Using breast cancer as an example, Fig. 3 demonstrates the tumor cell proliferation index determined by immunostaining for the MIB-1 clone of the Ki-67 proliferation marker. The labeling index for this case was 31%. This is a relatively high rate of proliferation for breast cancer and is associated with high-grade, high-stage disease with a propensity for recurrence after surgical or radiation therapy. Additional biomarkers studied by IHC that have predicted outcome in solid tumors include cyclin D1 and the cyclin-dependent kinase inhibitors p21 and p27 *(55–58).*

Although the studies of these markers have not been performed prior to treatment with proteasome inhibitors, preclinical evidence *(44)* suggests that their expression is regulated by the proteasome, indicating that they have the potential to serve as surrogate markers of drug efficacy.

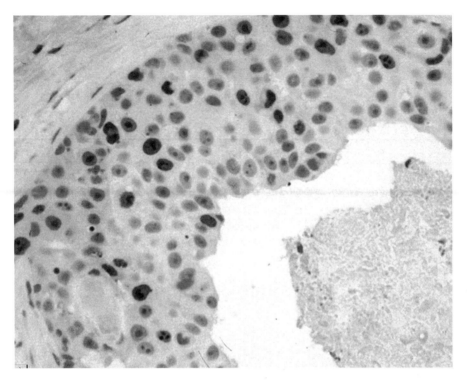

Fig. 3. Cell proliferation in breast cancer.

3.5. The Ubiquitin–Proteasome Pathway Target

Measurements of tumor proteasome activity by IHC or other techniques have not been reported, and proteasome activity levels have not been studied as prognostic or predictive factors. Future studies will attempt to link levels of total proteasome and proteasome subunit activity with responses to proteasome inhibitors such as bortezomib.

4. MOLECULAR DIAGNOSTICS AND PROTEASOME INHIBITION IN MULTIPLE MYELOMA

4.1. Standard Prognostic Factors in Myeloma

A series of prognostic factors designed to monitor the general responses to standard therapies and to predict the overall clinical course of the disease are summarized in Table 4. Although numerous additional chromosomal and molecular markers have been studied, the serum M-protein level remains the gold standard as a monitor of disease activity (59–61). Figure 4 shows that eight cycles of bortezomib treatment resulted in a major reduction in the serum clonal IgG M-protein concentration (left) and corresponding increases in the production of IgM and IgA.

4.2. Pharmacogenomics in Multiple Myeloma

The use of pharmacogenomics to predict response to chemotherapy is revolutionizing the drug development process and the patient health care industry. An example of the ongoing revolution in personalized medicine is the integration of pharmacogenomics

Table 4
General Prognostic and Predictive Factors
in Multiple Myeloma[a]

Bone marrow plasma cell counts
High-grade (plasmablastic) morphologic appearance
Number of osseous lesions
Serum M protein level
Serum β_2-microglobulin level
Serum immunoglobulin levels
Bone marrow plasma cell proliferation index
Cytogenetics: chromosome 13 deletions
Serum calcium level
Urine protein loss per 24 h
Bence Jones urine proteins
White blood cell, red blood cell,
    and platelet vounts
Renal function tests
Development of amyloidosis

[a]The factors reviewed include serum b_2-microglobulin, bone marrow plasma cell labeling index, cytogenetics, and plasmablastic morphology.

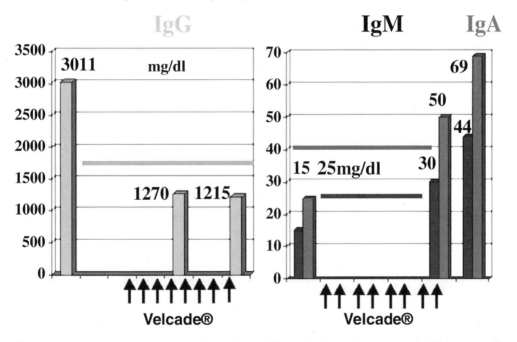

Fig. 4. Serum immunoglobulin levels in patients with multiple myeloma treated with bortezomib.

into the clinical development plans for bortezomib in the multicenter phase II trials of the investigational drug in patients with relapsed and refractory myeloma. Although it has been hypothesized that NF-κB signaling and bcl-2 overexpression play major roles in the

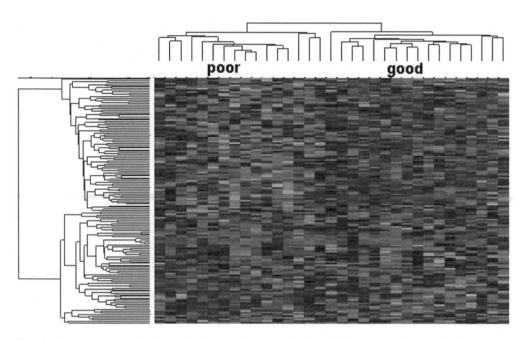

Fig. 5. Pharmacogenomics in multiple myeloma. prediction of short-term M-protein response to bortezomib-based proteasome inhibition using 150 genes identified through bortezomib phase II myeloma trials.

development of chemoresistance to standard agents used for myeloma treatment *(40–45)*, gene expression-based studies using transcriptional profiling have not as yet confirmed these concepts.

Through a collaborative effort with the clinical sites, patient bone marrow aspirates were subjected to a rapid negative selection enrichment protocol to purify myeloma cells from the aspirate before being frozen and shipped for analysis. Approximately 65% of the approx 220 patients enrolled in the phase II study volunteered an additional bone marrow biopsy for expression profiling analysis. The intrinsic gene expression patterns of these samples were captured on microarrays prior to treatment and are now being analyzed to look for prognostic markers correlating with clinical response to bortezomib as part of the trial. Bioinformatic marker selection algorithms have been used to identify statistically significant genes that differ between good and poor responders to treatment with bortezomib (Fig. 5). Additional analyses to build predictive marker sets and additional bioinformatics approaches designed to identify the relevant biologic pathways associated with response (Fig. 6), as well as putative regions of chromosomal loss or amplification, are also currently under way.

5. MOLECULAR DIAGNOSTICS AND PROTEASOME INHIBITION IN SOLID TUMORS

5.1. Standard Prognostic Factors in Solid Tumors

A wide variety of biomarkers have been studied for their ability to predict clinical outcome in the common solid tumors (Table 5). The College of American Pathologists

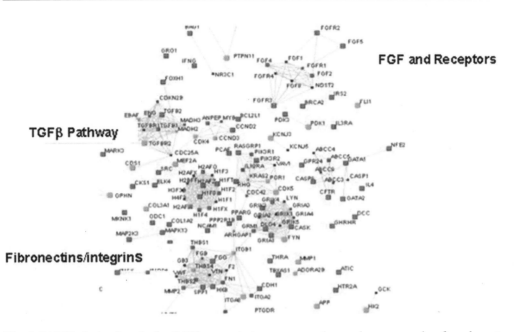

Fig. 6. PARIS-derived analysis of differences between responders and nonresponders for relevant biologic pathways associated with bortezomib response in patients with multiple myeloma. FGF, fibroblast growth factor; TGFβ, transforming growth factor β.

Table 5
Prognostic and Predictive Markers in the Major Solid Tumors

Biomarker	Breast cancer	Prostate cancer	Non-small cancer	Colorectal cancer
Proliferation: Ki-67	+++	++	+++	+++
Proliferation: cyclin D	+++	++	++	+++
Proliferation: p21	++	++	+	+
Proliferation: p27	++	+++	++	++
Hormone receptors: ER/PR	+++	−	−	−
Growth factor: EGFR	+	−	+	++
Growth factor: HER-2/neu	+++	+	++	+
Angiogenesis: VEGF	++	++	+	++
Angiogenesis: microvessel density	+++	+++	++	++
Apoptosis: bcl-2/bax	++	++	++	+++
Apoptosis: survivin	++	++	++	+++
Oncogene: RAS	+/−	−	+++	+++
Tumor suppressor gene: *p53*	++	+	+++	+++
Cell adhesion: E-cadherin	++	++	++	++
Cell signaling: NF-κB	Unknown	Unknown	Unknown	Unknown
Cell signaling: β-catenin	+	+	++	+++
Proteasome pathway	Unknown	Unknown	Unknown	Unknown

EGFR, epidermal growth factor receptor; ER, estrogen receptor; NF-κB, nuclear factor-κB; PR, progesterone receptor; VEGF, vascular endothelial growth factor.

has sponsored multiple studies to update the marker sets continuously based on publications confirming their accuracy, reliability, and clinical utility for each solid tumor type *(62)*. Studies of cell proliferation, tumor angiogenesis, and resistance to apoptosis in solid tumors as predictors of response in patients undergoing bortezomib-based combination chemotherapy in clinical trials are now under way. In addition, measurements of NF-κB and proteasome pathway biomarkers are also under evaluation for their ability to predict tumor responses to proteasome inhibitors as single agents and in combinations with standard of care cytotoxic drugs.

6. CONCLUSIONS

The introduction of proteasome inhibitors as potential anticancer drugs is in an early stage. Clinical molecular diagnostic approaches show significant promise in their ability to select individual cancer patients for treatment with drugs such as bortezomib and to integrate the use of existing biomarkers with newly discovered pharmacogenomic markers to optimize clinical response. Preliminary evidence suggests that pharmacogenomic tests may be helpful in customizing the use of proteasome inhibitors. Over the next several years, the impact on patient outcomes of this integration of molecular diagnostics with therapeutics will be better understood.

REFERENCES

1. Keesee SK. Molecular diagnostics: impact upon cancer detection. *Expert Rev Mol Diagn* 2002;2:91–92.
2. Poste G. Molecular diagnostics: a powerful new component of the healthcarevalue chain. *Expert Rev Mol Diagn* 2001;1:1–5.
3. Leonard DG. The present and future of molecular diagnostics. *Mol Diagn* 2001;6:71–72.
4. Vogel CL, et al. Efficacy and safety of trastuzumab as a single agent in first-line treatment of HER2-overexpressing metastatic breast cancer. *J Clin Oncol* 2002;20:719–726.
5. O'Dwyer ME, et al. STI571: an inhibitor of the BCR-ABL tyrosine kinase for the treatment of chronic myelogenous leukaemia. *Lancet Oncol* 2000;1:207–211.
6. Amos J, et al. Commercial molecular diagnostics in the U.S.: The Human Genome Project to the clinical laboratory. *Hum Mutat* 2002;19:324–333.
7. Ross JS, et al. Integrating diagnostics and therapeutics: revolutionizing drug discovery and patient care. *Drug Discov Today* 2002;7:859–864.
8. Morgan GJ, et al. Modern molecular diagnostics and the management of haematological malignancies. *Clin Lab Haematol* 1998;20:135–141.
9. Relling MV, et al. Pharmacogenetics and cancer therapy. *Nat Rev Cancer* 2001;1:99–108.
10. Taylor JG, et al. Using genetic variation to study human disease. *Trends Mol Med* 2001;7:507–512.
11. Diasio RB, et al. The role of pharmacogenetics and pharmacogenomics in cancer chemotherapy with 5-fluorouracil. *Pharmacology* 2000;61:199–203.
12. Relling MV, et al. Pharmacogenetics and cancer therapy. *Nat Rev Cancer* 2001;1:99–108.
13. Pullarkat ST, et al. Thymidylate synthase gene polymorphism determines response and toxicity of 5-FU chemotherapy. *Pharmacogenomics J* 2001;1:65–70.
14. Ingelman-Sundberg M. Genetic susceptibility to adverse effects of drugs and environmental toxicants. The role of the CYP family of enzymes. *Mutat Res* 2001;482:11–19.
15. Ingelman-Sundberg M. Pharmacogenetics: an opportunity for a safer and more efficient pharmacotherapy. *J Intern Med* 2001;250:186–200.
16. Rusnak JM, et al. Pharmacogenomics: a clinician's primer on emerging technologies for improved patient care. *Mayo Clin Proc* 2001;76:299–309.
17. Hess P, et al. Impact of pharmacogenomics on the clinical laboratory. *Mol Diagn* 1999;4:289–298.
18. Schena M, et al. Quantitative monitoring of gene expression patterns with a complementary DNA microarray. *Science* 1995;270:467–470.
19. Ramaswamy S, et al. DNA microarrays in clinical oncology. *J Clin Oncol* 2002;20:1932–1941.

20. Raetz EA, et al. Gene expression profiling. Methods and clinical applications in oncology. *Hematol Oncol Clin North Am* 2001;15:911–930.
21. Diasio RB, et al. The role of pharmacogenetics and pharmacogenomics in cancer chemotherapy with 5-fluorouracil. *Pharmacology* 2000;61:199–203
22. Los G, et al. Using mRNA expression profiling to determine anticancer drug efficacy. *Cytometry* 2002;47:66–71.
23. Slonim DK. Transcriptional profiling in cancer: the path to clinical pharmacogenomics. *Pharmacogenomics* 2001;2:123–136.
24. Lightcap ES, et al. Proteasome inhibition measurements: clinical application. *Clin Chem* 2000;46:673–683.
25. Adams J. Development of the proteasome inhibitor PS-341. *Oncologist* 2002;7:9–16.
26. Elliott PJ, et al. The proteasome: a new target for novel drug therapies. *Am J Clin Pathol* 2001;116:637–646.
27. Albanell J, et al. Pharmacodynamic studies of the epidermal growth factor receptor inhibitor ZD1839 in skin from cancer patients: histopathologic and molecular consequences of receptor inhibition. *J Clin Oncol* 2002;20:110–124.
28. Hamadeh HK, et al. Discovery in toxicology: mediation by gene expression array technology. *J Biochem Mol Toxicol* 2001;15:231–242.
29. Fielden MR, et al. Challenges and limitations of gene expression profiling in mechanistic and predictive toxicology. *Toxicol Sci* 2001;60:6–10.
30. Burchiel SW, Knall CM, Davis JW 2nd, Paules RS, Boggs SE, Afshari CA. Analysis of genetic and epigenetic mechanisms of toxicity: potential roles of toxicogenomics and proteomics in toxicology. *Toxicol Sci* 2001;59:193–195.
31. Hamadeh HK, et al. An overview of toxicogenomics. *Curr Issues Mol Biol* 2002;4:45–56.
32. Ross JS, et al. Techniques in oncology molecular diagnostics. In: *Cancer Molecular Diagnostics* (Nakamura R, Grody WW, eds). Humana, Totowa, NJ, 2003.
33. Baldwin AS. The NF-kappa B and I kappa B proteins: new discoveries and insights. *Annu Rev Immunol* 1996;14:649–683.
34. Rayet B, et al. Aberrant rel/nfkb genes and activity in human cancer. *Oncogene* 1999;18:6938-6947.
35. Wang C-Y, et al. Control of inducible chemoresistance: enhanced antitumor therapy through increased apoptosis by inhibition of NF-κB. *Nat Med* 1999;5:412–417.
36. Sunwoo JB, et al. Novel proteasome inhibitor PS-341 inhibits activation of nuclear factor-kappa B, cell survival, tumor growth, and angiogenesis in squamous cell carcinoma. *Clin Cancer Res* 2001;7:1419–1428
37. Lin ZP, et al. Prevention of brefeldin A-induced resistance to teniposide by the proteasome inhibitor MG-132: involvement of NF-κB activation in drug resistance. *Cancer Res* 1998;58:3059–3065.
38. Schenkein D. Proteasome inhibitors in the treatment of B-cell malignancies. *Clin Lymphoma* 2002;3:49–55.
39. Adams J. Preclinical and clinical evaluation of proteasome inhibitor PS-341 for the treatment of cancer. *Curr Opin Chem Biol* 2002;6:493–500.
40. Mitsiades N, et al. Biologic sequelae of nuclear factor-kappaB blockade in multiple myeloma: therapeutic applications. *Blood* 2002;99:4079–4086.
41. Berenson JR, et al. The role of nuclear factor-kappaB in the biology and treatment of multiple myeloma. *Semin Oncol* 2001;28:626–633.

22 Phase II Trials of Bortezomib for the Treatment of Multiple Myeloma

Kenneth C. Anderson

ABSTRACT

Multiple myeloma is incurable, and novel therapies are urgently needed. The proteasome inhibitor bortezomib targets both the tumor cell and the bone marrow microenvironment to overcome drug resistance in preclinical in vitro and in vivo models of human multiple myeloma. A recently completed phase II trial of bortezomib demonstrated durable responses and associated clinical benefit in patients with relapsed refractory myeloma, providing the basis for its Food and Drug Administration approval. Ongoing studies are evaluating bortezomib, alone and in combination, to treat patients earlier in the disease course.

KEY WORDS

Proteasome inhibitor, multiple myeloma, refractory relapsed disease, salvage therapy

1. INTRODUCTION

Bortezomib (Velcade™; formerly known as PS-341, LDP-341, and MLN341) was the first proteasome inhibitor to enter clinical trials. Preclinically, this agent has demonstrated antitumor activity in a variety of hematologic malignancies *(1–3)* and solid tumor models *(4–11)*. In 1998, a broad phase I program assessing the maximum tolerated dose (MTD) in advanced hematologic malignancies and solid tumors (*see* Chap. 21 for a review of phase I trials) was initiated. One of these trials, led by Dr. Robert Z. Orlowski at the University of North Carolina (UNC) and Steven Soignet at Memorial Sloan-

From: *Cancer Drug Discovery and Development: Proteasome Inhibitors in Cancer Therapy*
Edited by: J. Adams © Humana Press Inc., Totowa, NJ

Kettering Cancer Center (MSKCC), assessed bortezomib in advanced hematologic malignancies. Of the 27 patients enrolled in this trial, 12 had plasma cell dyscrasias *(12)*. Nine of these patients completed one full cycle of bortezomib and were assessable for response. Several patients showed stable disease or reductions in serum M-protein and/ or marrow plasmacytosis, and one patient had a complete response. This patient had initially responded to vincristine–doxorubicin (Adriamycin®)–dexamethasone (VAD) but subsequently relapsed and was refractory to VAD and topotecan–dexamethasone. She had a confirmed complete response after three cycles of bortezomib and went on to complete four cycles of therapy. Although evidence of recurrence (faint monoclonal band in immunofixation) occurred 6 mo later, she required no antimyeloma therapy for a year. These data provided the rationale for multicenter phase II trials (study 025 and study 024) of bortezomib in multiple myeloma.

2. MULTIPLE MYELOMA OVERVIEW

Each year in the United States approx 14,600 cases of multiple myeloma are diagnosed, and 10,800 patients die of this disease *(13)*. Multiple myeloma is a disease of the antibody-producing plasma cells. Myeloma typically invades the bone marrow, causing anemia, thrombocytopenia, and neutropenia, and subsequently may invade other sites, notably the bone and soft tissues, potentially causing pain, hypercalcemia, and paralysis (due to tumor involvement in the spine), as well as a host of other complications. Multiple myeloma is incurable, but temporary remissions or disease stabilization are relatively common with current treatment regimens, which include combination chemotherapy or stem cell transplantation with high-dose chemotherapy. Although some patients have refractory disease from the outset, a significant number of patients respond one or more times to treatment. Over time, however, the duration of remission becomes increasingly shorter; eventually, the patient's disease becomes refractory to all therapy, with death occurring within 6–9 mo. Myeloma patients thus span a spectrum from newly diagnosed patients who can expect to achieve one or more remissions with standard chemotherapy or transplantation over several years, to patients with refractory disease and no treatment options. New treatment options are urgently needed.

3. STUDY POPULATIONS OF PHASE II STUDIES

Patients in study 025 were relapsed *and* refractory to their most recent therapy—not only had their disease relapsed but the most recent therapy had failed to induce a response. Patients in study 024 were relapsed *or* refractory after front-line therapy. This population included relapsed patients whose disease had not shown evidence of unresponsiveness to chemotherapy as well as patients with refractory disease. Study 024 patients thus allowed for the enrollment of patients with relatively earlier stage disease, whereas study 025 patients were often heavily pretreated and were late in the course of their disease. As expected, study 025 enrolled more rapidly than study 024, as study 025 patients had exhausted all conventional treatment options.

4. TREATMENTS

Study 025 assessed 1.3 mg/m^2 bortezomib given on d 1, 4, 8, and 11 of a 21-d cycle (twice weekly with 10-d rest; d 12–21 are the rest period). Dexamethasone could be added in patients who demonstrated progressive disease after two cycles or stable disease after four cycles. In study 024, patients were randomized to receive either 1.0 or 1.3 mg/m^2 using the same schedule, with dexamethasone added if patients had progressive or stable disease. These doses were selected as the most reasonable doses for phase II trials based on an analysis of the MTDs reached in a variety of phase I studies in advanced hematologic and solid tumors; MTDs in these trials varied by dose intensity but ranged from 1.04 mg/m^2 in the most dose-intensive regimen (bortezomib twice weekly for 4 wk, followed by a 2-wk rest *[12]*) to 1.8 mg/m^2 in less dose-intensive schedules (once weekly for 4 wk, followed by a 2-wk rest) *(14)*. Moderate dose-intensity regimens—bortezomib twice weekly for 2 wk—showed an MTD of 1.56 mg/m^2 *(15)*. The dose range of 1.0–1.3 mg/m^2 twice weekly with a 10-d rest (d 12–21 are the rest period) seemed to provide the most reasonable balance between potential efficacy and toxicity and was chosen for further evaluation in phase II.

5. EFFICACY

The results of study 025 were recently reported *(16)*. A total of 202 patients were enrolled, the majority of whom (72%) had Durie-Salmon stage III disease. Mean age was 60 yr, and the median years from diagnosis were 4. Median β_2-microglobulin levels, hemoglobin levels, and platelet counts were 3.5 mg/L (range, 0.1–133 mg/L), 10.2 g/dL (range, 5.4–14.6 g/dL), and 162×10^9 (range, $11–479 \times 10^9$), respectively. Response criteria were based on those of Bladé and colleagues *(17)*. By these criteria, responses must be confirmed 6 wk after the initial observation. Parameters assessed were M-protein, urinary light chain (the κ or λ component of the M-protein, which is used if serum M-protein is not detectable), soft tissue plasmacytomas, lytic lesions in bone, and percentage of plasma cells in bone marrow. Using these criteria, a complete response requires complete absence of M-protein with immunofixation confirmation (i.e., negative immunofixation on two occasions), plasma cells in marrow less than 5%, no plasmacytomas, and stable skeletal disease. This degree of rigor has not commonly been employed in most myeloma trials. Traditional measures of response, such as the Southwest Oncology Group criteria, define complete response as a reduction in M-protein of at least 75% and plasma cells in marrow less than 5% confirmed 3 wk apart, but assessment of plasmacytomas and skeletal disease is not required (Table 1). All responses in study 025 were confirmed by an independent response committee (IRC), which comprised three independent oncologists who were not investigators in the trial.

Of 202 enrolled patients, 193 were evaluable; 92% had been treated with three or more of the major classes of agents for myeloma, and 91% were refractory to their most recent therapy. The response rate to bortezomib was 35%, including 10% immunofixation-negative and -positive complete responses (Table 2). The median overall survival was 16 mo, with a median duration response of 12 mo. Response was typically associated with improvements in hemoglobin levels, decreased transfusion requirements, improved quality of life, and improved levels of normal immunoglobulins.

The most common grade 3 adverse events were thrombocytopenia (28%), fatigue (12%), peripheral neuropathy (11%), and neutropenia (11%). Grade 4 events were uncommon (14%). The most clinically significant toxicity was cumulative dose-related peripheral sensory neuropathy. In 26% of patients, peripheral neuropathy occurred, or existing neuropathy worsened. There were no cases of grade 4 neuropathy. In most

Table 1
Comparison of Complete Response Criteria for Study 025[a]

	SPEP/UPEP (%) ↓	Immunofixation-negative	Plasma cells in marrow < 5%	No plasmacytomas	Stable skeletal signs	Confirmation (wk)
Bladé	100/100	✓	✓	✓	✓	6 wk
SWOG	≥75/90	NR	NR	NR	NR	3 wk

NR, not required; SPEP, serum protein electrophoresis; SWOG, Southwest Oncology Group; UPEP, urinary protein electrophoresis.
[a]Data based on Bladé et al. (17) and the Southwest Oncology Group (21).

Table 2
Responses to Bortezomib Monotherapy
in Study 025 (n = 193)

Response	%
CR[a]	10
Immunofixation negative	4
Immunofixation positive[a]	6
PR	18
MR	7
NC	24

CR, complete response; PR, partial response; MR, minimal response; NC, no change.
[a]Patients who fulfilled all Bladé criteria for CR except for positive immunofixation.

patients, neuropathy improved during the follow-up period. Only one patient without baseline neuropathy developed grade 3 neuropathy on treatment. It is hoped that in subsequent trials enrolling less heavily pretreated patients the incidence of neuropathy will be lower. Preliminary data from study 024 are consistent with this hypothesis (18).

6. FUTURE DIRECTIONS

Based largely on study 025, bortezomib received accelerated Food and Drug Administration approval in May of 2003 for the treatment of relapsed and refractory myeloma. An international, phase III trial (APEX) comparing bortezomib with high-dose dexamethasone in patients with relapsed or refractory multiple myeloma treated with one to three prior lines of therapy has currently enrolled over 400 patients, with a target of 600. This trial will provide important comparative data to confirm the activity of bortezomib and to clarify its adverse effect profile further.

The role of bortezomib in clinical practice is in its infancy. Its use in earlier stage disease and its use in combination are key clinical questions that will be actively studied over the next several years. Preclinical data suggest that activity may be improved in combination with other drugs, such as IMiDs, melphalan, doxorubicin, or dexamethasone. Preliminary phase I data combining bortezomib with melphalan *(19)* or doxorubicin *(20)* have suggested that these combinations are clinically feasible, with acceptable toxicities and evidence of antitumor activity. Phase II trials of these and other combinations are eagerly awaited. The emergence of bortezomib, along with the active investigation of other promising drugs in clinical development, represents a promising time in the field of myeloma research. Although a cure has still not been found, significant strides have been made.

REFERENCES

1. Hideshima T, et al. The proteasome inhibitor PS-341 inhibits growth, induces apoptosis, and overcomes drug resistance in human multiple myeloma cells. *Cancer Res* 2001;61:3071–3076.
2. LeBlanc R, et al. Proteasome inhibitor PS-341 inhibits human myeloma cell growth in vivo and prolongs survival in a murine model. *Cancer Res* 2002;62:4996–5000.
3. Pham L, et al. Antitumor activity of the proteasome inhibitor PS-341 in mantle cell lymphoma B cells. *Blood* 2001;98:465a.
4. Adams J, et al. Proteasome inhibitors: a novel class of potent and effective antitumor agents. *Cancer Res* 1999;59:2615–2622.
5. Teicher BA, et al. The proteasome inhibitor PS-341 in cancer therapy. *Clin Cancer Res* 1999;5:2638–2645.
6. Bold RJ, Virudachalam S, McConkey DJ. Chemosensitization of pancreatic cancer by inhibition of the 26S proteasome. *J Surg Res* 2001;100:11–17.
7. Shah SA, et al. 26S proteasome inhibition induces apoptosis and limits growth of human pancreatic cancer. *J Cell Biochem* 2001;82:110–122.
8. Cusack JC Jr, Liu R, Houston M, et al. Enhanced chemosensitivity to CPT-11 with proteasome inhibitor PS-341: implications for systemic nuclear factor-kappaB inhibition. *Cancer Res* 2001;61:3535–3540.
9. Sunwoo JB, et al. Novel proteasome inhibitor PS-341 inhibits activation of nuclear factor-κB, cell survival, tumor growth, and angiogenesis in squamous cell carcinoma. *Clin Cancer Res* 2001;7:1419–1428.
10. Russo SM, et al. Enhancement of radiosensitivity by proteasome inhibition: implications for a role of NF-κB. *Int J Radiat Oncol Biol Phys* 2001;50:183–193.
11. Pervan M, Pajonk F, Sun JR, Withers HR, McBride WH. Molecular pathways that modify tumor radiation response. *Am J Clin Oncol* 2001;24:481–485.
12. Orlowski RZ, et al. Phase I trial of the proteasome inhibitor PS-341 in patients with refractory hematologic malignancies. *J Clin Oncol* 2002;20:4420–4427.
13. *Cancer Facts & Figures 2002*. Publication 02-250M, no. 5008.02. 2002. American Cancer Society, Atlanta, GA, 2002.
14. Papandreou C, et al. Phase I study of intravenous (I.V.) proteasome inhibitor PS-341 in patients (Pts) with advanced malignancies. In: *Proceedings of the American Society of Clinical Oncology-37th Annual Meeting*, 2001;20:86a.
15. Aghajanian C, et al. A phase I trial of the novel proteasome inhibitor PS341 in advanced solid tumor malignancies. *Clin Cancer Res* 2002;8:2505–2511.
16. Richardson PG, et al. A phase 2 study of bortezomib in relapsed, refractory myeloma. *N Engl J Med* 2003;348:2609–2617.
17. Bladé J, et al. Criteria for evaluating disease response and progression in patients with multiple myeloma treated by high-dose therapy and haemopoietic stem cell transplantation. Myeloma Subcommittee of the EBMT. European Group for Blood and Marrow Transplant. *Br J Haematol* 1998;102:1115–1123.
18. Jagannath S, et al. A phase II multicenter randomized study of the proteasome inhibitor bortezomib (VELCADE™, formerly PS-341) in multiple myeloma (MM) patients (pts) relapsed after front-line therapy. *Blood* 2002;100:812a.
19. Yang HH, et al. A phase I/II study of combination treatment with bortezomib and melphalan (Vc+M) in patients with relapsed or refractory multiple myeloma (MM). Presented at the American Society of Clinical Oncology Annual Meeting, May 31–June 3, 2003m Chicago, IL.
20. Orlowski RZ, et al. Phase I study of the proteasome inhibitor bortezomib and pegylated liposomal doxorubicin in patients with refractory hematologic malignancies. Presented at the American Society of Clinical Oncology 2003 Annual Meeting, May 31–June 3, 2003, Chicago, IL.
21. Alexanian R, et al. Combination chemotherapy for multiple myeloma. *Cancer* 1972;30:382–389.

Index

About the Editor

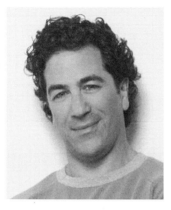

Dr. Adams has recently joined Infinity Pharmaceuticals, Inc. as Chief Scientific Officer. Prior to Infinity, Dr. Adams served as Senior Vice President, Drug Discovery and Development at Millennium Pharmaceuticals, Inc. (NASDAQ MLNM). Dr. Adams joined Millennium in December of 1999 following the company's merger with LeukoSite bringing with him the recently approved drug VELCADE™, a proteasome inhibitor for cancer therapy, and led drug discovery teams in producing drug candidates through lead optimization for preclinical development in both the U.S. and U.K. At LeukoSite, he served as Senior Vice President of Research and Development since July 1999. From 1994 to 1999, he served as Executive Vice President of Research and Development at Proscript, Inc., a biopharmaceutical company. In 1987, he joined Boehringer Ingelheim where he served in various positions including Director of Medicinal Chemistry. At Boehringer, he successfully discovered the drug Viramune® for HIV. From 1982 to 1987, he was a Medicinal Chemist at Merck in Montreal. Dr. Adams received a B.S. from McGill University and a Ph.D. from the Massachusetts Institute of Technology in the field of synthetic organic chemistry. He also received many awards, including the 2001 Ribbon of Hope Award for PS-341 (VELCADE™) from the International Myeloma Foundation. Dr. Adams has received over fifty patents and has authored over a hundred papers and book chapters in peer reviewed journals.